'Over the years, appropriate supports for autistic individuals have been vigorously debated. Now, within the pages of this long-awaited guide, individuals, caregivers and professionals have an excellent, trustworthy reference that helps to guide these decisions. Evidence based support and how to find what's right for an individual, has been a treasure marked X, but without the map! This book provides the map and is an essential aid to eliminating potential hurdles along the way.'

—***Wenn B. Lawson, PhD***

'As autism experts on many levels, Dr Goodall, Dr Nugent and Dr Bennett utilise their professional standing and knowledge with the "insider experience" in this long-awaited guide to navigating the minefield of purported autism supports. This book is sequential, logical and easily accessible for anyone who seeks to use current evidence and valuable autistic feedback as the basis for their decision making. In the style of the authors, I award this work a gold star!'

—***Ms Judy Brewer, AO****, former Chair, Autism CRC, and parent advocate*

'This volume provides a truly comprehensive overview of the range of treatments for individuals with ASD. In doing so it covers both well-established evidence-based treatments, treatments with a small but emerging evidence base, and some treatments with little to no evidence base (past the level of case report/anecdote). The system of rating the evidence available in support of treatments is extremely helpful and can be used by parents, teachers, and others in making informed decisions about programs and treatments. It also includes a summary of medications sometimes used for the treatment of associated problems like anxiety, depression, irritability, and sleep as well as other treatment approaches for these conditions. An invaluable guide for students, parents, and teachers this volume provides an extremely helpful overview of the current state of knowledge in treatments for autism.'

—***Fred Volkmar, MD****, Irving B. Harris Professor of Child Psychiatry, Pediatrics, and Psychology – Yale University School of Medicine, and Dorothy Goodwin Family Professor of Special Education, Southern Connecticut State University, New Haven, CT, USA*

Choosing Effective Support for People on the Autism Spectrum

This book is essential for anyone interested in learning about the therapeutic potential of orthodox and state-of-the-art supports for autistics. Using research evidence, supports are rated using a Gold, Silver, Bronze, and Tin category system. 'Gold' is extremely promising and use with confidence, whereas 'Tin' is extremely unsafe and potentially life threatening. This book, however, is more complex than just presenting literature reviews about supports for autistics and then rating the efficacy of the support. In addition to this, the insights and experiences of autistics about the autism supports examined are presented. Such testimonials provide an *insider perspective* from those who ultimately stand to benefit or suffer after receiving a support – namely autistics themselves.

Matthew Bennett is an Independent Researcher.

Emma Goodall is National Co-ordinator – Content and Resources at Positive Partnerships, and Consultant at Healthy Possibilities.

Jane Nugent was a qualified Medical Doctor and an experienced University Lecturer in Psychopharmacology, with diverse work experience in rural and remote health settings.

Choosing Effective Support for People on the Autism Spectrum

A Guide Based on Academic Perspectives and Lived Experience

Matthew Bennett, Emma Goodall, and Jane Nugent

Routledge
Taylor & Francis Group
LONDON AND NEW YORK

First published 2021
by Routledge
2 Park Square, Milton Park, Abingdon, Oxon OX14 4RN

and by Routledge
52 Vanderbilt Avenue, New York, NY 10017

Routledge is an imprint of the Taylor & Francis Group, an informa business

British Library Cataloguing in Publication Data
A catalogue record for this book is available from the British Library

Library of Congress Cataloging-in-Publication Data
A catalog record has been requested for this book

ISBN: 978-0-367-42126-7 (hbk)
ISBN: 978-0-367-42127-4 (pbk)
ISBN: 978-0-367-82197-5 (ebk)

Typeset in Times New Roman
by Taylor & Francis Books

We would like to acknowledge the contribution of Dr Jane Nugent to the medications chapter. Psychopharmacology was her speciality and passion and she particularly enjoyed empowering people to make informed decisions regarding their wellbeing. Prior to publication, sadly, Dr Jane Nugent unexpectedly and suddenly passed away. We would like to dedicate this book to her, in honour of her work in health care and education for people with complex needs.

Contents

Tables

Tables

Acknowledgements

Writing a book like this is a complex and time-consuming academic exercise, in which we were supported and guided by a number of people.

We would like to acknowledge and thank our family and friends for their support as we wrote this book.

We would also like to acknowledge and thank the professional assistance that we received from the following people:

- Dr Jessica Paynter, Senior Lecturer, School of Applied Psychology/The Hopkins Centre: Research for Rehabilitation & Resilience, Griffith University
- Dr Erin Leaf, Senior Lecturer – Educational Psychology and Applied Behaviour Analysis, Monash University
- Dr Wenn Lawson, Teaching Fellow, Birmingham University and co-chair of the Australian Autism Research Council.

This book would not have been written without the efforts of the many autistics and their families who have continued to raise their voice to challenge the prevalent perceptions and expectations of others. We hope that this book serves to help change preconceptions and give strength to autistic voices.

Chapter 1

Introduction

1.1 Introduction

As autistic researchers and writers, and a neurodiverse Medical Practitioner, we have some interesting interpretations of the direction of some autism research. We truly believe that all individuals thrive when given the right supports to enable them to feel valued, loved, and able to engage with the wider world. For us, this is what we mean by an effective support, one that enables an individual of whatever age to engage more easily and comfortably with the wider world, whilst feeling valued as an individual human being. Throughout this book the term autistic is used to describe individuals who are on the autism spectrum. For people who are more used to the terms 'with autism' or 'ASD', it is important to understand that the majority of autistics prefer to refer to themselves as autistic or neurodiverse. These are statements of pride and belonging, hinting at the core issue. Autistics do not need fixing, we require support to thrive.

When a parent learns that their child is autistic, it is often perceived of as a life changing event, or at the very least a momentous occasion, with many parents worrying that their child will not be able to thrive. In response to this diagnosis, families often seek strategies or programs that can help their autistic child to reach their potential. Although families have the best of intentions, the chance of them finding an effective strategy or program is hampered by the plethora of strategies marketed as evidence-based supports and therapeutic programs. We wanted to write this book to help people understand that picking a support or therapy is more complex than just assuming that a professional will be of benefit to an autistic. In addition, we wanted to highlight that the research evidence for a support/therapy does not always look at aspects that are important to the autistics participating in the support/therapy, so that a support seen as highly reputable may still be experienced as not useful to an individual autistic.

This complexity is further exacerbated when the family may only have a basic understanding about what makes a strategy or program effective. This point was illustrated by Green et al. (2006) who reported that, out of 111 potential support programs and strategies for autistics, 26.8% of parents had their autistic child on a Casein-free diet at the time of their study. This is despite many studies concluding that Casein-free diets do not help autistics unless they have issues with the digestion of casein (Elder et al., 2015).

In many countries, when someone becomes physically unwell, or displays atypical behaviours, they or their family members typically seek the advice of medical professionals. People often perceive that such professionals are familiar with all common conditions, including autism. Although the public's awareness of autism has increased, resulting in the creation of many public policies (Penner et al., 2018), regrettably there are still some medical and allied health professionals who do not fully understand autism or individual autistics (Taylor et al., 2016; Ward, Sullivan, & Gilmore, 2016). Their lack of knowledge about the autism spectrum can inhibit their ability to advise parents about suitable support programs and strategies for autistic children. It is our hope that both parents and professionals can use this book as a guide when making decisions about what autism supports are suitable for an individual and why.

Some parents regard the internet as a valuable source of information about the autism spectrum. Rhoades, Scarpa, and Salley (2007) found that 73% of caregivers raising autistic children reported that they used the internet to learn about the autism spectrum. Similarly, Mackintosh, Myers, and Goin-Kochel (2005) reported that parents often learned about the autism spectrum after reading books (88%), web pages/emails (86%), autism newsletters (69%), with only a minority consulting scientific or academic journals (44%). Despite its popularity, the internet contains a considerable amount of misinformation about the autism spectrum (Grant, Rodger, & Hoffmann, 2015; Reichow et al., 2012). Stephenson, Carter, and Kemp (2012) found that websites run by national autism associations sometimes give parents and teachers inaccurate information about supports for autistics. Such inaccuracies have added credence and proliferated the spread of ineffective and dangerous autism supports, such as holding therapy. We hope that the contents in this book will help dispel some of the inaccuracies that are commonly found on the internet.

The internet is not the only source of information that can influence a parent's decision about what types of supports and/or programs they choose to use on their autistic children. For some parents, a celebrity's opinion can influence such decisions. Perhaps the most noticeable example is Jenny McCarthy's views on curing autism. On 18 September 2007, McCarthy appeared on *The Oprah Winfrey Show* to talk about her book *Louder than Words – A Mother's Journey in Healing Autism*. During the show, McCarthy claimed that she was able to cure her son's autism by putting him on a Gluten-free and Casein-free (GFCF) diet. However, credible peer-reviewed studies do not support McCarthy's view (Elder et al., 2015). By giving Hollywood celebrities, like Jenny McCarthy, a public forum to argue the opposite view to that in the literature creates the perception that such diets can actually be beneficial for autistics who do not have food intolerances. In some ways, McCarthy's public endorsement of GFCF diets is akin to the autism-vaccination debate. The literature shows that vaccines do not contribute to the development of autism (Bennett et al., 2018). However, by giving a public platform to those who espouse the opposite view, this implies that concerns about vaccine safety are legitimate (Gottlieb, 2016). We hope that after reading this book readers will be in a position to critically evaluate the persuasive influence of celebrities and other cultural influences.

Sometimes, minimal knowledge about or awareness of an autism support can entice parents of autistic children, or even autistic people themselves, to try the support. Green (2007) found that, regardless of the amount of empirical evidence about its efficacy, parents often gravitated towards trying supports that they believed yielded benefits quickly with relatively little effort. However, not all supports can be implemented easily and quickly, nor can all supports produce immediate benefits. For example, an autistic may have to spend countless hours over many weeks participating in an exercise program before they notice any improvement in their physical fitness and/or gross motor coordination skills. Somewhat regrettably, as Green notes, the longer parents continue to subject their autistic children to ineffective supports the more inclined they are to believe that the support itself is beneficial when, in reality, it is actually producing either no benefits or the opposite outcome.

> Once a commitment has been made, it is perhaps not surprising that the longer parents use a treatment and invest both time and money there is an increased likelihood that they will report positive outcomes regardless of whether this is in fact true or not.
>
> (Green, 2007, p. 100).

Prolonged usage of ineffective supports and/or programs for autistics can not only result in parents believing that the strategy is effective, it can also prevent them from investigating and using other strategies that have a comprehensive evidence-base of proven benefits for autistics. For example, Vivanti, Dissanayake, and the Victorian ASELCC Team (2016) reported that the Early Start Denver Model (ESDM) was more effective in helping younger autistic children (i.e., 18–48 months) achieve greater verbal developmental quotients than older autistic children (i.e., 48–62 months). If a parent believes that an ineffective support is helping their autistic child, then they would be more inclined to continue using the support. As a consequence, the child may have aged to a point where they would have missed the opportunity to obtain the maximum benefits from the ESDM. We hope that after studying the contents of this book parents will choose not to use ineffective supports and will avoid falling into the trap explained in the given quote by Green (2007).

Another factor that can influence a parent's selection of supports for their autistic child is the marketing techniques used by those who sell unproven supports. Parents often contact such providers after learning about them from the television, internet, or word of mouth (Mackintosh, Myers, & Goin-Kochel, 2005). Often organisations that sell dubious supports for autistics, use slick and appealing advertising that boast sensationalist and grandiose results, such as promising 'quick fixes' and 'high success rates'. However, just because a person or an organisation expresses grandiose claims with conviction does not mean that the claims themselves are true. Regardless of their sincerity, those who sell ineffective supports for autistics typically obtain a parent's money by exploiting their legitimate concerns about their child's development (Finke et al., 2019). Once a parent has spent their savings and has not seen their child improve it is not only their funds that have been depleted but also their trust in professionals. Once this trust has been lost, it can be extremely difficult for a reputable professional to engage with these parents and help their autistic children. It is our intention that after reading this book parents of autistic children will take a more cautious approach when selecting possible supports. Additionally, parents and professionals might wish to use the questions listed in Appendix 1 to help them decide what supports to try.

1.2 The key features of this book

1.2.1 Philosophical stance about support programs for autistics

In our opinion, there is a distinction between support programs that are designed to enhance an autistic's abilities or manage comorbid conditions, to enable the individual to thrive, and support programs that are designed to 'iron out' autistic characteristics and tendencies, such as stimming or a focus on a topic of interest. In the interests of supporting the rights of autistics and appreciating their unique abilities, we do not endorse or evaluate supports that aim to remove autistic tendencies or characteristics, nor things that purport to cure autism. Autism is not a disease and therefore cannot be cured. It is a life-long neurodevelopmental difference that impacts the way autistics perceive and relate to themselves and the wider world. For these reasons, we only examine supports that can be used to improve the quality of life for autistics by either reducing the impact of their co-morbid conditions (i.e., insomnia, hyperactivity) or improving their existing skills (i.e., using an equine program to improve developing motor coordination and social skills).

Throughout this book we use identity-first language conventions because we do not endorse or evaluate supports that aim to 'cure autism', as we subscribe to the view that autism is not inherently problematic. In our view, what is problematic is a mismatch between the support needs and characteristics of autistics and the way most autistics are responded to by the systems around them, such as the health and education systems. To reflect this belief, we have used the terms 'autistics', 'autistic children', and 'autistic adults' instead of person-first language (e.g., person with autism). Our linguistic convention also echoes Kenny et al.'s (2016) view that people on the autism spectrum prefer to be referred to as 'autistics' or 'autistic people' because they view autism as an indispensable part of their identity that cannot, and should not, be cured. However, in the interests of accuracy, we use person-first language when a study examines a subsection of the autistic community, such as people with a diagnosis of autism or people with a diagnosis of Asperger syndrome.

1.2.2 Review of the literature

A scoping review of the literature was conducted to identify, quantify, and examine available peer-reviewed studies about supports and strategies that can help autistics. The first step in our scoping study involved us becoming familiar with the myriad of supports and programs available to autistics. This was accomplished by using the list of autism supports discussed in Green et al.'s (2006) study as a starting point. Using our academic and professional knowledge and experiences of the autism spectrum, along with our desire to explore a wide range of approaches (e.g., diets, assistive technology, early childhood programs, and animals), we selected from this list what we believed were the most common types of supports.

Once we finalised what supports would be assessed a search for relevant literature that was located on Springer, SAGE, Taylor & Francis, Google Scholar, and PubMed was conducted. We entered into the search field both the name and alternative names of the support along with the word 'autis*' and the term 'ASD'. For example, to search for studies about equine therapy for autistics we used the terms 'horse' OR 'equine' AND 'aut*' OR 'ASD'.

This literature search provided evidence of a myriad of studies about supports for autistics and that summarising this body of literature was going to be a herculean task. For efficiency key findings in peer-reviewed literature reviews and meta-analysis studies about specific supports for autistics were examined, as longs as they were peer-reviewed and published in English. The *JBI Critical Appraisal Checklist for Systematic Reviews and Research Synthesis* was used on potential studies to determine if it was of a suitable methodological standard (See Appendix 2). Those studies that scored more than six 'Yes' responses on this checklist were examined and included in this book.

At every opportunity, we examined and presented the contents of literature reviews and meta-analysis studies about specific supports for autistics. An exception to this is Chapter 10, where a purely pharmacological rationale was taken using common pharmacological guidelines in addition to relevant literature reviews. Peer-reviewed research was examined using the *McMaster Critical Review Form – Quantitative Studies* checklist (See Appendix 3). Those studies that scored more than seven 'Yes' responses on this checklist were examined and included in this book.

This approach of searching through mainstream and credible academic repositories using quality control processes and using methodological checklists ensured that only studies of the highest quality and robustness were examined and presented. This rigorous approach towards examining the literature was deemed vital, especially considering that sub-quality research can result in ineffective supports being endorsed.

1.2.3 Insights from autistics about autism supports

Qualitative experiences

When examining studies about supports for autistics, it became apparent that only a few studies presented insights from autistics about the support's efficacy. To some it may appear strange that autistics have not been given the opportunity to express their views, especially considering that they are the recipients of such supports and that they can provide us with an 'insider's perspective'. However, this gap in the research was considered a valuable discovery, since it provided the opportunity to include 'autistic voice' to explore the benefits and drawbacks of supports for autistics.

An online questionnaire was developed and distributed, in which autistics explained their perspectives about the autism supports being included in this book (See Appendix 4). Links to the questionnaire were posted on autistic-specific online forums. To participate the respondents had to have either self-identified as autistic or been diagnosed as autistic (i.e., DSM-5 ASD diagnosis, DSM-IV-TR Autistic Disorder diagnosis, or DSM-IV-TR Asperger syndrome diagnosis), and use the internet to complete the survey. Respondents did not receive any compensation for donating their time and effort to share their knowledge. Additionally, an experienced autistic psychologist and an experienced autistic education consultant were interviewed using the same questions as the survey questionnaire to seek more detailed answers than were provided in the online survey.

It is hoped that the perspectives provided will give the reader some insight into some of the often-unintended consequences that autistics have experienced during and after participating in specific supports. For example, before enrolling in an equine therapy program, an autistic or their parents might learn some unforeseen aspects of this therapy after reading the respondents' insights and experiences of this program. Alternatively, their insights might dispel a reader's misunderstanding about a support. For example, the academic literature and our rating of GFCF diets may not convince a reader that such diets are beneficial for autistics. However, after reading several autistic accounts about this support their stance might change. It is hoped that where the views of autistics were quite different to that of researchers, that this will prompt a number of actions. Firstly, that people will think carefully about what aspects of that support might or might not be helpful for a particular individual. Secondly that there are changes in the way future research is conducted, to take into account the lived experiences of autistics.

Quantitative ratings

Whilst completing our online survey, respondents were asked to rate the support's efficacy. The ratings that they could select were:

1. N/A – 0 stars
2. Did not enjoy or find useful – 1 star
3. Enjoyed but did not find useful – 2 stars
4. Did not enjoy but found useful – 3 stars
5. Enjoyed and found useful – 4 stars
6. Enjoyed, found useful and found that my wellbeing and mood were improved – 5 stars

These stars were chosen to reflect the importance placed by autistics on both the usefulness of a support or strategy and the need to not become distressed or stressed by a support or strategy. It is hoped that this will be particularly useful for families and professionals in deciding what supports to explore. As autism is so varied in the way it impacts individuals, no one person's experience will be exactly the same as another. This is clear in the lived experience sections, but not in the reviews of the literature.

After we finished receiving survey responses the average star rating for each support was calculated. However, a star rating was not given to a support when less than ten respondents (5% of the total number of respondents for our survey) rated the support. This is because we did not want the reader to be misled into believing that a support was endorsed by the respondents when there was such a low response rate.

Sample characteristics

Our survey was open to the public from 7 October 2019 until 28 October 2019. During this time we collected 206 responses. Of these, most disclosed that they had a formal autism diagnosis (n = 153, 74.27%) (See Table 1.1), with the rest being self-identified as autistic. Respondents who were neither self-identified nor diagnosed as on the autism spectrum were excluded from the survey after completing the initial age, location, and supports received or not questions. Most respondents stated that they were either aged between 36–45 years (n = 50, 24.39%) or aged between 46–55 years (n = 45, 21.95%). In contrast, only five respondents (2.44%) said that they were aged between 66 to 100 years of age (See Table 1.2). Most respondents noted that they had not received any therapies or supports for their autism (n = 104, 51.49%), whilst 98 (48.51%) said they had received one or more strategy or support specifically in relation to their autism (See Table 1.3). Finally, in terms of physical location most respondents lived in Australia (n = 85, 41.46%), followed by the United States of America (n = 36, 17.56%), and the United Kingdom (n = 30, 14.63%) (See Table 1.4).

Table 1.1 Do you have a formal autism diagnosis?

Answer choices	*Responses*	*%*
Yes	153	74.27
No	12	5.83
No, but I self-identify as autistic	41	19.90
TOTAL	**206**	**100**
Number of respondents who skipped this question	0	

Table 1.2 How old are you?

Answer choices	*Responses*	*%*
Under 18	19	9.27
18–25	22	10.73
26–35	39	19.02
36–45	50	24.39
46–55	45	21.95
56–65	25	12.20
66–100	5	2.44
TOTAL	**205**	**100**
Number of respondents who skipped this question	1	

1.2.4 Rating autism supports

One of the defining features of this book is that we rated each support's efficacy for autistics, using the findings in the literature about a particular support to rate its effectiveness for autistics using a five-category rating system (See Table 1.5). At this point it is important to acknowledge that every autistic is unique and that a single support cannot help every autistic with every comorbidity or support need. Thus, you should not view our ratings as absolute truisms but subjective judgments that are based on our interpretations of the results in the studies reviewed and our clinical and academic experience of the autism spectrum. To emphasise this point we have conveyed our judgments in a generalist sense (e.g., may, might, possibly) and placed caveats on our opinions (e.g., provided an autistic doesn't have...). For example, we stated that acupuncture 'may' help autistics provided they 'do not have sensory sensitivities to touch'.

Table 1.3 Have you ever received any therapies or supports because of your autism?

Answer choices	*Responses*	*%*
Yes	98	48.51
No	104	51.49
TOTAL	**202**	**100**
Number of respondents who skipped this question	4	

Table 1.4 Where do you live?

Answer choices	*Responses*	*%*
Australia	85	41.46
United States of America	36	17.56
United Kingdom	30	14.63
New Zealand	27	13.17
Europe (Country not specified)	13	6.34
Canada	5	2.44
Ireland	4	2.00
Netherlands	2	1.00
Chile	1	0.50
South Africa	1	0.50
Norway	1	0.50
TOTAL	**205**	**100**
Number of respondents who skipped this question	1	

1.2.5 Outlining future research directions

Our book is more than just rating the effectiveness of supports for autistics and presenting a synergy between autistic and academic perspectives about such supports. After rating the support's effectiveness, we offer the reader some suggestions about where more research into the support could be conducted in the future. We based our recommendations on the suggestions explained in the examined literature. For example, in Section 3.5.3 we discuss Matson and Konst's (2013) claim that most studies about the efficacy of Early Intensive Behavioural Intervention (EIBI) for autistics have used the term *follow-up* to describe what is actually *post-test data* (i.e., data collected immediately after the conclusion of the study). Due to this confusion in terminology, Matson and Konst have suggested that in the future more research about the long-term efficacy of EIBI programs for autistics should be published.

1.3 The intended audience for this book

1.3.1 University students

In a range of countries there are undergraduate and post-graduate students studying the autism spectrum in their education, psychology, and health sciences courses. This book will enhance their knowledge about the autism spectrum by presenting the evidence on the effectiveness of a broad range of conventional and cutting-edge strategies used to support autistics. After reading this book they should enter professional practice equipped with a wide range of knowledge about how best to support their autistic clients.

1.3.2 Professionals

Healthcare professionals who assist autistic clients will find this book helpful for three reasons. First, they will be able to recommend effective supports after reading the research cited and our rating (i.e., Gold, Silver, Bronze, Tin, or Insufficient information). Second, after reading the future research section they will be able to understand

Table 1.5 Five ratings used to evaluate autism interventions and supports

Rating	*Definition*
Gold – Extremely promising and use with confidence	The highest rating used in this book was 'Gold – Extremely promising and use with confidence'. Those who use Gold-rated supports can have a **high degree** of confidence that they will most likely benefit from such supports.
Silver – Usually promising	The second-highest rating used in this book was 'Silver – Usually promising'. Those who use Silver-rated supports can have a **reasonable degree** of confidence that they will most likely benefit from such supports. However, caution needs to be advised since there is still some uncertainty about its efficacy.
Bronze – Safe but ineffective	The third-highest rating used in this book was 'Bronze - Safe but ineffective'. Supports were given this rating to reflect the fact that most of the peer-reviewed literature has concluded that they are safe but that they do not provide any benefits to autistics.
Tin – Extremely unsafe and potentially life-threatening	The lowest rating used in this book was 'Tin – Extremely unsafe and potentially life-threatening'. For a support to receive this rating a large volume of peer-reviewed research had to show that it was dangerous and that in certain circumstances it was life-threatening. **Tin rated supports should not be used under any circumstances.**
Insufficient information to make a recommendation	The final rating used in this book was 'Insufficient information to make a recommendation'. This rating was given when there were less than five studies about the efficacy of a support for autistics.

some of the limitations of the support that they are recommending. Third, after reading the 'autistic perspective' section they will be able to explain to their autistic clients some of the consequences that they might experience when using the support.

1.3.3 Parents of autistic children

Parents can make a more informed choice about a support they may wish their autistic children to try after reading the information contained in this book and our rating of the support's efficacy for autistics. They can also learn what their autistic children might experience during the delivery of the support after reading the autistic perspective section about the support.

1.3.4 Autistics

Autistics can obtain several benefits after reading this book. First, our rating of a support can help them make an informed decision about if they would like to use the support to help them improve their skills. For example, if they are interested in improving their social skills, perhaps in the hope of performing well at a job interview, then they might choose to participate in a social skills group after reading the research and recommendations about this support. Conversely, the ratings can also help them avoid choosing dangerous and ineffective supports. For example, after reading the evidence and our rating of Chelation therapy they might refuse to try this. Second, autistic adults can use the contents of this book to facilitate a discussion between themselves and their parents and/or their healthcare providers or other support providers, about suitable supports that they might wish to try to help them achieve optimum outcomes in life.

References

Bennett, M., Webster, A. A., Goodall, E., & Rowland, S. (2018). Challenging the public's perception of life on autism spectrum: The impact of the vaccination myth. In *Life on the Autism Spectrum* (pp. 37–60). Springer, Singapore. doi:10.1007/978-981-13-3359-0_3.

Elder, J. H., Kreider, C. M., Schaefer, N. M., & de Laosa, M. B. (2015). A review of gluten-and casein-free diets for treatment of autism: 2005–2015. *Nutrition and Dietary Supplements*, 7, 87. doi:10.2147/NDS.S74718.

Finke, E. H., Kremkow, J. M., Drager, K. D., Murillo, A., Richardson, L., & Serpentine, E. C. (2019). "I would like for my child to be happy with his life": Parental hopes for their children with ASD across the lifespan. *Journal of Autism and Developmental Disorders*, 49(5), 2049–2068. doi:10.1007/s10803-019-03882-9.

Gottlieb, S. D. (2016). Vaccine resistances reconsidered: Vaccine skeptics and the Jenny McCarthy effect. *Biosocieties*, 11(2), 152–174. doi:10.1057/biosoc.2015.30.

Grant, N., Rodger, S., & Hoffmann, T. (2015). Evaluation of autism-related health information on the Web. *Journal of Applied Research in Intellectual Disabilities*, 28(4), 276–282. doi:10.1111/jar.12127.

Green, V. A. (2007). Parental experience with treatments for autism. *Journal of Developmental and Physical Disabilities*, 19(2), 91–101. doi:10.1007/s10882-007-9035-y.

Green, V. A., Pituch, K. A., Itchon, J., Choi, A., O'Reilly, M., & Sigafoos, J. (2006). Internet survey of treatments used by parents of children with autism. *Research in Developmental Disabilities*, 27(1), 70–84. doi:10.1016/j.ridd.2004.12.002.

Kenny, L., Hattersley, C., Molins, B., Buckley, C., Povey, C., & Pellicano, E. (2016). Which terms should be used to describe autism? Perspectives from the UK autism community. *Autism*, 20(4), 442–462. doi:10.1177/1362361315588200.

Mackintosh, V. H., Myers, B. J., & Goin-Kochel, R. P. (2005). Sources of information and support used by parents of children with autism spectrum disorders. *Journal on Developmental Disabilities*, 12(1), 41–51.

Matson, J. L., & Konst, M. J. (2013). What is the evidence for long term effects of early autism interventions? *Research in Autism Spectrum Disorders*, 7(3), 475–479. doi:10.1016/j.rasd.2012.11.005.

Penner, M., Anagnostou, E., Andoni, L. Y., & Ungar, W. J. (2018). Environmental scan of Canadian and UK policies for autism spectrum disorder diagnostic assessment. *Paediatrics & Child Health*, 24(3), e125–e134. doi:10.1093/pch/pxy107.

Reichow, B., Halpern, J. I., Steinhoff, T. B., Letsinger, N., Naples, A., & Volkmar, F. R. (2012). Characteristics and quality of autism websites. *Journal of Autism and Developmental Disorders*, 42(6), 1263–1274. doi:10.1007/s10803-011-1342-6.

Rhoades, R. A., Scarpa, A., & Salley, B. (2007). The importance of physician knowledge of autism spectrum disorder: Results of a parent survey. *BMC Pediatrics*, 7(1), 37. doi:10.1186/1471-2431-7-37.

Stephenson, J., Carter, M., & Kemp, C. (2012). Quality of the information on educational and therapy interventions provided on the web sites of national autism associations. *Research in Autism Spectrum Disorders*, 6(1), 11–18. doi:10.1016/j.rasd.2011.08.002.

Taylor, L. J., Eapen, V., Maybery, M. T., Midford, S., Paynter, J., Quarmby, L., ... & Whitehouse, A. J. (2016). Diagnostic evaluation for autism spectrum disorder: A survey of health professionals in Australia. *BMJ Open*, 6(9), e012517. doi:10.1136/bmjopen-2016-012517.

Vivanti, G., Dissanayake, C., & Victorian ASELCCTeam. (2016). Outcome for children receiving the Early Start Denver Model before and after 48 months. *Journal of Autism and Developmental Disorders*, 46(7), 2441–2449. doi:10.1007/s10803-016-2777-6.

Ward, S. L., Sullivan, K. A., & Gilmore, L. (2016). Practitioner perceptions of the assessment and diagnosis of autism in Australia. *Australian Psychologist*, 51(4), 272–279. doi:10.1111/ap.12211.

Chapter 2

Strategies involving social interactions

2.1 Introduction

This chapter presents the literature about possible therapeutic benefits that autistics may obtain from social skills groups (SSGs) and peer-mediated activities. These two strategies predominantly involve autistics socially interacting with others. This chapter begins by presenting the contents of three literature reviews in which studies about the efficacy of SSGs for autistics have been examined. It then rates the efficacy of this support for autistics, provides several recommendations about where more research could be conducted in the future, and presents a series of insights and experiences from autistics about SSGs. It then examines the same elements about peer-mediated activities for autistics. It should be noted that social skills groups are most often run by non-autistics with the goal of 'improving' social skills. What improvement means in this context is not always made clear by providers, and may or may not be in tune with what individual autistics and/or their families deem useful. Peer mediated activities are usually organised by and for autistics themselves with the goal of socialising or engaging in activities of mutual interest. They can also be mentoring based, in which case the peer may or may not be autistic, but the activity is usually agreed on by both people.

2.2 Social skills groups (SSGs)

2.2.1 Social skills groups (SSGs)

The term 'social skills groups' (SSGs) refers to groups of people who meet and discuss various topics or undertake activities that they find, or are assumed to find, interesting. After reviewing the broader literature about support programs for autistics we found three literature reviews in which the researchers examined studies about SSGs for autistics (Gates, Kang, & Lerner, 2017; Hotton & Coles, 2016; Spain & Blainey, 2015).

Spain and Blainey (2015) reviewed five studies about the effectiveness of SSGs for autistic adults with low support needs, whom they described as 'high-functioning'. They believed that they were the first to examine the efficacy of SSGs for this subgroup of autistics. They found that SSGs helped participants develop their knowledge of appropriate social skills but not their actual social skills. In their words:

> To date, five studies have investigated the effectiveness of group-based SSI [Social Skills Interventions] to reduce social skill deficits in adults with hf-ASD [high functioning – autism spectrum disorder]. Study findings provide preliminary support for these interventions. Yet, overall, interventions were more effective for enhancing knowledge and understanding rather than increasing specific social skills.
>
> (Spain & Blainey, 2015, p. 884).

While their literature review has enhanced our understanding about the potential value that SSGs can give some autistics, Spain and Blainey disclosed several limitations in their review that could have undermined the integrity of their conclusions. These limitations were that they did not examine, studies in which SSGs were delivered in an alternative format to face-to-face (e.g., online communication), or studies in which the SSG was used in conjunction with other supports or therapies (e.g., psychological supports). If Spain and Blainey had examined these types of studies then they might have reached a different conclusion about the efficacy of SSGs for autistics.

In 2016, Hotton and Coles published a literature review in which they examined 13 studies about the benefits that SSGs might bring to autistic adolescents and adults. They reviewed the literature published over the past 20 years that examined the impact of group-based social skills training in improving the social abilities of autistic adults and adolescents. After reviewing the collected literature, they concluded:

> … group-based social skills training was generally effective at improving social skills, with some students observing transfer effects to improvements in wider psychological wellbeing.
>
> (Hotton & Coles, 2016, p. 68).

While their conclusion appears to show that autistics can obtain benefits from SSGs, Hotton and Coles's study does have several limitations. First, all the studies that they examined had sampled participants who were, as assessed by intelligence tests, to be cognitively average or above. Consequently, they did not examine the potential benefits or issues with SSGs for autistics with intellectual disabilities (i.e., defined as an intelligence quotient below 70 points). Second, they excluded commentaries and other literature reviews, which meant that they may have missed information that confirmed or invalidated their findings about the efficacy of SSGs for autistics.

Gates, Kang, and Lerner (2017) conducted a two-stage search of the literature about the potential efficacy or benefits of SSGs for autistics. They reviewed 21 studies and despite not finding any longitudinal studies, since most of the research that they examined did not include any follow-up assessments, they concluded that:

> GSSI [Group Social Skills Interventions] lead to moderate overall improvements in social competence in youth with ASD [Autism Spectrum Disorder] relative to non-treatment or waitlist controls. This study also indicates that parents and observers report small effects of GSSIs, and task-based measures yield medium effects. Teachers appear not to see effects of GSSIs. While youth with ASD self-report large effects, these changes appear entirely attributable to changes in social knowledge.
>
> (Gates, Kang, & Lerner, 2017, p. 175).

Their findings show the complexity of evaluating anything that is being implemented to impact on the social skills of any individual or group. The individual or group may perceive that they are benefiting greatly whilst their peers or others around them may have different perceptions. It may be that Spain and Blainey's (2015) observation that SSGs appear to increase knowledge and understanding of social skills explains Gates, Kang, and Lerner's (2017) finding that *some* autistic youth believe SSGs are effective.

2.2.2 *Evaluation of social skills groups (SSGs)*

Gold – Extremely promising and use with confidence

Based on the literature examined we have rated SSGs for autistics as 'Gold – Extremely promising and use with confidence'. We have given SSGs this rating because most of the literature has concluded that SSGs can offer autistics multiple benefits. For example, the studies reviewed by Hotton and Coles (2016) showed that they can help improve an autistic's knowledge about social skills, social responsiveness, communication, and motivation. Additionally, Spain and Blainey (2015) claimed that SSGs can equip autistics with greater knowledge about social skills but not necessarily greater social abilities. However, in our opinion, increased knowledge about social skills may be an incentive for some autistics to increase social competence as they feel more confident about what to do when and why. We believe if autistics develop greater knowledge and understanding of social situations and appropriate social etiquette in their wider community setting, then this increased knowledge can help them to feel more comfortable engaging in conventional social situations which can enhance their social skills.

2.2.3 *Directions for research in the future about social skills groups (SSGs)*

Despite multiple literature reviews concluding that SSGs can be of benefit to some autistics, there remains three areas where more research can be conducted about this topic. These three areas are outlined here.

First, Gates, Kang, and Lerner (2017), Spain and Blainey (2015), and Hotton and Coles (2016) were unable to find any studies that evaluated long-term benefits of SSGs for autistics. None of the studies that they examined had follow-up data collection. Longitudinal research into this topic could provide researchers with several opportunities. For example, such research could address the question 'Do SSG programs that are long in duration (e.g., over six months or a year) produce more long-term benefits than SSGs that are short in duration (e.g., less than three months in duration)?' Similarly, longitudinal research might also determine if SSGs that occur more frequently (e.g., three one-hour sessions per week) might provide more long-term benefits than SSGs that rarely meet (e.g., two one-hour sessions per month), or if it might be that another factor entirely is the key to providing long-lasting benefits, such as involvement in picking activities or discussion topics.

Second, Hotton and Coles (2016) noted that since the autistic participants in the research that they reviewed were not consulted about their perceptions and experiences of SSGs, researchers and clinicians were unlikely to be providing customised, person-centered SSGs. It could be that for some autistics the topics discussed in the SSG could be uncomfortable or of no interest. For example, some may feel uncomfortable discussing their experiences of friendships. Their discomfort may be further exacerbated if the facilitator does not accommodate their apprehension. By listening to the views of autistics, SSGs with more interesting topics and outings for the autistic group members might be created. Anecdotally these types of groups do exist and are usually autistic created and led. However, they have not been the subject of research.

Third, Miller et al. (2014) found that many studies about SSGs for autistics did not compare the efficacy of smaller and larger SSGs. It appears that SSGs typically have between four to six participants. This group size may be most common because it gives the group the flexibility to explore different topics, or because this is more acceptable to autistics or their families or funding organisations. However, comparisons of the effectiveness of larger and smaller SSGs for autistics has not been extensively researched, nor has the rationale for group size been reviewed. This research would be valuable since the size of the SSG might be an important factor in determining the most effective way to develop confidence and competence in social interactions. For example, teaching autistic children appropriate classroom etiquette might be more easily conveyed and learned in a large SSG than a small SSG. In contrast, employment skills might be more effectively taught in a small SSG than a large SSG. Irrespective of these examples, the relationship between the size of the SSG and the complexity of the social skills that are being taught or discussed would benefit from further research.

2.2.4 *Autistic views about social skills groups (SSGs)*

Have you personally been part of a social skills group for autistics?

Of the 206 respondents who completed the online survey, 65 (31.55%) answered the question 'Have you personally been part of a social skills group for autistics?' Of those who answered this question, 55 (84.62%) explained that they had not participated in a social skills group, seven (10.77%) that they had been in such a group when they were an adult, and three (4.62%) stated that they had participated in such a group when they were children.

Respondents' ratings of the efficacy of social skills groups (SSGs)

When rating the efficacy of social skills groups, most respondents selected the option 'did not enjoy or find useful' (n = 5, 8.77%), followed by 'enjoyed but did not find

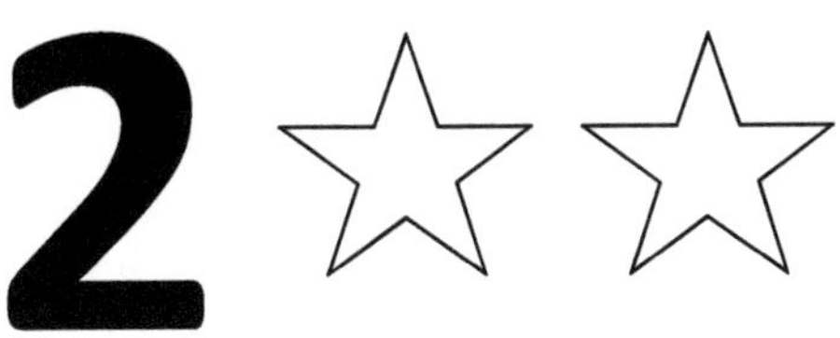

Figure 2.1 2 stars

useful' (n = 4, 7.02%). Since most selected one of these two options, the efficacy of social skills groups for autistics as perceived by autistics was calculated as two stars.

Respondents' comments about social skills groups (SSGs)

Out of the respondents who completed the online survey, 13 answered the question 'How was your experience of social skills groups?' Our examination of their comments showed three believed SSGs were beneficial, three believed they were useless, and seven provided answers that contained minimal information.

One respondent explained that while they learnt social skills during their participation in SSGs, they were not able to generalise these skills to other environments.

> "To be clear, it was a social skills group but not specifically for autistics (no diagnosis at that time). I enjoyed it because the other kids were awkward and had a hard time making friends, like me, so there was some solidarity there. But ultimately, I wasn't able translate those skills into real life."

While some autistic respondents found that SSGs provided them with benefits, others did not express this view. One respondent found the idea 'patronising'.

> "Found the idea so patronising and unappealing that I have never taken part."

Another respondent explained that if the activities in the SSGs focused on their special interests then their social skills might have been improved.

> "There were elements of it that were ok but I wouldn't go so far as to say I enjoyed it. The only thing we had in common was that we were all women with a diagnosis of ASD but I didn't really have a lot in common with the others apart from that. It would have been more useful if it had been focused on my special interests."

In interviewing an autistic psychologist who runs an autistic adult support group, not as part of their clinical practice, which is in effect a naturalistic social space and peer support group, run by and for autistics, it was clear that *peer mediated/run* social groups can be hugely beneficial for adult autistics. This group uses consensus organisation to arrange dates, times, and activities via a private Facebook group. Topics discussed are of mutual interest to those attending. Attendees report that they have somewhere where they can 'just be themselves'. In practical terms, the group provides a 'no judgement environment' where people can feel safe around others. The group is highly valued by all the members. Some of the members now meet up outside of the group to go walking, which has increased their interactions with the wider world significantly.

Other adult autistics who attend autistic led and run groups, commented in text interviews that autistic space is easy to be in, welcoming, and non-judgemental.

> "Autistic space can be really hard initially as we are not connected to who we are, but once this is uncovered in conversation, everything changes. People say we are not social, but in autistic space, you can't shut us up. It's like we trust we have permission to be ourselves and then we are up and running."

The respondents' insights and experiences of SSGs showed that some found such groups beneficial, particularly when autistic led/run, while SSGs that were run by non-autistics were not enjoyed as much and not perceived of as useful. Based on the experiences presented, it appears crucial that for the SSG to be successful potential participants should feel comfortable and not patronised. Making participants feel relaxed can be accomplished by using social skills activities that are based on their passions and interests. Such interests can also create a more comfortable atmosphere for social skills development.

2.3 Peer-mediated activities

2.3.1 Peer-mediated activities

Peer-mediated activities are, in a general sense, activities that are conducted in dyads with one person peer supporting the other person to develop or practise skills, understanding or knowledge. Peer-mediated activities have been extensively used in education; for example, to help school students with reading disabilities improve their literacy skills (Calhoon, 2005). Peer-mediated activities have also been used to help autistics develop skills. We identified five literature reviews in which studies about the efficacy of peer-mentoring activities for autistics were examined.

In 2011, Wang, Cui, and Parrila published a meta-analysis in which they compared case studies about the effectiveness of peer-mediated social skills versus video-modelling activities for teaching autistic children social skills. They examined 13 studies: four about the effectiveness of video-modelling and nine about the effectiveness of peer-mediated activities. They found that peer-mediated and video-modelling activities were equally effective in improving the social behaviours of autistic children. However, they acknowledged that they did not review studies that included participants who were older than ten years. Due to this limitation, they were not able to determine if video-modelling or peer-mediated activities can benefit autistics who are over ten years old.

In 2014, Bene, Banda, and Brown published a meta-analysis in which they examined 14 studies that examined academic peer-mediated activities (e.g., co-operative learning, peer tutoring, peer-mediated learning, and group learning). Most of the studies that they examined measured if peer-mediated activities improved academic skills, such as reading, word recognition, and specific classroom tasks (e.g., poetry writing, art, and social engagement). However, three studies investigated the impact of peer-mediated activities on non-academic skills, including social communication skills, prosocial behaviours, and communication. Based on the literature that they reviewed, they concluded that:

> peer-mediated instructional arrangements may be viable methods for teaching and improving academic and social skills. Peer-mediated instructional arrangement strategies facilitated maintenance and generalization of learned skills in several of the participants.
>
> (Bene, Banda, & Brown, 2014, p. 141).

In 2016, Chang and Locke published a literature review in which they examined five studies about the benefits that peer-mediated activities offered autistic children. To evaluate the methodological quality of these studies they used Reichow, Volkmar, and Cicchetti's

(2008) *Evaluative Method for Determining Evidence-Based Practices in Autism* protocol. A 'strong' quality rating was given to three studies, one was rated as 'adequate', and one was rated as 'weak'. Based on the literature reviewed, Chang and Locke (2016, p. 1) concluded:

> PMI [Peer-medicated Instructions] is a promising approach to address social skills in children with ASD, and this approach can be conducted in meaningful real-world contexts, such as schools ...

Although Chang and Locke's study has improved our understanding of peer-mediated activities for autistics it does have two limitations. First, each study that they reviewed examined the impact of peer-mediated activities for autistic children who had above average cognitive abilities. They did not examine studies that measured if such activities were beneficial for autistics with lower cognitive abilities or those with high support needs. Due to this gap, they were not able to suggest who on the autism spectrum would or would not benefit from peer-mediated activities. Second, they found that there were no studies that used randomised controlled group designs or control groups to measure or compare the impacts of peer-mediated activities with developments that would happen over the same period. It is very difficult to ascertain whether social skills improve due to peer-mediated activities or other interactions and contextual factors that are happening over the same period of time.

In 2015, Watkins and colleagues examined studies that explored if peer-mediated activities improved the social interaction skills of autistic students in inclusive educational settings. Like in Chang and Locke's (2016) study, they too also applied Reichow, Volkmar, and Cicchetti's (2008) *Evaluative Method for Determining Evidence-Based Practices in Autism* protocol to examine the study's quality. Using this protocol, they found that three studies fitted the criteria for 'strong' quality research, nine were deemed as being of 'adequate' quality because they had minor flaws in design and procedure, and two were rated as being of 'weak' quality due to low ratings for experimental control. They found that out of the 14 studies examined, 10 reported positive interventions for all the variables measured (i.e., generalisation, maintenance, fidelity, and social validity measures). Based on these findings, Watkins et al. (2015, p. 1079) concluded:

> The positive outcomes reported in these 14 studies suggest that PMI [Peer-Mediated Interventions] is a promising intervention for promoting social interaction between students with ASD [Autism Spectrum Disorder] and their peers in inclusive settings.

Watkins and colleagues stressed that their results should be interpreted with some caution because of the small number of participants across the 14 studies reviewed and the predominant use of single-subject designs. These limitations made it difficult to generalise the efficacy of peer-mediated activities for the entire autistic population.

In 2016, Zagona and Mastergeorge examined 17 studies that examined the benefits of peer-mediated activities for autistics. They found that in most of the reviewed studies participants demonstrated an increased ability to engage in social-communication skills, including skills related to initiations, responses, and continuations during peer-mediated activities. However, they stressed that in the future studies should include more robust measures of generalisation and include greater numbers of participants.

2.3.2 Evaluation of peer-mediated activities

Gold – Extremely promising and use with confidence

Based on the literature that we examined, we have rated peer-mediated activities for autistics as 'Gold – Extremely promising and use with confidence'. There are two reasons why we have ascribed this rating to such activities. First, Chang and Locke (2016) and Watkins et al. (2015) used Reichow, Volkmar, and Cicchetti's (2008) *Evaluation Method for Determining Evidence-Based Practices in Autism* protocol to determine the methodological quality of the studies that they examined. They found that most studies that they examined were methodologically sound. Second, Bene, Banda, and Brown (2014) showed that peer-mediated activities can provide autistics with many different benefits including reading, maintaining attention, communication abilities, and motor skills development.

2.3.3 Directions for research in the future about peer-mediated activities

Although there are many studies about the benefits that peer-mediated activities might deliver for individual autistics, there are two areas where additional research could be conducted. For example, with the exception of Watkins et al.'s (2015) literature review, the other literature reviews examined in the previous section based their conclusions on studies that had samples of autistic children (Bene, Banda, & Brown, 2014; Chang & Locke, 2016; Wang, Cui, & Parrila, 2011; Zagona & Mastergeorge, 2016). As a consequence, not much research has been conducted into the benefits that autistic adults could obtain from peer-mediated activities. In the future, it would be useful to evaluate the value of such activities for autistic adults, especially since they often encounter more complex social situations than autistic children, such as participating in the workforce or engaging in romantic relationships.

2.3.4 Autistic views about peer-mediated activities

Have you personally had peer-mentoring for autistics or taken part in any peer mediated activities?

Of the 206 respondents who completed the online survey, 61 (29.61%) answered the question 'Have you personally had peer mentoring for autistics or taken part in any peer mediated activities?' Of those who answered this question, most (n = 41, 67.21%) said that they had never participated in a peer-mentoring program, 19 (31.15%) stated that they had participated in such activities as an adult, and one (1.64%) noted that they had participated in such activities when they were a child.

Respondents' ratings of the efficacy of peer-mentoring activities

When rating the efficacy of peer mediated activities for autistics, most respondents (n = 11, 20.00%) selected the option 'enjoyed and found useful', followed by six (10.91%) who selected the option 'enjoyed, found useful and was able to apply skills learnt to other situations'. Based on the distribution of responses, the efficacy of peer-mentoring activities for autistics as perceived by autistics was calculated as 3.9 stars.

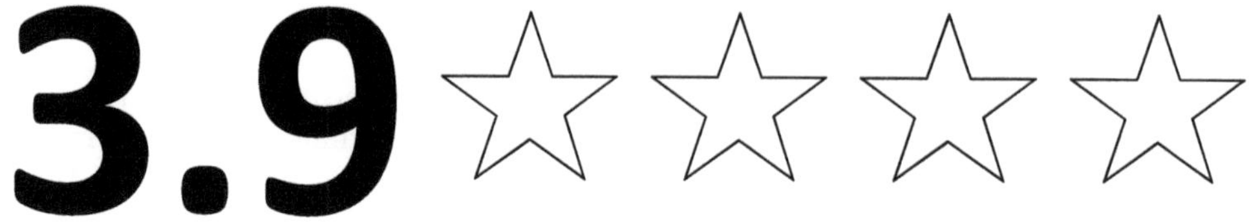

Figure 2.2 3.9 stars

Respondents' comments about peer-mentoring activities

When asked 'How was your experience of peer mentoring and/or peer mediated activities?' 15 respondents provided a comment. Out of these comments we identified seven that provided comments related to the question. Of which, five believed that peer-mentoring activities were beneficial and two that they were not beneficial.

Of those respondents who believed peer-mentoring activities were beneficial, one believed such activities were more valuable than clinical interventions.

> "I actually think that peer mentoring provides a holistic intervention where healing can and is taking place for many autistic adults who have only realised that they are autistic after seeking professional support for their autistic children and teens. The lived experience wisdom exceeds anything that I have observed in any clinical practice setting or any textbook that has been written by professionals without the lived experience of identifying as autistic themselves. I have noticed, through listened to autistic conversations in social media as well as face to face, that other autistic adults are similarly seeking out autistic mentors themselves and finding this type of 'intervention' to be the most effective support / intervention that they have experienced."

Other respondents explained that peer-mentoring activities gave them the opportunity to make friends.

> "I found other people like me with whom I could relate and make friends. People who understood my challenges."

Finally, one respondent explained that peer-mentoring gave them a sense of 'belonging'.

> "Been [a] peer mentor and had peer mentoring, both are very empowering and create a sense of belonging and being mentored gave me the confidence and skills to be the best autistic I can be."

This quote that follows, from an interview highlights that peer mentoring can be from same age, same gender, same ethnicity and/or same neurology. The interviewee noted that one of the successes of the iCAN network is their peer mentoring of young adult autistics by slightly older autistics. Other more formal peer mentoring in Australia, the 'Future Leaders' program, was found to be highly effective as a way to drive empowerment of autistics. Future Leaders program is sponsored by Autism Spectrum Australia and led by Autism CRC which receives funding from the Australian Government.

> "Being supported by an autistic peer comes across differently to being told what you are doing wrong by a non-autistic peer. There is understanding and the information is provided in a way that I can access."

However, not all respondents found peer-mentoring activities beneficial, one explained that "just sharing problems made me stressed and tired" while another stated "I felt like the mentor was gaslighting me." This last comment highlights the need for peer mentors to be carefully selected to ensure that the individuals get on and are respectful of each other.

Our analysis of the comments collected showed that some respondents found peer-mentoring activities beneficial, with these mainly being autistic led activities. The two who did not enjoy it, clearly had not been given the opportunity to choose what they would do during the session. Based on this point, it is important to take into consideration the views of autistic people before placing them into peer-mentoring activities. One of the key considerations in thinking about peer-mediated activities is, will I (or the autistic individual for who I am thinking about peer-mediated activities), get on with the peer? It is possible that a peer mentor with whom there is not a positive, mutually respectful relationship, may be damaging. In contrast, a positive peer relationship may provide a rich source of learning and confidence.

2.4 Conclusion

This chapter presented the contents of literature reviews about the efficacy of SSGs and peer-mediated activities for autistics. Both of these strategies were rated as 'Gold – Extremely promising and use with confidence'. For people considering these support strategies it is worth considering if the offered options are a good fit for you (or your child or client). Things to consider are:

- Will the SSG cover topics or activities that you (or your child or client) find interesting?
- Is the SSG held somewhere that is accessible and not anxiety provoking?
- Are specific sensory needs catered for sensitively?
- Can you (or your child or client) choose what activities to do during peer-mediated activities?
- Can you (or your child or client) set the goals for the peer-mediated activities?
- Are the supports offered in a positive, proactive manner or are they being presented as something that will 'fix' something that is wrong or 'defective', as this is unlikely to be as helpful or effective.
- Is the group run by or facilitated by autistics?

It was recommended that, in the future, studies about the efficacy of SSGs for autistics should take into consideration the views of autistics (i.e., what they think has or has not worked for them), as well as determining the optimum size of the SSG for different social tasks to be learned. However, for peer-mediated activities it was recommended that, in the future, studies should examine if such activities are beneficial for autistic adults since most of the research has examined their efficacy for autistic children. The views of a small sample of autistic adults were also presented. They explained their perceptions of the benefits and drawbacks of peer-mediated activities and SSGs.

References

Bene, K., Banda, D. R., & Brown, D. (2014). A meta-analysis of peer-mediated instructional arrangements and autism. *Review Journal of Autism and Developmental Disorders*, 1(2), 135–142. doi:10.1007/s40489-014-0014-9.

Calhoon, M. B. (2005). Effects of a peer-mediated phonological skill and reading comprehension program on reading skill acquisition for middle school students with reading disabilities. *Journal of Learning Disabilities*, 38(5), 424–433. doi:10.1177/00222194050380050501.

Chang, Y. C., & Locke, J. (2016). A systematic review of peer-mediated interventions for children with autism spectrum disorder. *Research in Autism Spectrum Disorders*, 27, 1–10. doi:10.1016/j.rasd.2016.03.010.

Gates, J. A., Kang, E., & Lerner, M. D. (2017). Efficacy of group social skills interventions for youth with autism spectrum disorder: A systematic review and meta-analysis. *Clinical Psychology Review*, 52, 164–181. doi:10.1016/j.cpr.2017.01.006.

Hotton, M., & Coles, S. (2016). The effectiveness of social skills training groups for individuals with autism spectrum disorder. *Review Journal of Autism and Developmental Disorders*, 3(1), 68–81. doi:10.1007/s40489-015-0066-5.

Miller, A., Vernon, T., Wu, V., & Russo, K. (2014). Social skill group interventions for adolescents with autism spectrum disorders: A systematic review. *Review Journal of Autism and Developmental Disorders*, 1(4), 254–265. doi:10.1007/s40489-014-0017-6.

Reichow, B., Volkmar, F., & Cicchetti, D. (2008). Development of the evaluative method for evaluating and determining evidence-based practices in autism. *Journal of Autism and Developmental Disorders*, 38(7), 1311–1319. doi:10.1007/s10803-007-0517-7.

Spain, D., & Blainey, S. H. (2015). Group social skills interventions for adults with high-functioning autism spectrum disorders: A systematic review. *Autism*, 19(7), 874–886. doi:10.1177/1362361315587659.

Wang, S. Y., Cui, Y., & Parrila, R. (2011). Examining the effectiveness of peer-mediated and video-modeling social skills interventions for children with autism spectrum disorders: A meta-analysis in single-case research using HLM. *Research in Autism Spectrum Disorders*, 5 (1), 562–569. doi:10.1016/j.rasd.2010.06.023.

Watkins, L., O'Reilly, M., Kuhn, M., Gevarter, C., Lancioni, G. E., Sigafoos, J., & Lang, R. (2015). A review of peer-mediated social interaction interventions for students with autism in inclusive settings. *Journal of Autism and Developmental Disorders*, 45(4), 1070–1083. doi:10.1007/s10803-014-2264-x.

Zagona, A. L., & Mastergeorge, A. M. (2018). An empirical review of peer-mediated interventions: Implications for young children with autism spectrum disorders. *Focus on Autism and Other Developmental Disabilities*, 33(3), 131–141. doi:10.1177/1088357616671295.

Chapter 3

Developmental and behavioural supports and programs

3.1 Introduction

This chapter presents the literature about the efficacy of support programs for autistics that are based on developmental and behavioural principles. It begins with an overview of the history of Løvaas's research on applied behaviour analysis (ABA), a set of principles that are the foundation of all the programs and supports that are addressed in this chapter. It then examines the efficacy of the Picture Exchange Communication System (PECS) for autistics, a 'focused intervention program' designed to teach participants one skill; namely communication. It then examines the efficacy of Pivotal Response Training (PRT), Early Intensive Behavioural Intervention (EIBI), and the Early Start Denver Model (ESDM) in helping autistics. These programs are regarded as 'comprehensive programs' or 'Naturalistic Developmental Behavioural Interventions' (NDBIs) since they aim to teach autistics multiple skills in naturalistic settings. After reviewing this literature, a rating of the support's efficacy for autistics is then provided, followed by recommendations for where research in the future could be conducted and a selection of views and experiences from a sample of autistics about the supports and programs evaluated.

3.2 History of applied behaviour analysis (ABA) and the autism spectrum

Dyer (2013, pp. 225–226) has defined applied behaviour analysis (ABA) as:

> … a science that identifies variables that meaningfully and lawfully influence socially significant behaviour in real-world settings. This is done by using principles of behavior to successful teach and support the learning of adaptive, constructive behavior and by reducing excessive problem behavior.

One of the earliest applications of ABA for autistics occurred during the early 1960s when Wolf, Risley, and some of their colleagues at the University of Washington attempted to help a three-year-old autistic boy wear his glasses. This boy lived in a psychiatric facility and risked going blind after receiving cataract surgery because he refused to wear his glasses. He also displayed problems with communication, insomnia, self-destructive behaviours, and eating problems. Sedatives, tranquilizers, and restraints did not provide any benefits. They got this child to wear his glasses by offering him the opportunity to eat small amounts of his preferred food after he wore them (Dyer, 2013).

Dr Ole Ivar Løvaas (8 May 1927–2 August 2010) has published one of the largest bodies of literature about ABA's application with autistics. Before Løvaas's work, it was commonly assumed that autistic children were not capable of learning. Løvaas's major contribution was creating a system that helped autistic children improve their skills and reduce behavioural challenges by providing rewards for desirable behaviour (i.e. reinforcement) and consequences or removal of privileges for undesirable behaviour (i.e. negative reinforcement or punishment) (Smith & Eikeseth, 2011).

Throughout most of his career, Løvaas encouraged positive reinforcement. However, there were occasions when he and several of his colleagues recommended and used physical punishments. During the 1960s, they used low-intensity electric shocks to discourage institutionalised children with autism from exhibiting self-injurious behaviours and physical aggression. Løvaas discovered that physical punishments not only reduced disruptive behaviours but that it also disproved the widespread consensus that children with autism were incapable of understanding or adjusting their behaviours to avoid negative consequences. As Løvaas progressed through his career, he used less physical punishment. For instance, during the 1970s and 1980s he used to slap children with autism on the thigh for challenging behaviours. However, by the late 1980s he had stopped using physical punishments altogether in favour of non-physical forms of punishment, such as removing toys or time out. Although he stopped using physical punishments, his endorsement of them over many years of his career remains a controversial aspect of his legacy (Smith & Eikeseth, 2011) and indeed such aversive former practices are often highlighted in broader critiques and concerns around ABA.

Before the 1980s, there was not much research about the long-term effects that exposure to ABA had on autistics. However, in 1987 this changed when Løvaas published the article "Behavioural Treatment and Normal Educational and Intellectual Functioning in Young Autistic Children" in the *Journal of Consulting and Clinical Psychology*. In this paper, he reported that 47% of children with autism who participated in his ABA program developed typical language and academic skills by the age of seven. He also reported that children with autism who received ABA when they were very young achieved better outcomes than those with similar backgrounds and abilities who received little or no ABA (Løvaas, 1987). However, Løvaas' findings have rarely been replicated (Dawson & Gernsbacher, 2010). Research aiming to replicate Løvaas' research was published in 2000 found that the difference in language performance between the children receiving ABA and the children not receiving ABA was not significant. In addition, there were no differences in adaptive behaviour or intensity of self-regulation issues post intervention between the two groups (Smith, Groen, & Wynn, 2000).

To improve the outcomes of future generations of autistic children, Løvaas and his colleagues proposed several modifications to increase the effectiveness of ABA. These modifications included starting the ABA intervention during the child's preschool years rather than during later childhood or adolescence, involving parents during ABA sessions, and delivering ABA sessions in an environment familiar to the subject (e.g., their home) instead of an environment that is unfamiliar to them (e.g., institutional setting). At the time, these recommendations were controversial. This was illustrated when Løvaas and his colleagues submitted a manuscript that listed these recommendations to the *Journal of Applied Behavior Analysis*. After much negotiation with the editor, their article was published but it had to include a disclaimer which explained the significance of their article and emphasised that there was only a small amount of evidence that supported their recommendations (Smith & Eikeseth, 2011).

When Løvaas was researching and practicing ABA other professionals and some autistics and some of their allies started to criticise programs that relied heavily on ABA methods. Kohn (2020) has listed several common criticisms that are often levelled against ABA, such as that the usage of rewards can communicate the notion of conditional acceptance:

> With endless "Good jobs!" and other expressions of enthusiasm offered only conditionally — You [autistic child] must submit to my will [ABA practitioner] in order to get a big smile, a thumbs up, a high-five — ABA by its very nature makes care transactional and leads children to infer that they're worthwhile only when they do what is demanded of them.

Another criticism of Løvaas's ABA technique is that it can incentivise autistics to become dependent on prompts to guide their learning and development, otherwise known as 'prompt dependency'. Wilson et al. (2014) reported that spouses disclosed that their partners with Asperger syndrome who were exposed to ABA practices when they were children acknowledged that they developed prompted dependency. This dependency created a lack of self-motivation and constant stress within their relationship. Those on the "lower functioning end" of the autism spectrum can also develop prompt dependency after participating in programs that have used classical ABA techniques and settings. They often do not develop the skills to initiate activities since they have been trained to wait for a nudge or command first before engaging in an activity. As Sandoval-Norton and Shkedy (2019, p. 4) have stated:

> A lifetime or punishment and reward without an understanding of the task that is being asked, can create individuals who are compliant and conditioned to obey others, independent of a task. It creates individuals without intrinsic motivation, self-confidence, or self-esteem to successfully engage in any task. A lifetime of having food, candy, toys, and other objects being withheld without an understanding as to why, can create learned helpless, anxiety, and stress.

The prospect that ABA can lead to autistics developing Post-Traumatic Stress Disorder (PTSD) has been examined. Kupferstein (2018) analysed 460 survey responses from autistic adults (n = 243) and caregivers of autistic children (n = 217) about their experiences with ABA programs. Kupferstein discovered that respondents of all ages that participated in ABA programs were 86% more inclined to meet the diagnostic criteria for PTSD than respondents who were not exposed to ABA. Although to some their results might appear controversial, there has not yet been a replication of their results.

In response to these and other criticisms, Naturalistic Development Behavioural Interventions (NDBIs) were developed. Unlike traditional programs based on ABA principles, NDBIs incorporate principles of ABA into naturalistic settings. According to Schreibman and colleagues (2015, p. 2416) NDBIs:

> reflect a developmental systems approach, in which the goal is to ensure that development of a skill in one domain (e.g., learning a symbol, such as a new word

or gesture, in one activity) will be integrated with development of skills in other domains (e.g., using the word or gesture to sustain engagement with another person and in other activities) from the beginning. Thus, in the NDBI approaches, skills are usually not taught discretely or in isolation, but rather in the course of the child's typical daily interactions, experiences, and routines, with multiple materials and by multiple people.

Most NDBIs share the following eight elements.

1 They all use a three-part contingency (i.e., antecedent-response-consequence) to help the participant understand when they are expected to respond to an instruction and when they can expect feedback.
2 The procedures to implement the program are clearly documented. Such documentation helps professionals and other treatment providers, such as parents, understand how to implement the NDBI effectively.
3 They all have a clear fidelity of implementation criteria that explains the way in which a treatment is supposed to be implemented.
4 They all have treatment goals which are clear, specific, and measurable and which are individualised to the participant's skills, circumstances, and needs.
5 They all have mechanisms for measuring ongoing progress. Such measurements may be made at specific intervals during an NDBI session or could be curriculum-based assessments performed at the end of the NDBI program. The method of data collection is usually tailored to the intervention program used and the participant's goals.
6 In all NDBIs the participant initiates the teaching activity. Often the participant indicates what they are interested in doing or engages in a familiar routine and then the instructor incorporates and presents the teaching opportunity in the activity.
7 In NDBIs the instructor arranges the environment so that the participant has to interact with the instructor. For example, using items a participant desires but that are out of their reach so that they have to ask the instructor for assistance.
8 During an NDBI instructors use natural reinforcers that are intrinsically appealing to the participant instead of an arbitrary reward. For example, if a child successfully completes a task and expresses a desire to play with a car toy, then the instructor would give them the toy instead of a reward that they do not consider intrinsically appealing, such as a break or food (Schreibman et al., 2015).

Currently a wide range of naturalistic and developmental approaches are available in community settings for use from early infancy through to adulthood. These may target a specific goal over the short term (focused practices) or multiple domains over an extended period (comprehensive intervention packages) (Wong et al., 2015). In this chapter the literature about PECS, a focused intervention approach to teaching communication, is outlined along with a rating of its efficacy and the views of autistics.

'Pure' ABA supports have not been reviewed in this book for a number of reasons. In reality, it is very hard for families to ascertain when supports are ABA or not as providers and therapists do not necessarily declare the theory behind their therapy. Additionally, it is difficult to find comprehensive literature reviews on ABA that are not based on goals of decreasing 'autistic symptomology'. As this book is reviewing strategies and supports that might enable autistics to thrive, supports were reviewed that were offering autistics access to learning in naturalistic settings or ways to communicate when they have no speech. Naturalistic settings may be significantly less stressful for autistics and may facilitate generalisation of skills more easily.

3.3 The Picture Exchange Communication System (PECS)

3.3.1 The Picture Exchange Communication System (PECS)

In 2009, Bondy and Frost developed the Picture Exchange Communication System (PECS), which is an augmentative and alternative communication system. The PECS teaching protocol is based on Skinner's book *Verbal Behavior*, which is based on ABA principles. As its name suggests, a key component of PECS is picture cards, also called icons, that represent objects (e.g., cup, pen), people (e.g., doctor, teacher, mother, father, brother, sister), and activities (e.g., walking, hugging). A user selects icons from either a computer program or a physical catalogue. They then combine the picture card with a sentence item, such as 'I want' or 'I hear'. Such combinations form statements or requests that can be as simple or complex as the person using PECS wants (or is able to make) them to be. For example, by combining the sentence item 'I want' with the picture card 'mother' a user can convey the request 'I want mother'. Furthermore, a user of PECS may just offer the picture of milk to request a drink of milk. However, as their familiarity with PECS increases, they may start to make responsive and spontaneous comments, such as stating that the milk yesterday was off, and they want a glass of fresh milk to drink.

PECS has a number of advantages. First, the materials required to create a PECS system are relatively inexpensive, making it accessible to people without access to high levels of disposable income. Second, PECS is easy to transport so it can be used in many different settings, including school and the workplace. Third, icons can be easily created which means that it can be tailored to a user's interests and circumstances. Fourth, paper-based PECS programs are technologically simple which can eliminate the issue of technological failure. Fifth, the meanings of the picture cards do not change and they directly correspond with an object, person, or activity. Since the meanings are static, instances of misinterpretation and miscommunication are reduced (Ganz, Simpson, & Lund, 2012).

PECS has been used to help children with many different disabilities communicate with others (Walker & Snell, 2013). However, for the purposes of this book, only the research about the utility of PECS for autistics is reviewed. During our literature search we identified three literature reviews in which studies about the benefits of PECS for autistics were examined (Flippin, Reszka, & Watson, 2010; Sulzer-Azaroff et al., 2009; Tien, 2008).

Flippin, Reszka, and Watson (2010) published a meta-analysis in which they examined 11 studies about the utility of PECS in helping autistic children communicate. Their main objective was to examine the benefits that PECS had on the communication abilities of autistic children. They also used guidelines developed by Wolf (1978) to examine the quality of the literature collected. Based on the research collected, along with an assessment of its quality, they concluded that:

> the overall effectiveness of the PECS approach for communication outcomes with children with ASD is promising although not yet established … Further empirical

> research is now needed to directly examine the generalizablity of speech and communication gains following PECS and to examine and identify child characteristics that may account for the variance in outcomes.
>
> (Flippin, Reszka, & Watson, 2010, p. 190)

Although their findings have paved a way for future research their conclusions need to be interpreted with caution. Flippin, Reszka, and Watson found that two of the three group design studies and four of the eight single-subject design studies did not explain clearly the procedures used to implement the PECS program, including descriptions of what training personnel received to deliver the PECS program. Due to this lack of detail, it is difficult to replicate these studies in order to validate the results articulated.

In 2008, Tien published a literature review of studies about the impact that the PECS program had on the communication abilities of autistics. They examined the contents of 11 articles, which collectively examined 13 studies and 125 participants. Based on the literature that they reviewed, Tien concluded that PECS is an effective tool for enhancing the communication skills of autistics who use little or no verbal speech.

> Taken as a whole, therefore, results of the studies reviewed provide evidence for the effectiveness of PECS; specifically, PECS is effective in enhancing functional communication skills of individuals with ASD. Therefore, PECS is recommended as an evidence-based intervention for this purpose.
>
> (Tien, 2008, p. 74).

In 2009, Sulzer-Azaroff and colleagues echoed Tien's (2008) view after examining 34 studies. They concluded:

> The controlled single-case studies and group experimental reports reviewed in this article suggest that PECS has enabled hundreds of individuals to effectively express their wants, needs, and observations. Though not directly designed to teach speech or to reduce aggression, a number of individuals who use PECS have begun to speak and/or to diminish maladaptive behaviors.
>
> (Sulzer-Azaroff et al., 2009, p. 101).

3.3.2 Evaluation of the Picture Exchange Communication System (PECS)

Rating: Gold – Extremely promising and use with confidence

We have rated the efficacy of PECS for autistics who have limited speech as 'Gold – Extremely promising and use with confidence'. PECS received this rating because most of the studies examined by the three literature reviews presented in Section 3.3.1 have provided a positive endorsement of PECS. On a side note, despite considering teaching PECS to an autistic child a time-consuming exercise, the practitioners interviewed for Alsayedhassan et al.'s (2019) study believed that autistic children found PECS an easy and effective way for them to develop their communication skills. Additionally, PECS has been found to reduce the stress that autistics experience when they are not able to express themselves (Sulzer-Azaroff et al., 2009). Finally, since PECS is a symbol-based communication system, computer programs (e.g., prologquo2go) can hold a large number of symbols to facilitate communication across a range of contexts.

3.3.3 *Directions for research in the future about the Picture Exchange Communication System (PECS)*

Although PECS can help some autistics who use no or minimal verbal speech to express themselves, there are additional areas where more research can be conducted; namely a need to conduct additional research about the long-term efficacy of PECS, and examining if the efficacy of PECS can be enhanced when combined with other supports.

Whether or not the benefits of PECS are maintained long-term remains a subject of inquiry. This point was expressed by Tien (2008) who reported that out of the 12 single-subject participant studies that they examined, only three (25%) reported follow-up data after the discontinuation of their study. Similarly, Flippin, Reszka, and Watson (2010) reported that 50% of single-subject studies that they examined incorporated a follow-up assessment to examine if PECS produced any long-term benefits. Due to the lack of studies that have used follow-up procedures, knowledge about the long-term benefits that PECS provides for autistics remains unknown. To explore this topic, studies should incorporate into their research designs follow-up assessments. Incorporating such assessments will not only increase our knowledge about PECS, it will also help us understand if PECS is a viable long-term strategy to help autistics who use no or minimal verbal speech to communicate more effectively with others.

Currently, few studies have explored if PECS's efficacy can be enhanced by combining it with another support program. For example, it is possible that the communication skills an autistic develops with PECS could be enhanced if they apply these newly acquired skills in a social skills group. In other words, by combining PECS with a social skills group an autistic child may gain the confidence to use PECS around others. Additionally, such usage can also help others in the social skills group acclimatise to autistics using PECS.

3.3.4 *Autistic views about the Picture Exchange Communication System (PECS)*

Have you personally used the Picture Exchange Communication System (PECS)?

Most respondents (n = 51, 82.26%) selected the option 'No' when asked 'Have you personally used the Picture Exchange Communication System (PECS)?' However, 11 reported that they had used PECS; two (3.23%) noted that they have used it to communicate with others, and nine (14.52%) stated they had used it to communicate with someone else who communicates using PECS.

Respondents' ratings of the efficacy of the Picture Exchange Communication System (PECS)

Most respondents (n = 10, 19.61%) who reported that they had used PECS stated that it was 'easy and useful'. Based on the distribution of responses, the efficacy of PECS as rated by autistics was four stars.

Respondents' comments about the Picture Exchange Communication System (PECS)

Ten participants answered the question 'How did you, or do you, find using PECS?' Of these responses, eight explained that PECS was 'easy to use'.

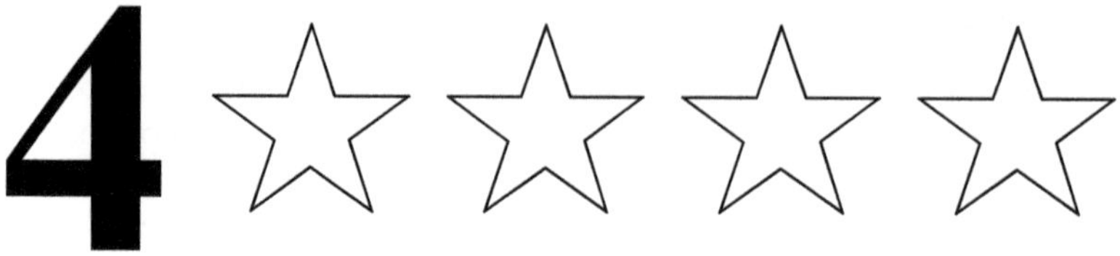

Figure 3.1 4 stars

> "Easy and useful."
>
> "Easy and somewhat useful. I find that I can be more expressive with communication in ASL, though, so where possible I do favour sign language."
>
> "My son is also autistic and non-verbal so once learnt this was an easy way for us to communicate and required less mental energy for me also."
>
> "easy to use at a basic level, much harder when doing the full on PECS with grammar."

Additionally, one participant explained that PECS was also a useful communication tool when they were experiencing a 'meltdown'.

> "Useful during meltdown when verbal ability disappears and nobody knows sign language."

None of the responses collected indicated that participants thought PECS was complex or unusable. Taking into account the positive feedback collected, it is clear that when deciding if PECS is an appropriate tool for communication, people may want to take into account the visual skills of the individual as poor visual discrimination or visual impairments where an individual cannot tell the difference between pictures or symbols would be an impediment to implementing PECS. PECS is seen as easy to use and useful by both the autistic respondents and the research literature. The literature notes that the use of PECS may also help develop spoken language (Sulzer-Azaroff et al., 2009), whereas many of the autistics suggested that PECS was useful whether or not they used speech at any times.

3.4 Pivotal Response Training (PRT)

3.4.1 Pivotal Response Training (PRT)

Pivotal Response Training (PRT) involves autistic children learning skills in naturalistic settings (e.g., their family home or school) instead of settings that they find unfamiliar (e.g., a clinical setting). PRT focuses on children developing four pivotal skills (i.e., motivation for social communication, self-initiation, responding to multiple cues, and self-management). What follows are two examples of PRT for autistic children (See Table 3.1).

Table 3.1 Two examples of Pivotal Response Training (PRT) for autistic children

Situation	*Steps in Pivotal Response Training (PRT)*
A learning opportunity for the target behaviour three-word sentence in a young child with ASD	1. The child chooses to play with a ball (PRT technique: Following the child's interests) 2. The therapist holds the ball after the child rolls the ball (PRT technique: Catching the child's attention) 3. The therapist prompts the child by saying a three-word sentence: 'Roll the ball' (PRT technique: Providing a clear learning opportunity with appropriate help) 4. If the child responds with 'roll ball', the therapist rolls the ball (PRT techniques: Providing a natural reward and rewarding attempts).
A learning opportunity for the target behaviour asking an informative question in an adolescent with ASD	1. The adolescent enjoys playing different video games and the therapist brings a new video game (PRT technique: Following the adolescent's interests) 2. The video game is on the table but is still wrapped in paper (PRT technique: Catching the adolescent's attention) 3. The therapist prompts the adolescent first by waiting for a response. If the adolescent does not respond, the therapist prompts the adolescent again by saying: "You can ask now: Which game did you bring?" (PRT technique: Providing a clear learning opportunity with appropriate help) 4. If the participant says, "which game is it?", the therapist answers the question and unwraps the paper (PRT techniques: Providing a natural reward and rewarding attempts).

Source: Smeekens et al., 2017, p. 14.

The research suggests that PRT programs can help autistics of varying ages, developmental levels, and verbal abilities. For very young autistic children, PRT can teach them how to begin a conversation. For autistic adolescents, PRT can teach age-appropriate social behaviours in typical settings, such as a family home, with parents and siblings. PRT can occur in different environments (e.g., school classrooms, playgrounds, family home) and involve different people (e.g., teachers, parents, peers) (Smeekens et al., 2017).

3.4.2 Pivotal Response Training (PRT) and autistic children

There are three literature reviews in which studies about the efficacy of PRT programs for autistics have been examined (Boudreau et al., 2015; Verschuur et al., 2014; Wong et al., 2015). In 2014, Verschuur and colleagues published a literature review of studies about the efficacy of PRT for autistic children. They evaluated the success of PRT for improving the skills of autistic children and to evaluate the certainty of evidence arising from the studies. Based on the studies they collected, they concluded that:

> The majority of the reviewed studies (56.4 %) had serious methodological limitations. However, the reviewed studies that provided conclusive or preponderant evidence (43.6 %) indicated that PRT results in increases in self-initiations and

> collateral improvements in communication and language, play skills, affect and reductions in maladaptive behavior for a number of children.
>
> (Verschuur et al., 2014, p. 34).

In 2015, Boudreau and colleagues applied Reichow et al.'s (2008) *Evaluative Method for Determining Evidence-Based Practice in Autism* to five single-case studies about the effectiveness of peer-mediated PRT in helping autistic children improve their social-communication skills. They found that while most studies reported positive outcomes, the research did not meet Reichow et al.'s criteria and that more research is needed before PRT can be considered an evidence-based practice for helping autistic children improve their social-communication abilities.

In contrast to Boudreau et al.'s findings, Wong et al. (2015) reported that PRT met the criteria for being an evidence-based practice. After examining this evidence, they concluded that:

> Most studies of PM-PRT [Peer-Mediated - Pivotal Response Training] observed positive outcomes. However, the existing research base did not meet criteria for classification as promising or established evidence-based practice (EBP) for improving social skill deficits in children with ASD. More research is required for PM-PRT to be considered formally as EBP.
>
> (Boudreau et al., 2015, p. 218).

3.4.3 Evaluation of Pivotal Response Training (PRT)

Rating: Silver – Usually promising

Based on an examination of the studies in Verschuur et al.'s (2014), Wong et al.'s (2015), and Boudreau et al.'s (2015) literature reviews we have rated the efficacy of PRT for autistics as 'Silver – Usually promising'. We ascribed this rating because Verschuur et al. and Boudreau et al. did not definitively conclude that PRT yielded benefits for autistics. For example, several studies in Verschuur et al.'s literature review concluded that PRT yielded mixed results for autistics (Bernard-Opitz, Ing, & Kong, 2004; Coolican, Smith, & Bryson, 2010; Huskens et al., 2012; Lydon, Healy, & Leader, 2011; Randolph et al., 2011; Robinson, 2011; Steiner et al., 2013).

3.4.4 Directions for research in the future about Pivotal Response Training (PRT)

Despite there being many researchers that have evaluated the efficacy of PRT for autistics, there are three areas where more research in the future can be conducted. First, most studies that Verschuur et al. (2014) investigated (56.4%) contained methodological flaws which resulted in them being classified as having a 'suggestive' level of evidence. To validate the results discovered, studies should adopt a higher standard of research design, including using blinded rating systems. Second, to understand more about the efficacy of PRT for autistics, studies should compare the effectiveness of PRT against other types of supports. This can be accomplished by comparing the benefits that autistic children in a PRT group receive to the benefits that autistic children receive from another type of support, or to a group who are not receiving any formal supports. Groups should be matched on age, gender, intelligence and cognitive abilities, language abilities, and autistic diagnosis. Third, studies should examine the perspectives and views of verbal autistics about what they think they have obtained from PRT programs. Such insights could provide further inroads into designing effective PRT programs for autistics.

3.4.5 Autistic views about Pivotal Response Training (PRT)

Have you personally experienced Pivotal Response Training (PRT) as a group on 1:1 with a therapist?

Since no respondent rated the efficacy of PRT its efficacy was not rated. It is possible that respondents did not select an option because they either did not experience or did not know that supports received were PRT.

3.5 Early Intensive Behavioural Intervention (EIBI)

3.5.1 Early Intensive Behavioural Intervention (EIBI)

EIBI is a comprehensive intervention that is most closely aligned to the work of Løvaas. In 2018, Reichow and colleagues published a literature review in which they evaluated five studies about the benefits of EIBI for autistics. A total of 219 autistic children were sampled across these studies; of which, 116 were in the EIBI group and 103 were in the treatment-as-usual group. Regarding the intervention, three studies provided 24 months of EIBI support and two studies provided 36 months. They found that EIBI improved adaptive behaviour, communication skills, expressive and language abilities, social competence skills, and daily living skills. Their findings are similar to those published in other studies about this topic (Eldevik et al., 2009; Makrygianni & Reed, 2010; Virués-Ortega, 2010). Despite Reichow et al.'s study validating the findings in the literature, they stressed that their conclusions should be interpreted with caution since they:

> found weak evidence that children receiving the EIBI treatment performed better than children in the comparison groups after about two years of treatment on scales of adaptive behavior, intelligence tests, expressive language (spoken language), and receptive language (the ability to understand what is said) … or a child's problem behavior.
>
> (Reichow et al., 2018, p. 3).

Studies have examined if the benefits which EIBI programs give autistics can be sustained long-term (Kovshoff, Hastings, & Remington, 2011; Perry et al., 2019; Rivard et al., 2018). Perry et al. (2019) examined if EIBI programs maintained cognitive abilities and adaptive skills. They evaluated these outcomes at four time points; Time Point 1 was conducted prior to the start of the EIBI program, Time Point 2 was conducted after the EIBI program finished, Time Point 3 was conducted at follow-up one to six years after the completion of the EIBI program, and Time Point 4 occurred at a follow-up point which was on average ten years after the EIBI program finished. Out of a maximum of 36 participants, seven had relocated and could not be contacted at follow-up, seven refused to participate and one could not participate because of their location. Their final sample was comprised of 21 youths (19 males, two females). Based on the diagnostic instruments they used and the data collected, Perry et al. (2019, p. 199) concluded:

> We found generally stable scores and classifications of outcome about 10 years after cessation of EIBI. Such long-term benefits have not previously been documented and are a crucial piece of evidence justifying the extensive resources required to mount this intervention.

Although Perry et al.'s findings have contributed to our understanding about the long-term benefits that EIBI programs can give autistics their study does have some limitations, with no reasons given for the refusal to participate by almost a quarter of the individuals, in the follow up. Additional limitations relate to the *Childhood Autism Rating Scale* (CARS), which was used at all time points in the study. However, the raters who completed this test at Time Points 1 and 2 did not receive the same training, whereas all raters from Time Points 3 and 4 received the same training and completed the ratings in a consistent manner. Compounding this lack of standardisation was that the CARS test is not ideal for detecting very subtle changes in the characteristic signs of autism. Thus, the reduction in autism severity at follow-up may be overstated, which may have given the impression that EIBI was effective. In addition, Perry et al.'s findings do not consider whether the same reduction would be found long-term in autistic children who had more naturalistic supports than EIBI, as suggested by Reichow et al. (2018).

Rivard and colleagues (2018) assessed the outcomes of 32 autistic children (21 males, 11 females) at post-treatment and one-year follow-up after they attended a low to moderate intensity of EIBI (i.e., ten to 20 hours per week). To measure if EIBI produced long-term benefits for reducing the severity of autism symptoms, they used several tests, including the French versions of the *Gilliam Autism Rating Scale-Second Edition* and the *Wechsler Preschool and Primary Scale of Intelligence-Third Edition*, CARS, and the *Adaptive Behavior Assessment System-II*. Based on the data collected they concluded:

> Overall, children with ASD who received low-to-moderate intensity EIBI showed improvements in several areas of intellectual functioning that were generally maintained over the year following the cessation of treatment, when these children were enrolled in school. Despite these encouraging findings, it should be noted that some children continued to present substantial difficulties in terms of AB [Adaptive Behavior].
>
> (Rivard et al., 2018, pp. 21–22).

Despite the importance of these results, Rivard et al.'s study had several limitations which may have influenced the results. First, due to the small sample size, of 32 autistic participants, it is difficult to reach any definitive conclusions due to the limited statistical power. Second, the EIBI program was universally accessible to all eligible children who lived in the area where the study was conducted. Due to its accessibility, it was not feasible to form a control group of autistic children who did not receive EIBI support over the same time and in the same location. Since there was no control group it was not possible to compare the efficacy of EIBI against a group that either received another support or no support at all. Third, long-term data has shown that autistics have fairly stable development over time, which suggests that changes may not be entirely due to an intervention itself. An example of this can be found in Howlin et al.'s (2014) 40-year follow-up study of cognitive and language skills in autistic adults. They found that:

> For the majority of participants (N=45, 75%), who were testable both as children and adults, IQ remained very stable and language also improved over time.
> (Howlin et al., 2014, p. 49).

3.5.2 Evaluation of Early Intensive Behavioural Intervention (EIBI)

Rating: Bronze – Safe but ineffective

The literature about the benefits autistics obtain from EIBI programs has not universally concluded that they can help autistics. For example, Reichow et al. (2018) concluded that autistic children who received EIBI treatment for two years did not show improvements in adaptive behaviour intelligence tests, spoken language, and the ability to understand what is said in comparison to autistic children who did not receive EIBI treatment. Due to such limitations, we have rated such programs as 'Bronze – Safe but ineffective'. However, it is possible that some autistics may not enjoy participating in EIBI, particularly if they are not able to indulge in their passions and interests because of the participation requirements of the program.

3.5.3 Directions for research in the future about Early Intensive Behavioural Intervention (EIBI)

While there is an extensive amount of literature about the possible efficacy of EIBI programs for autistic children, there are two areas where more research can be conducted in the future. Currently, there are not many studies that have measured the long-term benefits that autistic children have obtained from EIBI, particularly in comparison with supportive parenting and effective communication supports. This point has been expressed by Matson and Konst (2013) who examined 22 studies about the long-term efficacy of EIBI programs for autistic children which used the term 'follow-up'. Of these, 19 studies actually did not conduct any follow-up evaluations, they instead used post-test data. The remaining three studies used follow-up instruments to determine the long-term efficacy of EIBI programs. They concluded that most studies that used the term 'follow-up' should have instead used the term 'post-test data'. In the future studies should use appropriate terminology so that the long-term benefits of EIBI for autistic children can be clearly understood. The term 'follow-up' should be used to refer to the measurement of EIBI efficacy after a prolonged period of time has elapsed since the ending of the EIBI program. However, any data collected soon after the EIBI program has stopped should be referred to as 'post-test data'. By clarifying these terms, the long-term benefits of EIBI for autistic children will be clearly defined.

Another area where research can be conducted in the future is in examining the environmental and cost factors that can influence the efficacy of EIBI programs with matched control groups. This point was expressed by Howlin, Magiati, and Charman (2009) who explained that in the future family factors (i.e., parental marital status, financial and employment circumstances of the family, and parental well-being and support) should be documented. Recording such factors and then comparing the effectiveness of EIBI versus naturalistic supports only, such factors could reveal what family dynamics might compromise or enhance the efficacy of EIBI programs versus naturalistic supports. There is a need for cost effectiveness research and understanding how many hours are sufficient for balancing benefit to the child with the broader impact on the family in terms of time, energy, and money when they or a professional are delivering the EIBI. The positives and negatives of one-to-one versus group EIBI programs would benefit from being researched within this wider context. Furthermore, by measuring the impact of family factors on the efficacy of EIBI for autistic children it will be possible to target EIBI more effectively within the autistic community.

3.5.4 Autistic views about Early Intensive Behavioural Intervention (EIBI)

Have you personally experienced Early Intensive Behavioural Intervention (EIBI)?

Out of the 206 respondents who completed the online survey, 62 (30.09%) answered the question 'Have you personally experienced early intensive behavioural intervention (EIBI)?' Most (n = 55, 88.71%) said that they had not participated in an EIBI program when they were children. However, six (9.68%) stated that they had participated in a one-on-one EIBI session with a therapist when they were under 18 years old, and one respondent stated that they had participated in a group EIBI program when they were a child.

Respondents' ratings of the efficacy of Early Intensive Behavioural Intervention (EIBI)

Since there are less than ten responses, the efficacy of EIBI programs for autistics was not rated.

Respondents' comments about Early Intensive Behavioural Intervention (EIBI)

An analysis of the collected responses revealed that no respondents provided sufficient details to explain their experiences of EIBI. It is possible that not many were able to answer this question because they were unaware that they had participated in an EIBI program. However, two autistic adults contacted the authors to discuss the toll they felt the EIBI placed on autistics. Both of these felt that high intensity EIBI placed a higher priority on 'fixing autistics' than on 'children being allowed to play and explore and be children'. One of the respondents talked about the misuse of requiring autistic children's compliance in EIBI providers, whilst the other mentioned 'unintended side-effects' of some of the methods in a therapy that said it was EIBI. In this case the child was rewarded for saying 'hello' repeatedly whilst maintaining eye contact, the result was a young adult who would say 'hello' repeatedly. In thinking about if EIBI is right for a child, it is important to ask how it will fit into family life and how the therapist will work with the child to build confidence and competence and not "break the child down so they can be built up again" as a respondent reported that they had been told by an EIBI provider.

3.6 Early Start Denver Model (ESDM)

3.6.1 Early Start Denver Model (ESDM)

Sally Rogers and her colleagues at the University of Colorado developed the Early Start Denver Model (ESDM) during the early 1980s. ESDM is considered an NDBI since it incorporates principles of ABA in a natural environment. ESDM is a comprehensive program that focuses on helping autistic children improve their communication and social learning. There are two variants of the ESDM; a parent-mediated version where parents are trained as therapists to deliver at home, and a group-based program that is delivered in early childhood settings. Typically, autistic children who are aged between 12 to 60 months participate in ESDM programs. These programs are usually delivered in play and caregiving environments and focus on developing skills. ESDM approaches are highly individualised and can be delivered in many settings, such as a family home or school, and can involve anyone who is proficient in ESDM principles and practices (Rogers, Vivanti, & Rocha, 2017). However, it is of note that the parent and therapist manual are available for purchase but both parents and therapists are encouraged to do expensive and time-consuming training to provide ESDM services. Due to these costs it is possible that some people may be offering EDSM without having done training but having purchased the manual only. Therefore, if considering this program, it might be useful to ask for guidance from the therapist who has training and experience with EDSM.

There are four literature reviews in which studies about the efficacy of ESDM for autistics have been examined (Baril & Humphreys, 2017; Ryberg, 2015; Waddington, van der Meer, & Sigafoos, 2016; Warren et al., 2011). In 2015, Ryberg published a literature review in which they reviewed peer-reviewed studies about the use of the ESDM as an intervention for autistic children. They located eight studies which met their inclusion criteria; of which, two were randomised controlled trials, four were controlled trials, and two were observational cohort studies (See Table 3.2). Despite the diversity of different methodological designs, Ryberg (2015, p. 327) concluded that:

> The ESDM is an effective intervention that improves cognition, language, and adaptive behavior. ESDM strategies delivered in community group settings and in the home by parents have potential to be efficacious and feasible.

While the conclusions drawn by Ryberg supports the notion that autistic children would benefit from ESDM, their literature review has several limitations that could undermine their conclusions. First, they examined a small number of studies and the overall quality of evidence was small as only one randomised controlled trial was examined. Second, Ryberg limited the articles collected to those studies that were published in the last five years. It is possible that studies published earlier could have challenged the conclusions reached.

Table 3.2 Summary of studies examined by Ryberg (2015)

Author and year published	*Study type*	*Population*	*Intervention*	*Outcomes*	*GRADE* [a]
Dawson et al., 2010	RCT	Toddlers 18–30 months of age with ASD	This two-year study involved random assignment of 48 children diagnosed with ASD or PDDNOS to an ESDM intervention group or an A/M group. For the A/M group, referrals to community interventions were provided.	Compared to the A/M group, children assigned to the ESDM intervention demonstrated significant gains in IQ, adaptive behavior, and autism diagnosis.	High
Dawson et al., 2012	Controlled trial	Toddlers 48–77 months of age with ASD and typical children of same age	In association with Dawson et al. (2010) study, EEG activity was measured after two-year study during presentation of social (faces) and nonsocial (toys) stimuli.	ESDM improves a child's social behavior, and subsequently, brain activity related to social attention and engagement becomes normalised and comparable to typical children.	Moderate
Eapen, Črnčec, and Walter, 2013	Observational cohort study	Preschool, mean age 49.6 months, children with ASD	26 children with ASD received 15–20 hours of group-based and two 30-minute individual ESMD intervention per week by trained therapists while attending a childcare centre. Average period was ten months. No comparison group was used.	Participants made significant improvements in DQ, visual reception, receptive language, and expressive language. Significant increases were noted in receptive communication and motor skills, and there was a significant decrease in autism specific features.	Low

Author and year published	*Study type*	*Population*	*Intervention*	*Outcomes*	*GRADE* [a]
Estes et al., 2014	Controlled trial	Toddlers aged 12–24 months at risk for ASD and their parents	In association with the Rogers et al. (2012) study, parenting stress (77 families) and sense of competence (83 families) were assessed at the start and end of the 12-week intervention.	P-ESDM caregivers reported lower parenting stress. Community group reported an increase in stress. There was no significant difference between groups with parent sense of competence, and the number of intervention hours had no significant relationship to parent stress or sense of competence.	Moderate
Rogers et al., 2012	RCT	Toddlers aged 12–24 months at risk for ASD and their families	98 children with ASD were randomly assigned to either a 12-week, one-hour per week of therapist contact, parent-delivered intervention (P-ESDM) or to community treatment as usual for 12 weeks	There was no difference in the parent-child interaction or in any of the child outcomes with either group. Regardless of group, parent interaction skills improved and children exhibited an increased attainment of developmental skills and a decrease in symptoms. The community group received twice as many hours.	High
Rogers et al., 2014	Controlled trial	Symptomatic infants aged 7–15 months	Seven infants were matched to four comparison groups and engaged in a 12-week, low intensity treatment based on parental delivery of the ESDM.	At nine months of age, the treatment group demonstrated significantly more symptoms than most of the comparison groups but were significantly less symptomatic than the two most affected groups between 18 and 36 months. At 36 months, the treated group had much lower rates of both ASD and DQs under 70 than a similarly symptomatic group who did not enrol in the treatment study.	Low

(*continued*)

Table 3.2 (*coninued*)

Author and year published	*Study type*	*Population*	*Intervention*	*Outcomes*	*GRADE* [a]
Vivanti et al., 2014	Controlled trial	Toddlers aged 18–60 months diagnosed with ASD	To investigate the effectiveness and feasibility of the ESDM program delivered in a long-day care community service, 57 preschoolers with ASD received either 15–25 hours per week of ESDM (n = 27) or a community-based educational program in a similar setting with a similar level of intensity (n = 30).	Both groups showed significant improvement in cognitive skills, adaptive functioning, and social communication. Children in the ESDM intervention demonstrated significantly greater increases in developmental rate, receptive language, and cognitive abilities. Analysis of feasibility indicators suggests that the ESDM has the potential to be implemented under real-world conditions.	Moderate
Vismara, Young, and Rogers, 2013	Observational cohort study	24 community based EI practitioners	EI practitioners engaged in a four-day workshop to learn the ESDM. Fidelity was measured at the start and end of the workshop, and again at four months postworkshop.	At the end of the four-day workshop, participants were delivering the ESDM interactive procedures at 80% or better fidelity. After the four-month time frame, only 46% of participants submitted data. Those that did send data demonstrated high levels of fidelity to ESDM practices and generalisation of skills to new children with ASD.	Low

Source: Ryberg, 2015, pp. 330–331.

[a] GRADE is a system for grading quality of evidence and strength of recommendation. Its four levels of evidence quality are very low, low, moderate, and high. Its strength of recommendation is strong or weak.

One of the most recent literature reviews of studies about the efficacy of ESDM programs for autistic children was published in 2017 by Baril and Humphreys. They reviewed ten studies and found that there was a variability in methodological designs, participant and intervention characteristics, and research rigor. They also found that it is not fully known to what extent ESDM programs alone can help autistic children. Despite these findings, they found that:

> The ESDM shows promise as an evidence-based practice for young children with ASD and there is preliminary evidence to support implementation of the ESDM.
> (Baril & Humphreys, 2017, p. 321).

The question as to whether the ESDM is more effective for children younger or older than 48 months of age was examined by Vivanti, Dissanayake, and members of the Victorian ASELCC Team (2016). They compared the outcomes of 32 children aged between 18 to 48 months who received one year of 20 hours per week of ESDM training against 28 children who were aged between 48 to 62 months who also received the same amount of ESDM training. They found that autistic children in the 18 to 48 months group exhibited superior verbal developmental quotients than their older counterparts. However, there were no differences between both age groups regarding non-verbal developmental quotients and adaptive behaviour or changes with the presentation of autistic symptomology, as indicated by both groups not showing improvements in scores from the *Autistic Diagnostic Observation Schedule.*

3.6.2 Evaluation of Early Start Denver Model (ESDM)

Rating: Silver – Extremely promising and use with confidence

The literature that we reviewed showed that the ESDM program can provide some autistic children with multiple benefits, including improved cognitive performance and language abilities (Warren et al., 2011). The literature reviewed also showed that the benefits that some autistics obtained from the ESDM can be generalised to other settings (Ryberg, 2015). Thus, we have rated it as 'Gold – Extremely promising and use with confidence'.

3.6.3 Directions for research in the future about the Early Start Denver Model (ESDM)

Despite the large amount of literature that concludes that the ESDM can give autistic children many benefits, there remains two areas where more research can be conducted in the future.

First, although the research shows that autistic children can obtain beneficial outcomes after participating in an ESDM program, whether these benefits continue long-term remains a source of conjecture. It is possible that the skills acquired during the ESDM program are not sufficiently complex for use as an autistic child ages and enters more socially complex and challenging environments. Alternatively, it is possible that the skills developed also evolve to meet the demands of the social environment. Despite these hypothetical outcomes, studies should examine if the skills learned during ESDM intervention continue to show benefits for the child as the child ages.

Second, most studies about the efficacy of ESDM programs for autistic children have reported overall group differences; for example, the benefits that a group of autistic children obtained from their ESDM program against the benefits that a group of autistic children obtained from other supports. This focus has meant that we do not know what individual characteristics an autistic possesses makes them more receptive to obtaining benefits from an ESDM program. Hypothetically, it is possible that autistic children with average cognitive abilities will derive more benefits from ESDM programs than autistic children who have below-average cognitive abilities. Understanding what characteristics contribute to the efficacy of ESDM programs can help therapists make better judgements about which autistics should participate in ESDM programs.

3.6.4 Autistic views about Early Start Denver Model (ESDM)

Have you personally taken part in the Denver Early Start Model?

Of the 206 respondents who completed the online survey, 60 (29.12%) answered the question 'Have you personally taken part in the Denver Early Start Model?' Of those who answered this question, all (n = 60, 100%) said that they had never taken part in an ESDM program.

Respondents' ratings of the efficacy of the Early Start Denver Model (ESDM)

Since there are less than ten responses, the efficacy of ESDM programs for autistics was not rated.

Respondents' comments about the Early Start Denver Model (ESDM)

Out of the 206 respondents who completed our survey, no one explained their experiences or views of ESDM programs. The lack of responses to this question may reflect the fact that the ESDM is a fairly recent program outside the United States of America; for example mainstream implementation of the ESDM program started in Australia in 2011.

3.7 Conclusion

This chapter reviewed several prominent support programs that are based on the main elements of ABA. It began by examining the efficacy of PECS, a focused intervention program. It then examined three comprehensive programs; PRT, EIBI, and ESDM. Based on the literature examined, the efficacy of PRT and EDSM were 'Silver – Usually promising', PECS was 'Gold – Extremely promising and use with confidence', and EIBI was rated as 'Bronze – Safe but ineffective'. Several recommendations for where more research can be conducted as well as the experiences and insights from autistics was then presented. The majority of respondents did not have personal experience of these supports, possibly because they were exposed to these programs when they were children and could not recall such programs.

References

Alsayedhassan, B., Lee, J., Banda, D. R., Kim, Y., & Griffin-Shirley, N. (2019). Practitioners' perceptions of the picture exchange communication system for children with autism. *Disability and Rehabilitation*, 1–6. doi:10.1080/09638288.2019.1620878.

Baril, E. M., & Humphreys, B. P. (2017). An evaluation of the research evidence on the Early Start Denver Model. *Journal of Early Intervention*, 39(4), 321–338. doi:10.1177/1053815117722618.

Bernard-Opitz, V., Ing, S., & Kong, T. Y. (2004). Comparison of behavioural and natural play interventions for young children with autism. *Autism*, 8(3), 319–333. doi:10.1177/1362361304045212.

Boudreau, A. M., Corkum, P., Meko, K., & Smith, I. M. (2015). Peer-mediated pivotal response treatment for young children with autism spectrum disorders: A systematic review. *Canadian Journal of School Psychology*, 30(3), 218–235. doi:10.1177/0829573515581156.

Coolican, J., Smith, I. M., & Bryson, S. E. (2010). Brief parent training in pivotal response treatment for preschoolers with autism. *Journal of Child Psychology and Psychiatry*, 51(12), 1321–1330. doi:10.1111/j.1469-7610.2010.02326.x.

Dawson, G., Jones, E. J., Merkle, K., Venema, K., Lowy, R., Faja, S., … & Webb, S. J. (2012). Early behavioral intervention is associated with normalized brain activity in young children with autism. *Journal of the American Academy of Child & Adolescent Psychiatry*, 51(11), 1150–1159. doi:10.1016/j.jaac.2012.08.018.

Dawson, G., Rogers, S., Munson, J., Smith, M., Winter, J., Greenson, J., … & Varley, J. (2010). Randomized, controlled trial of an intervention for toddlers with autism: The Early Start Denver Model. *Pediatrics*, 125(1), e17–e23. doi:10.1542/peds.2009-0958.

Dawson, M., & Gernsbacher, M. A. (2010). Effectiveness of intensive autism programmes. *The Lancet*, 375(9716), 722–723. doi:10.1016/S0140-6736(10)60299-1.

Dyer K. (2013) Applied behavior analysis. In: Volkmar, F.R. (ed) *Encyclopedia of Autism Spectrum Disorders.* Springer, New York, NY doi:10.1007/978-1-4419-1698-3.

Eapen, V., Črnčec, R., & Walter, A. (2013). Clinical outcomes of an early intervention program for preschool children with autism spectrum disorder in a community group setting. *BioMed Central Pediatrics*, 13(3). doi:10.1186/1471-2431-13-3.

Eldevik, S., Hastings, R. P., Hughes, J. C., Jahr, E., Eikeseth, S., & Cross, S. (2009). Meta-analysis of early intensive behavioral intervention for children with autism. *Journal of Clinical Child & Adolescent Psychology*, 38(3), 439–450. doi:10.1080/15374410902851739.

Estes, A., Vismara, L., Mercado, C., Fitzpatrick, A., Elder, L., Greenson, J., … & Dawson, G. (2014). The impact of parent-delivered intervention on parents of very young children with autism. *Journal of Autism and Developmental Disorders*, 44(2), 353–365. doi:10.1007/s10803-013-1874-z.

Flippin, M., Reszka, S., & Watson, L. R. (2010). Effectiveness of the Picture Exchange Communication System (PECS) on communication and speech for children with autism spectrum disorders: A meta-analysis. *American Journal of Speech-Language Pathology.* doi:10.1044/1058-0360(2010/09-0022).

Ganz, J. B., Simpson, R. L., & Lund, E. M. (2012). The picture exchange communication system (PECS): A promising method for improving communication skills of learners with autism spectrum disorders. *Education and Training in Autism and Developmental Disabilities*, 47(2), 176–186.

Howlin, P., Magiati, I., & Charman, T. (2009). Systematic review of early intensive behavioral interventions for children with autism. *American Journal on Intellectual and Developmental Disabilities*, 114(1), 23–41. doi:10.1352/2009.114:23-41.

Howlin, P., Savage, S., Moss, P., Tempier, A., & Rutter, M. (2014). Cognitive and language skills in adults with autism: A 40-year follow-up. *Journal of Child Psychology and Psychiatry*, 55(1), 49–58. doi:10.1111/jcpp.12115.

Huskens, B., Reijers, H., & Didden, R. (2012). Staff training effective in increasing learning opportunities for school-aged children with autism spectrum disorders. *Developmental Neurorehabilitation*, 15(6), 435–447. doi:10.3109/17518423.2012.705910.

Kohn, A. (2020). Autism and behaviorism: New research adds to an already compelling case against ABA. Retrieved from https://www.alfiekohn.org/blogs/autism/?fbclid=IwAR23hObda3iyyTn8M7JfoeCiiRcPxTBI5qvjnCis75XAH1AEelGhZ_6fxwM.

Kovshoff, H., Hastings, R. P., & Remington, B. (2011). Two-year outcomes for children with autism after the cessation of early intensive behavioral intervention. *Behavior Modification*, 35(5), 427–450. doi:10.1177/0145445511405513.

Kupferstein, H. (2018). Evidence of increased PTSD symptoms in autistics exposed to applied behavior analysis, *Advances in Autism*, 4(1), 19–29. doi:10.1108/AIA-08-2017-0016.

Løvaas, O. I. (1987). Behavioral treatment and normal educational and intellectual functioning in young autistic children. *Journal of Consulting and Clinical Psychology*, 55(1), 3–9.

Lydon, H., Healy, O., & Leader, G. (2011). A comparison of video modeling and pivotal response training to teach pretend play skills to children with autism spectrum disorder. *Research in Autism Spectrum Disorders*, 5(2), 872–884. doi:10.1016/j.rasd.2010.10.002.

Makrygianni, M. K., & Reed, P. (2010). A meta-analytic review of the effectiveness of behavioural early intervention programs for children with autistic spectrum disorders. *Research in Autism Spectrum Disorders*, 4(4), 577–593. doi:10.1016/j.rasd.2010.01.014.

Matson, J. L., & Konst, M. J. (2013). What is the evidence for long term effects of early autism interventions? *Research in Autism Spectrum Disorders*, 7(3), 475–479. doi:10.1016/j.rasd.2012.11.005.

Perry, A., Koudys, J., Prichard, A., & Ho, H. (2019). Follow-up study of youth who received EIBI as young children. *Behavior Modification*, 43(2), 181–201. doi:10.1177/0145445517746916.

Randolph, J. K., Stichter, J. P., Schmidt, C. T., & O'Connor, K. V. (2011). Fidelity and effectiveness of PRT implemented by caregivers without college degrees. *Focus on Autism and Other Developmental Disabilities*, 26(4), 230–238. doi:10.1177/1088357611421503.

Reichow, B., Hume, K., Barton, E. E., & Boyd, B. A. (2018). Early intensive behavioral intervention (EIBI) for young children with autism spectrum disorders (ASD). *Cochrane Database of Systematic Reviews.* https://www.cochranelibrary.com/cdsr/doi/10.1002/14651858.CD009260.pub3/full.

Reichow, B., Volkmar, F. R., & Cicchetti, D. V. (2008). Development of the evaluative method for evaluating and determining evidence-based practices in autism. *Journal of Autism and Developmental Disorders*, 38(7), 1311–1319. doi:10.1007/s10803-007-0517-7.

Rivard, M., Morin, M., Mello, C., Terroux, A., & Mercier, C. (2018). Follow-up of children with autism spectrum disorder 1 year after early behavioral intervention. *Behavior Modification*, 43(4), 490–517. doi:10.1177/0145445518773692.

Robinson, S. E. (2011). Teaching paraprofessionals of students with autism to implement pivotal response treatment in inclusive school settings using a brief video feedback training package. *Focus on Autism and Other Developmental Disabilities*, 26(2), 105–118. doi:10.1177/1088357611407063.

Rogers, S. J., Estes, A., Lord, C., Vismara, L., Winter, J., Fitzpatrick, A., … & Dawson, G. (2012). Effects of a brief Early Start Denver Model (ESDM)–based parent intervention on toddlers at risk for autism spectrum disorders: A randomized controlled trial. *Journal of the American Academy of Child & Adolescent Psychiatry*, 51(10), 1052–1065. doi:10.1016/j.jaac.2012.08.003.

Rogers, S. J., Vismara, L., Wagner, A. L., McCormick, C., Young, G., & Ozonoff, S. (2014). Autism treatment in the first year of life: A pilot study of infant start, a parent implemented intervention for symptomatic infants. *Journal of Autism and Developmental Disorders*, 44(12), 2981–2995. doi:10.1007/s10803-014-2202-y.

Rogers, S. J., Vivanti, G., & Rocha, M. (2017). Helping young children with autism spectrum disorder develop social ability: The early start Denver model approach. In: Leaf, J.F. (ed)

Handbook of Social Skills and Autism Spectrum Disorder (pp. 197–222). Springer. doi:10.1007/978-3-319-62995-7_13.

Ryberg, K. H. (2015). Evidence for the implementation of the Early Start Denver Model for young children with autism spectrum disorder. *Journal of the American Psychiatric Nurses Association*, 21(5), 327–337. doi:10.1177/1078390315608165.

Sandoval-Norton, A. H., & Shkedy, G. (2019). How much compliance is too much compliance: Is long-term ABA therapy abuse? *Cogent Psychology*, 6(1), 1–8. doi:10.1080/23311908.2019.1641258.

Schreibman, L., Dawson, G., Stahmer, A. C., Landa, R., Rogers, S. J., McGee, G. G., … & McNerney, E. (2015). Naturalistic developmental behavioral interventions: Empirically validated treatments for autism spectrum disorder. *Journal of Autism and Developmental Disorders*, 45(8), 2411–2428. doi:10.1007/s10803-015-2407-8.

Smeekens, I., Oosterling, I. J., den Boer, J. C., Buitelaar, J. K., Staal, W. G., & van Dongen-Boomsma M. (2017). *Pivotal Response Treatment for autism spectrum disorder (ASD). Cochrane Database of Systematic Reviews* 2017(12). Art. No.: CD012887. doi:10.1002/14651858.CD012887.

Smith, T., & Eikeseth, S. (2011). O. Ivar Lovaas: Pioneer of applied behavior analysis and intervention for children with autism. *Journal of Autism and Developmental Disorders*, 41(3), 375–378. doi:10.1007/s10803-010-1162-0.

Smith, T., Groen, A.D., & Wynn, J.W. (2000). Randomized trial of intensive early intervention for children with pervasive developmental disorder. *American Journal on Mental Retardation*, 105, 269–285. doi:10.1352/0895-8017.

Steiner, A. M., Gengoux, G. W., Klin, A., & Chawarska, K. (2013). Pivotal response treatment for infants at-risk for autism spectrum disorders: A pilot study. *Journal of Autism and Developmental Disorders*, 43(1), 91–102. doi:10.1007/s10803-012-1542-8.

Sulzer-Azaroff, B., Hoffman, A. O., Horton, C. B., Bondy, A., & Frost, L. (2009). The Picture Exchange Communication System (PECS) what do the data say? *Focus on Autism and Other Developmental Disabilities*, 24(2), 89–103. doi:10.1177/1088357609332743.

Tien, K. C. (2008). Effectiveness of the Picture Exchange Communication System as a functional communication intervention for individuals with autism spectrum disorders: A practice-based research synthesis. *Education and Training in Developmental Disabilities*, 43(1), 61–76.

Verschuur, R., Didden, R., Lang, R., Sigafoos, J., & Huskens, B. (2014). Pivotal response treatment for children with autism spectrum disorders: A systematic review. *Review Journal of Autism and Developmental Disorders*, 1(1), 34–61. doi:10.1007/s40489-013-0008-z.

Virués-Ortega, J. (2010). Applied behavior analytic intervention for autism in early childhood: Meta-analysis, meta-regression and dose–response meta-analysis of multiple outcomes. *Clinical Psychology Review*, 30(4), 387–399. doi:10.1016/j.cpr.2010.01.008.

Vismara, L. A., Young, G. S., & Rogers, S. J. (2013). Community dissemination of the Early Start Denver Model: Implications for science and practice. *Topics in Early Childhood Special Education*, 32(4), 223–233. doi:10.1177/0271121411409250.

Vivanti, G., Dissanayake, C., & Victorian ASELCCTeam. (2016). Outcome for children receiving the Early Start Denver Model before and after 48 months. *Journal of Autism and Developmental Disorders*, 46(7), 2441–2449. doi:10.1007/s10803-016-2777-6.

Vivanti, G., Paynter, J., Duncan, E., Fothergill, H., Dissanayake, C., & Rogers, S. J., & Victorian ASELCC Team. (2014). Effectiveness and feasibility of the Early Start Denver Model implemented in a group-based community childcare setting. *Journal of Autism and Developmental Disorders*, 44(12), 3140–3153. doi:10.1007/s10803-014-2168-9.

Waddington, H., van der Meer, L., & Sigafoos, J. (2016). Effectiveness of the Early Start Denver Model: A systematic review. *Review Journal of Autism and Developmental Disorders*, 3(2), 93–106. doi:10.1007/s40489-015-0068-3.

Walker, V. L., & Snell, M. E. (2013). Effects of augmentative and alternative communication on challenging behavior: A meta-analysis. *Augmentative and Alternative Communication*, 29(2), 117–131. doi:10.3109/07434618.2013.785020.

Warren, Z., McPheeters, M. L., Sathe, N., Foss-Feig, J. H., Glasser, A., & Veenstra-Vander Weele, J. (2011). A systematic review of early intensive intervention for autism spectrum disorders. *Pediatrics*, 127(5), e1303–e1311. doi:10.1542/peds.2011-0426.

Wilson, B., Beamish, W., Hay, S., & Attwood, T. (2014). Prompt dependency beyond childhood: Adults with Asperger's syndrome and intimate relationships. *Journal of Relationships Research*, 5. doi:10.1017/jrr.2014.11.

Wolf, M. (1978). Social validity: The case for subjective measurement or how applied behavior analysis is finding its heart. *Journal of Applied Behavioral Analysis*, 11, 203–214. doi:10.1901/jaba.1978.11-203.

Wong, C., Odom, S. L., Hume, K. A., Cox, A. W., Fettig, A., Kucharczyk, S., … & Schultz, T. R. (2015). Evidence-based practices for children, youth, and young adults with autism spectrum disorder: A comprehensive review. *Journal of Autism and Developmental Disorders*, 45(7), 1951–1966. doi:10.1007/s10803-014-2351-z.

Chapter 4

Assistive technology

4.1 Introduction

This chapter presents an overview of meta-analyses and literature reviews on the benefits that assistive technology may provide for autistics. 'Assistive technology' is a broad term and in the context of this chapter it applies to portable devices that are used to enhance academic performance, augmentative and alternative communication (AAC) devices, robots, and video-modelling. Once this literature has been reviewed, a rating of each technological approach in assisting autistics and an explanation of where research could be conducted in the future are presented. Throughout this chapter the views and experiences from autistics about the potential benefits and suitability of different assistive technology devices and strategies are also presented.

4.2 Portable devices

We discovered that portable devices can provide autistics with two types of benefits. First, they can help them achieve greater rates of academic success (Kagohara et al., 2013; Larwin & Aspiranti, 2019; Ledbetter-Cho et al., 2018). Second, they can give some autistics who have limited or no speech, the opportunity to communicate effectively with others (Alzrayer, Banda, & Koul, 2014; Lorah et al., 2015).

4.2.1 Academic benefits that portable devices can give autistic students

Our review of the broader literature about supports for autistics revealed three literature reviews that contained studies about the utility of portable devices in helping autistics achieve greater academic success (Kagohara et al., 2013. Larwin & Aspiranti, 2019; Ledbetter-Cho et al., 2018). Kagohara et al. (2013) examined 15 studies that assessed the utility of portable devices (e.g., iPods®, iPads®, and related devices such as iPhones®) in helping autistics achieve greater functionality in five different domains; academic, communication, employment, leisure, and transitions across school settings. They found that portable devices helped autistics perform better in these five domains. In terms of the influence that portable devices had on specific academic achievement, they claimed that iPads helped students with Asperger syndrome learn how to correctly spell words (Kagohara et al., 2012).

In 2018, Ledbetter-Cho and colleagues examined the academic benefits that autistic students in school obtained from portable devices and the quality of the academic literature. To determine the quality of the studies they collected they used the *Evaluative Method for Determining Evidence-Based Practices in Autism* (Reichow, Volkmar, & Cicchetti, 2008). In total, they examined 19 studies that they divided into two categories; studies that examined the utility of portable devices in helping autistic school students acquire academic skills and knowledge (n = 8), and studies which examined how portable devices can help autistic school students improve their classroom behaviours (n = 11). In terms of academic skills development, Ledbetter-Cho et al. discovered that portable devices can help autistic school students solve mathematical problems (Jowett, Moore, & Anderson, 2012; Yakubova, Hughes, & Hornberger, 2015), and can improve their confidence and ability to answer science questions (Smith, Spooner, & Wood, 2013). Regarding classroom behaviours, portable devices were shown to improve on-task behaviours in school settings (Hart & Whalon, 2012; Xin, Sheppard, & Brown, 2017). Based on the studies examined, Ledbetter-Cho et al. (2018, p. 3033) concluded:

> This meta-analysis suggests that touch screen devices are useful in improving academic skills and academic engagement in students with ASD. However, these devices should be viewed as a supplement to carefully-planned instruction involving evidence-based teaching practices. Finally, given the promising outcomes from interventions in which pretraining was conducted, educators should consider training the student to use the device and its software prior to introducing the targeted skill.

Recently, Larwin and Aspiranti (2019) published a meta-analysis in which they attempted to determine if autistic school students benefited from academic interventions that involved using an iPad. They examined seven studies and concluded that:

> ... iPads are a promising intervention modality for students with ASD. Practitioners are encouraged to consider investigating whether the use of iPads would be beneficial for their students, particularly given the opportunities to individualise the experience for each child. However, the use of an iPad for academics should be accompanied by evidence-based curriculum and not used as the predominant teaching method. (Larwin & Aspiranti, 2019, p. 240).

Although their study has provided valuable insights into the effectiveness of iPads in helping autistics achieve academic success, their study does have some limitations. First, many studies in their meta-analysis did not take into consideration how other demographic information about the participants (e.g., socioeconomic status, language functioning, adaptive behaviour and social skills, and attention span). By not including these details, it was not possible to conclude if iPads were the key factor in determining academic improvement or if other factors played a part. Second, they only examined the academic benefits that autistic school students obtained from programs that were a combination of iPads and other academic strategies. By combining the usage of an iPad with other academic strategies it was difficult to determine if it was the iPad itself that was responsible for increasing academic performance or if it was specific quality teaching strategies.

4.2.2 Evaluation of portable devices for helping autistic students improve their academic skills

Rating: Gold – Extremely promising and use with confidence

Larwin and Aspiranti (2019), Ledbetter-Cho et al. (2018), and Kagohara et al. (2013) have all highlighted the academic benefits that portable devices can give autistic school students. However, as stressed by Ledbetter-Cho et al., such devices should not be used in isolation but should be used as supplementary strategies to enhance teaching instructions. Since such devices are reliable and have produced positive results we have rated them as 'Gold – Extremely promising and use with confidence'.

4.2.3 Directions for research in the future about the academic benefits of portable devices

Some may regard the finding that portable devices can help autistics improve at academic tasks a promising development in creating strategies that can improve an autistic's academic outcomes. However, it is unknown if devices benefit all autistics, or only those with additional learning needs such as dyslexia or hand-eye co-ordination difficulties. Also, whether or not the academic benefits that portable devices seemly deliver to autistics are maintained long-term is currently a source of speculation. Thus, longitudinal research should be conducted to see if these benefits are maintained as autistic students transition from school to higher education. In addition, currently most studies about this subject have based their findings on samples of autistic children. Consequently, it is unknown if autistic adults can obtain academic benefits from portable devices whilst in higher education. Thus, to address this gap in our knowledge about this topic, it would be advantageous to conduct studies with adult autistics about this topic. Additionally, such studies should contain control groups so that the possible academic benefits are clearly highlighted. Further research should also be conducted on the use of portable devices to support academic achievement for autistic adults and children who have poor motor control and/or dyspraxia. This research could examine the benefits of both text to speech (reading) and speech to text (writing) as well as more traditional forms of usage such as typing.

4.2.4 Autistic views about the academic benefits of portable devices

Have you used technology to support your access to learning or study or the wider community?

Out of the 206 respondents who completed the online survey, 60 (29.12%) answered the question 'Have you used technology to support your access to learning or study or the wider community?' Of those who answered this question, 40 (66.67%) selected the option 'Yes' and 20 (33.33%) selected the option 'No'.

Respondents' ratings of the efficacy of using technology to access learning, study or the wider community

Most respondents (n = 27, 46.55%) selected the option 'technology is very helpful and I can use it in a range of situations' to describe their view about the usefulness of technology in helping them access learning, study or the wider community. This was followed by respondents selecting the options 'technology was helpful' (n = 10, 17.24%) and 'helpful sometimes but not other times' (n = 3, 5.17%). Since most respondents selected one of these favourable options, the efficacy of using technology to access learning, study or the wider community for autistics as perceived by autistics averaged out to 4.4 stars.

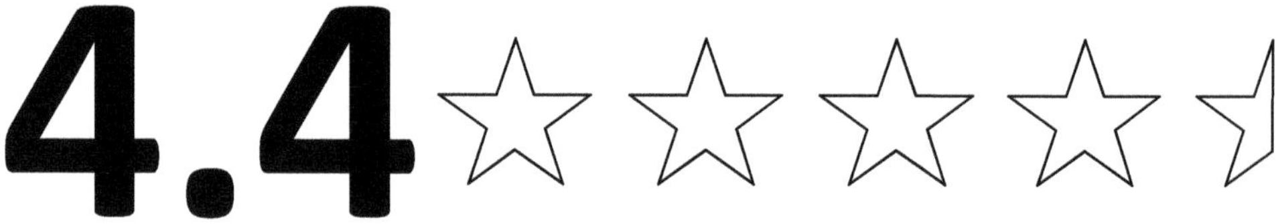

Figure 4.1 4.4 stars

Respondents' comments about using technology to access learning, study, or the wider community

Participants who completed our online survey were asked 'What is your experience with technology to support your access to learning or study or the wider community?' When asked this question 20 respondents provided a comment. Our analysis of these comments showed that 11 noted that technology was an important tool in helping them in accessing learning and studying opportunities. In particular, five participants stated that technology helped them access educational opportunities and other social services.

> "Allows me to access education and services in the manner of my choosing."
>
> "Again, it depends what you mean by technology but I found doing distance education much better than attending university on campus because it meant I could stay in my home city where all my support networks are."
>
> "I am currently doing a completely online course for which technology is crucial. It also eliminates the need for unnecessary social interaction for which I am very grateful."
>
> "I use online learning platforms, online library etc. to study online as I prefer studying online than in person so I can self-pace."
>
> "Online study – great for when you can't cope (anxiety) with education."

However, one respondent had mixed experiences with technology.

> "Being the only one using a computer in Year 11 & 12 was hard and time consuming but better than writing essays out by hand. I have tried using voice assistance on my phone but have real trouble interacting with it."

Two respondents explained that technology allowed them to communicate with other members of the autistic community.

"I use social media a lot to establish and maintain contact with social networks, especially the autistic community."

"Since my self-test and then diagnosis I am almost entirely dependent on the internet and Facebook groups to help me and to discuss Aspie and neurotypical stuff."

Interviewing an autistic researcher and academic, they were clear that technology for autistics can mitigate exclusion in education.

> "Technology takes away the pressure of immediacy and the need to give instant answers, so you can think first. Both autistic students and autistic lecturers can be kept on track by using technology in ways that work for them. I personally never write notes on my PowerPoints, but my putting together of the PowerPoint for my students, not only consolidates my learning, but guides me through the giving of a lecture."

The comments collected support the notion that technology can help autistics access social, learning and studying opportunities. However, despite its utility, some autistics found technological approaches helpful in some but not other contexts. Therefore, when making decisions about giving autistics technology to access learning and study opportunities, it is important that they are asked if they would like the opportunity to use a technological approach and to look at what other supports they may need to succeed.

4.2.5 Augmentative and alternative communication (AAC) devices

Portable devices that can help autistics who use no or minimal speech to express themselves are called 'augmentative and alternative communication' (AAC). We identified two literature reviews that examined studies examining the effects that AAC devices may have for autistics who did not use speech to communicate with others (Alzrayer, Banda, & Koul, 2014; Lorah et al., 2015).

Lorah et al. (2015) examined 17 studies about the utility of off-the-shelf handheld devices, such as tablet computers (i.e., iPad®, Samsung Galaxy Pad®), and portable multimedia players (i.e, iPods) in helping autistics communicate with others. Based on the studies that they reviewed, they concluded that:

> Studies comparing these devices to picture exchange or manual sign language found that acquisition was often quicker when using a tablet computer and that the vast majority of participants preferred using the device to picture exchange or manual sign language.
>
> (Lorah et al., 2015, p. 3792).

It should be noted that 15 out of the 17 studies they evaluated explored autistics using speech-generating devices in making requests. However, only three studies investigated the ability of such devices in facilitating more complex communication exchanges, such as an autistic responding to another's questions or requests (Strasberger & Ferreri, 2014; van der Meer et al., 2013). Thus, due to a lack of studies on complex communication, it was difficult to ascertain if AAC devices can assist autistics to develop complex communication skills, such as a sustained two-way interactions. In addition, nearly all studies examined the utility of iPad® or iPod Touch® and the Proloqu2Go software. Consequently, other types and brands of technology that may help autistics communicate were not explored.

In 2014, Alzrayer, Banda, and Koul reviewed the contents of 14 articles that measured the utility of iPad and iPods for speech generation communication. They reported that autistics exhibited a decrease in challenging behaviours after they started using an AAC device. For example, one participant in Sigafoos et al.'s (2013) study exhibited a decrease in physical aggression (i.e., hitting) after an iPad-based speech-generating device was introduced. This finding supports existing theories that propose that speech-generating devices can enhance a participant's ability to communicate with others and can mitigate the need to resort to using unconventional methods of expression (i.e., challenging behaviours or physical aggression) in order to have their needs met or communicate their wants (Walker & Snell, 2013).

Alzrayer, Banda, and Koul highlighted several limitations with their study; for instance, their results were based on studies that had samples of participants between three to 17 years of age. Thus, the benefits that these devices may provide autistic adults with were not measured. Additionally, several studies in their review contained samples of participants who were already familiar with iPad/iPod Touch technology before the start of the study (van der Meer et al., 2013). Thus, it is unknown if those who were not already familiar and proficient with the usage of such devices would have achieved the same outcomes in terms of exhibiting increased communication skills and reduced aggression. Finally, several of the studies that were examined did not clearly describe if the autistic participants were receiving other supports that helped them reduce their aggression in conjunction with the usage of an AAC device, such as art therapy or peer-mediated activities.

4.2.6 Evaluation of augmentative and alternative communication (AAC) devices

Rating for adults: Silver – Usually promising

Rating for children: Gold – Extremely promising and use with confidence

Alzrayer, Banda, and Koul (2014) reported that in certain situations autistics who have no or limited speech will exhibit a reduction in physical aggression while using an AAC device. Lorah et al. (2015) reported that autistics who have difficulties verbally communicating with others often gravitate towards using AAC devices instead of other options for communication and expression, such as manual sign language or paper-based picture exchange communication systems. The rationale for their choice was not examined. However, it is plausible that the interactive nature of AAC devices was appealing to users and made communication attempts more efficient. Based on this finding, practitioners can confidently recommend AAC devices to autistics who require assistance with communication. However, they are not able to recommend which AAC device will be of most benefit, since research has not explore if several types of AAC devices (e.g., Android pad) have also helped autistics communicate (Lorah et al., 2015).

As described in the previous section the cost of AAC devices, along with the costs associated with buying auxiliary equipment and software, can prevent some families and individuals from considering this technical option. While some may be able to access this technology through a subsidy program this is not an option for everyone. Due to this financial barrier, it may not be possible to provide expensive AAC devices to all autistics who need help to communicate with others. However, there are some free apps available for users who already have devices, which can offer AAC type benefits.

In summary, based on our appraisal of the current body of literature we have rated AAC devices as 'Silver – Usually promising' for adult autistics since their utility has not been proven and 'Gold – Extremely promising and use with confidence' for autistic children.

4.2.7 Directions for research in the future about augmentative and alternative communication (AAC) devices

A review of the literature showed that portable devices have helped autistics who use no or minimal verbal speech to communicate. Despite this potential benefit, there are still several questions yet to be answered by research. First, it is unknown if devices other than iPads, such as Android Pad or Microsoft Surface, can also help autistics communicate. The potential utility of these devices should be examined so that practitioners and autistics can make an informed choice about the utility of other AAC devices aside from iPads. Second, most of the studies about the benefits of portable devices for autistics have based their results on samples of autistic children. For example, out of the 17 studies examined in Lorah et al.'s literature review only one study contained adult participants (van der Meer et al., 2011). It may be that autistic adults might have a greater need for portable devices than autistic children, especially for adults that are living in situations where they do not receive any day to day supports.

The literature has also shown that portable devices can help autistics achieve academic tasks. While some may regard these potential benefits as promising developments in creating strategies to help autistics, they should be treated with caution since the findings in existing studies have not been replicated. Thus, additional research is required so that the potential academic benefits explained by Kagohara et al. (2013) can be validated.

4.2.8 Autistic views about augmentative and alternative communication (AAC) devices

Have you used technology to communicate?

Out of the 206 respondents who completed our survey, 61 (29.61%) answered the question 'Have you used technology to communicate?' Of these, most (n = 45, 73.77%) stated that they had used technology to communicate with others, and 16 (26.23%) noted that they have not used this approach.

Respondents' ratings of the efficacy of technology to communicate

The option 'technology is very helpful and I can use it in a range of situations' was selected by most respondents (n = 24, 42.86%) when rating the effectiveness of technology to communicate with others. This was followed by ten (17.86%) selecting the option 'Helpful sometimes but not other times' and nine (16.07%) selecting the option 'Technology is helpful'. Based on the distribution of responses, the efficacy of technology to communicate with others as perceived by autistics was calculated as 4.3 stars.

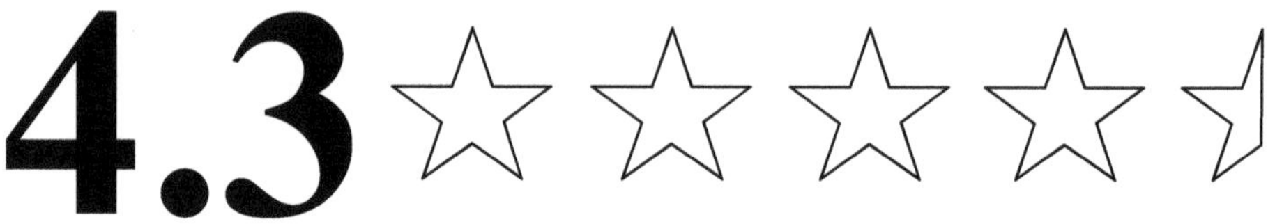

Figure 4.2 4.3 stars

Respondents' comments about using technology to communicate

When asked 'What is your experience with technology to communicate?' 24 respondents provided a comment. Our examination of their comments showed that ten respondents expressed positive views about using technology to communicate. In contrast, no respondents articulated a reservation or concern about using technology to communicate with others. Of those who endorsed the usage of technology as a tool to aid communication, two explained that it was helpful when they were anxious and not able to use verbal communication.

> "It is much easier for me to type responses in high-anxiety complex situations when my speech is limited."
>
> "I am mostly verbally fluent but sometimes lose speech, e.g. during meltdown/shutdown, and at those times technology is helpful to communicate by typing instead of speaking. I generally find I can communicate better in writing than in speech, even when I do have access to my speech."

Two respondents endorsed technology to communicate with others because it gave them time to develop their responses to other people's questions.

> "Using mail or chat gives me time to process and put an answer together. Especially with strangers this is important."
>
> "Asynchronous communication – I have time to get it right in my own time … easier to communicate this way."

Finally, four participants expressed a preference for using technology to communicate rather than the traditional face-to-face method for communicating.

> "I am able to communicate my wants and needs by text when I find it difficult to engage in face to face communication."
>
> "This is a broad question. To clarify, I've heavily relied on the Internet to make friends and communicate with people. It's far, far easier than real life."
>
> "I'm not sure exactly what you mean by technology, but I generally find communicating in writing easier so email is great!"
>
> "Communicating via email/text/video is highly useful and easier for me than the whole social communication."

When an autistic educational consultant was interviewed about their thoughts on AAC in autism, they felt that AAC opens the ordinary everyday world to non-verbal children and adults in ways that are not otherwise available to them.

> "Using something like proloquo2go we can go to McDonalds and order a burger and everyone gets it, AAC increases understanding across that gap between verbal and non-verbal in ways that other things don't. For people who are sometimes non-verbal once they have learnt and feel confident with AAC, their communication partners should also be trained in that AAC. Communication devices should be mobile, lightweight, and you need to be able to use them with other people. Just sitting next to someone and typing can be good. Learning to communicate in these various ways needs to be built into the curriculum."

Most respondents expressed the view that technology was a useful tool in helping them to communicate with others. Our analysis of the collected responses failed to find any participants who expressed the opposite view, demonstrating that access to AAC or texting/typing is worthwhile for many autistics as a communication tool.

4.3 Robots

4.3.1 Robots

With advances in technology and decreasing prices, robots have become more common. Today, robots can autonomously build products, such as cars or mobile phones, whilst other types of robots help the elderly and those with physical disabilities (Hersh, 2015; Sharkey, 2014; Sparrow & Sparrow, 2006). The potential benefits of robots for autistics have not gone unnoticed, with a number of literature reviews on this subject (Diehl et al., 2012; DiPietro et al., 2019; Pennisi et al., 2016). These studies will be examined to follow.

Perhaps one of the earliest systematic literature reviews exploring the potential benefits that autistics can obtain from robots was published in 2012 by Diehl and colleagues. They examined 15 peer-reviewed studies and five conference papers and concluded that in clinical settings robots can provide autistics with many potential benefits. For example, the predictable nature of robots in producing simplistic and predictable social behaviours repeatedly with no deviation from pre-programmed actions, seemed to result in a high level of comfort in autistic-robot interactions. They also noted that robots can be programmed and tailored to suit each child's unique characteristics and support goals.

Another literature review of studies about the utility of robots for autistics was published in 2016 by Pennisi and colleagues. The studies which they examined were divided into five categories; social behaviours, joint attention, imitation, language, and stereotyped behaviours. They concluded that:

> We found many positive implications in the use of social robots in therapy as for example: ASD subjects often performed better with a robot partner rather than a human partner; sometimes, ASD patients had, toward robots, behaviors that TD patients had toward human agents; ASDs had a lot of social behaviors toward

> robots; during robotic sessions, ASDs showed reduced repetitive and stereotyped behaviors and, social robots manage to improve spontaneous language during therapy sessions.
>
> (Pennisi et al., 2016, p. 165).

While Pennisi et al. concluded that autistics can obtain many benefits from interacting with robots, their findings need to be interpreted with some caution. They found that most of the studies which they examined for their systematic literature review did not contain a control group. A control group can help researchers measure the benefits that robots can give autistics because they can compare the benefits that they obtain from robots against the progress of skills development of autistics over a similar time frame who did not interact with robots. This would demonstrate whether the same benefits can be seen without any robotic intervention being provided.

Recently, in 2019, DiPietro and colleagues examined the contents of 18 studies; 11 studies about the benefits autistics obtained after interacting with robots and seven studies about the benefits they obtained after interacting with computer games. They identified many benefits that robot-interactions gave autistic children, including the opportunity to learn and apply new words (Saadatzi et al., 2018). However, Huskens et al. (2015) found that robots did not help autistic children improve their collaborative behaviours, such as interaction initiations, responses, and playing with others, demonstrating that the benefits may be specific to the type of robot-individual interactions.

DiPietro et al. reported that the studies they reviewed contained many strengths. First, most had robust research designs in terms of incorporating control groups and some degree of participant randomisation. Second, as an outcome measure, many examined the generalisation of a new skill. Generalisation is the ability to apply a skill across multiple settings or situations. They found that most of the studies that they examined measured the generalisation of a skill from a clinical setting to an environment familiar to the participant (i.e., home or a playground). Furthermore, several studies examined if over time the skill learned was maintained. By recording generalisation and maintenance measurements it was possible to determine if the skills that autistic children learned from robots were maintained long-term and could continue beyond the clinical/study setting itself. Third, many incorporated into their protocol the subject's real-world environment. Such environments not only helped generalise the skills learned, they also helped reduce the potential of autistic children being placed into situations where they could feel anxious. By reducing their anxiety, this emotion was not able to influence the results.

DiPietro et al. also reported several noteworthy limitations that the studies they reviewed shared. First, with the exception of de Vries et al.'s (2015) study, which sampled 121 participants, all of the studies that they examined based their results on fewer than 50 participants. Unlike larger samples, within small samples individual differences between participants are more pronounced, which makes it difficult to study a homogeneous group of participants. Second, in many studies, the results were based on subjective observations from researchers and parents instead of more scientifically validated and reliable diagnostic instruments. With such an approach there is an increased prospect of different members of the research team formulating different conclusions than collectively referring to one objective result. Despite these limitations, DiPietro et al. concluded that:

> These interventions show considerable promise, but more effectiveness and cost effectiveness research of high quality should be carried out with larger numbers of children. Also, further studies are necessary to evaluate these technologies' effectiveness amongst adults with ASD and within unique subsets of the … autism population. (2019, p. 1).

4.3.2 Evaluation of robots

Rating: Silver – Usually promising

Undoubtedly, there are many studies that have concluded that robots can provide autistics with a wide variety of benefits. However, despite these promising results, many studies on this topic still contain serious methodological flaws, such as small sample sizes and subjective and biased observations as to an autistic's developmental progress with a robot instead of more robust and objective assessments. It cannot be claimed with a high degree of confidence that robots are an effective tool for helping autistics learn new skills until more methodologically robust research reaches this conclusion. Thus, we have rated support programs which contain robots as teaching tools for autistics as 'Silver – Usually promising'.

4.3.3 Directions for research in the future about robots

Since the usage of robots to help autistics learn new skills is a contemporary and emerging field there are several areas where more research about this topic can be conducted. In their study, Diehl et al. (2012) explained that so far studies have examined what type of robot produces the best results for autistic children. However, currently, it is unknown whether such benefits occur for all individuals on the spectrum, regardless of their abilities, or if they are more useful for just some autistics. It could be, as a hypothetical example, that an autistic with average cognitive and language abilities and mild sensory sensitivities might obtain more benefits from robotic interactions than an autistic with a different set of characteristics. Until this research is conducted the following sentiment, that was expressed by Pennisi et al. (2016, p. 181), remains relevant:

> It most clearly emerges from this review that the studies conducted so far in this area are still insufficient. It is necessary to clarify whether the sex, IQ and age of participants affect the outcome of the therapy …

Diehl et al. (2012) found that some studies that they examined had two to four personnel in the room along with the robot and the autistic individual, with one of these staff often in control of the robot. This amount of staff is most likely not logistically or financially sustainable if the robot-autistic interaction needs to be long-term. This amount of staff may also obscure the results as it would not be possible to know if the autistic's interaction with the other people in the room, or the robot, or both the robot and the other people in the room produced the most beneficial outcomes. Diehl et al. recommended that studies in future should minimise the number of staff per robot-autistic interactive session not only so that the financial sustainability of the program can be optimised but so it is possible to know if the robot actually contributed to the support program's objectives.

Diehl et al. have pointed out that in the future research about the benefits that autistics can obtain from interacting with robots should examine more than just behavioural outcomes. The role which robots can play in influencing the development of cognitive processes, such as executive functioning, should also be examined in the future. For example, robot interactions might be able to help autistics plan and execute tasks or improve their confidence in decision-making. However, since studies about robot-autistic interactions have not focused on cognitive development such outcomes are hypothetical.

4.3.4 Autistic views about robots

Have you used robots to support your access to learning or study or the wider community?

All respondents (n = 59, 100%) who answered the question 'Have you used robots to support your access to learning or study or the wider community?' selected the 'No' option. We believe that no respondent selected the 'Yes' option because at the time of completing our survey robots were a relatively new and generally expensive support. Consequently, not many autistics would have used these devices. However, we did find an autistic adult who had worked with researchers who had been researching the use of robots in schools in a social skills group. This autistic adult described the group interactions with the robots in the same way as the literature adding that;

> "The exaggerated expressions on the robot's face helped the autistic students more easily identify the robot's emotions. However, the children preferred the company of the robot to their classmates!"

4.4 Video-modelling strategies

4.4.1 Video-modelling strategies

There are meta-analysis studies and literature reviews on the benefits which video-modelling, or variants of this approach, can offer autistics (Fragale, 2014; Shukla-Mehta, Miller, & Callahan, 2010). One of the earliest literature reviews on this topic was published in 2010 by Shukla-Mehta, Miller, and Callahan. They looked at the impact which different video-based instruction strategies had on the social and communication behaviours of autistic children. In their review they examined 26 studies, which were catalogued under the following six categories:

1 Studies where video-modelling was the only intervention component.
2 Studies where video-modelling was the primary intervention with additional intervention components.
3 Studies where video-modelling was a component of a multi-element intervention.
4 Studies where video-modelling was compared to another intervention strategy so that the relative effects of each intervention could be determined.
5 Studies in which only a video self-modelling intervention was used.

6 Studies in which only a point-of-view video-modelling intervention was used.
7 Studies where video-modelling was the only intervention component.

Video-modelling is an activity that involves a person watching a brief video clip that depicts a task or social behaviour in its entirety, such as one person introducing themselves, and then performing the task or behaviour which they have just viewed. For example, an autistic child can watch a video clip of a person waving and saying 'hello' and then they imitate the same task. Alternatively, video-modelling can involve a person watching a brief clip of a single component of a task or behaviour and then performing this single component before watching and performing the next component. This process continues for each single step component of a task in sequence until the social behaviour is mastered. For example, a participant watches a brief video clip of one person waving to another and then they practice this action before watching the next brief video clip of one person saying hello to another person before they practice this action. Generally, three- to five-minute video clips are regarded as appropriate (Buggey, 2005; Mayes & Calhoun, 2007).

Out of the 26 studies included in their literature review, Shukla-Mehta, Miller, and Callahan found that four of them used video-modelling to help teach target skills without any other components, these studies, therefore, did not contain any instructional prompts or reinforcers (D'Ateno, Mangiapanello, & Taylor, 2003; MacDonald et al., 2005; Nikopoulos & Keenan, 2004, 2007) (See Table 4.1). D'Ateno, Mangiapanello, and Taylor (2003) and MacDonald et al. (2005) found that video-modelling for communication led to the development of scripted but not unscripted verbal responses. In other words, video-modelling led to the children being able to reproduce exactly what they saw, but it did not lead to skills that generalised across to other situations. One benefit of these four studies was that they provided clarity around the efficacy that video-modelling can have on the development of target communication skills, as there were no other interventions used which could have distorted the outcomes. In contrast, Nikopoulos and Keenan (2004, 2007) found that for autistic children video-modelling in general improved social initiation, reciprocal play, object management, and imitation. They also found that these benefits were generalised across peers and settings and were maintained at follow-up.

Studies where video-modelling was a component of a multi-element intervention

Shukla-Mehta, Miller, and Callahan found five studies that used video-modelling in conjunction with instructional prompts and reinforcers to teach target skills (See Table 4.2). In these studies, the video-modelling task was accompanied by instructional prompts (Paterson & Arco, 2007) or a review of the video content after viewing the task or behaviour being taught (Charlop-Christy & Daneshvar, 2003; Taylor, Levin, & Jasper, 1999). They found that video-modelling in conjunction with prompts and reinforcers helped autistic children increase and maintain their conversations skills, perspective talking skills (Charlop-Christy & Daneshvar, 2003), appropriate play along with a decrease in repetitive behaviour (Paterson & Arco, 2007), and scripted and unscripted comments during play activities with their siblings or peers (Kroeger, Schultz, & Newsom, 2007; Taylor, Levin, & Jasper, 1999).

Table 4.1 Studies where video-modelling was the only intervention component

Study	*Design*	*Participants*	*Target Skills*	*Model*	*Setting*	*Intervention Components*	*Outcome*
D'Ateno, Mangiapanello, and Taylor, 2003	MBL across responses	One child, three years	Play behaviour (verbal and motor responses)	Adult	School	VM alone (without prompting, correction, or reinforcement procedures)	VM led to acquisition of scripted verbal and modelled motor responses but not generalised for unscripted verbal and nonmodeled motor responses.
MacDonald et al., 2005	Multiple Probe within child across play sets	Two children, four and seven years	Scripted and unscripted actions and verbalisations for pretend play	Adult	School	VM alone (no prompts or reinforcers except to cue play time)	Both children acquired scripted verbalisations and play actions during VM with maintenance during follow-up. Zero or low occurrence for unscripted responses was noted.
Nikopoulos and Keenan, 2004	MBL across participants	Three children, 7.5 to 10.5 years	Social initiation, reciprocal play, object engagement, and others	Unknown adult and peer	School	VM alone without any instructional prompts or reinforcers, but response to participant initiations were provided	Target skills were acquired and generalised across toys and settings; effects were maintained at follow-up.
Nikopoulos and Keenan, 2007	MBL across participants in the first experiment	Three children, 6.5 and 7 years	Social initiations, reciprocal play, and imitation	Peer	School	VM alone wherein different videos showed engagement in increasing number of play activities. Responses to participant initiations were provided.	VM enhanced acquisition of target skills that generalised across peers and maintained at follow-up. Results of Experiment 2 not noted because the design was non-experimental (AB).

Source: Shukla-Mehta, Miller, and Callahan, 2010, p. 27.

Table 4.2 Studies where video-modelling intervention included instructional prompts and/or reinforcers

Study	*Design*	*Participants*	*Target Skills*	*Model*	*Setting*	*Intervention Components*	*Outcome*
Charlop and Milstein, 1989	MBL across participants	Three children, six to seven years	Conversation skills	Adult	Home and clinical	VM with instructional prompts and tangible reinforcers from four to 20 presentations for effect	Conversational skills of children generalised and maintained over a 15-month period
Charlop-Christy and Daneshvar, 2003	MBL across children and within child	Three children, six to nine years	Perspective taking skills	Adult	Clinical	VM with prompts and training in target skills; reviewed content with child after two viewings	Positive outcomes for both stimulus and response generalisation
Kroeger, Schultz, and Newsom, 2007	Matched random group comparison	25 children, four to six years (13 in experimental group)	Social and communication skills	Peter	PDD clinic	Direct instruction during VM with prompts and edible reinforcers followed by prompts to display target skills during play	Both groups increased prosocial behaviour, but the experimental group (VM) showed higher gains in initiating, responding, and interacting with peers
Paterson and Arco, 2007	MBL across toys and a reversal	Two children, six to nine years	Verbal and motor play behaviour	Young adult	School	VM plus instructional prompts, redirection, and reinforcers (verbal and tangible)	Appropriate play increased, repetitive behaviour decreased; generalized play with related toys
Taylor, Levin, and Jasper, 1999	MBL probe design across activities	Two children, six and nine years	Scripted, unscripted play comments	Adult and sibling	Home	Three video viewings; repeated prompts until correct response was made. Reinforcers for correct responding to adult's comments.	VM resulted in a slow or variable but steady increase in play comments or statements for both children during play activities with their respective siblings.

Source: Shukla-Mehta, Miller, and Callahan, 2010, p. 28.

Note. MBL = Multiple Baseline design; PDD = Pervasive Developmental Disorder; VM = Video-modelling

Studies where video-modelling was compared to another intervention strategy so that the relative effects of each intervention could be determined

Out of the 26 studies that Shukla-Mehta, Miller, and Callahan catalogued, three compared video-modelling to another intervention strategy to determine which intervention was more effective (Charlop-Christy, Le, & Freeman, 2000; Gena, Couloura, & Kymissis, 2005; Sherer et al., 2001) (See Table 4.3). Gena, Couloura, and Kymissis (2005) and Charlop-Christy, Le, and Freeman (2000) compared the effectiveness of video-modelling followed by imitation against an autistic watching a clip and then recording their observations and possible lessons learnt. In their study, the children in the group who took part in video-modelling also experienced at least one demonstration of a person modelling the action live. This exposure technically did not make it possible for a comparison of the effectiveness of person modelling the action or video-modelling to be conducted. Charlop-Christy, Le, and Freeman found that video-modelling was more time and cost-efficient than modelling by a person. The third study, published by Sherer et al. (2001), compared the effectiveness of video-modelling against video self-modelling on achieving the goal of being able to produce a goal behaviour. They found that four out of the five children in their study achieved skill acquisition with either video-modelling or video self-modelling or both.

Studies in which only a video self-modelling intervention was used

With video self-modelling the participant is videotaped doing an action perfectly, often by editing the recording and splicing it together to showcase the child doing the required task/action. The child then watches the recording of themselves completing the task or behaviour that they are learning. The video is usually spliced together from several different videos so that no errors or mistakes are seen in the product. Instead, the individual sees themselves already being successful, which can then lead to the self-fulfilling prophecy where you can do something. Out of the 26 studies which Shukla-Mehta, Miller, and Callahan examined, four examined video self-modelling as the sole intervention without any instructional prompts or reinforcers (Bellini, Akullian, & Hopf, 2007; Buggey, 2005; Buggey et al., 1999; Wert & Neisworth, 2003) (See Table 4.4). In each of these four studies, participants were shown video clips between two to five minutes of themselves performing tasks or behaviours. Shukla-Mehta, Miller, and Callahan found that all four studies showed that video self-modelling increased desired behavioural responses, such as increased social initiations and interactions. Bellini, Akullian, and Hopf (2007) found that video self-modelling resulted in autistic children demonstrating more unprompted social engagements with peers and that the level of these social engagements was maintained after the video self-modelling sessions ended. Buggey (2005) found that after the introduction of video self-modelling all five autistic children exhibited increases in social initiations and responses to questions and a decrease in problem behaviours. However, during the maintenance phase, the acquisition of these skills started to decline for two of the five participants. Buggey et al. (1999) found that for all three autistic children in their study, video self-modelling resulted in increasing verbal responses to questions asked by an adult. Finally, Wert and Neisworth (2003) found that three out of the four children who participated in their video self-modelling program demonstrated large increases in spontaneous requesting. This behaviour was maintained for three of the four children.

Table 4.3 Studies where video-modelling was compared with another intervention

Study	*Design*	*Participants*	*Target Skills*	*Model*	*Setting*	*Intervention Components*	*Outcome*
Charlop-Christy, Le, and Freeman, 2000	MBL across children and within child	Five children, seven to 11 years	Social, communication, and functional responses	Adult	Clinical	VM and in-vivo with prompts and reinforcers for attending to the model but not for target skills; prompt was used to evoke imitation of model's behaviour	VM rather than in-vivo modeling led to faster acquisition and generalisation of target responses for four of five children.
Gena, Couloura, and Kymissis, 2005	MBL with ABAC with generalisation where B was VM and C was in-vivo instruction	Three children, four to six years	Affective behaviours	Peer	Home	VM included prompts, error correction, and reinforcement for attending; in-vivo included prompts, correction, and reinforcement for accurate target responses.	Both VM and in-vivo were relatively effective in the acquisition and generalisation of affective responses. A steady pattern during in-vivo might have been produced through contingent reinforcement for target responses.
Sherer et al., 2001	MBL with alternating treatments (peer vs. self as model)	Five children, ages four to 11 years	Response to conversation questions (asked by adult)	Peer	Home and clinical	Each child watched the videotape thrice in the evening before going to bed. Subsequently the therapist conversed with child to assess learning.	Skill acquisition for four of five students occurred with one or the other or both types of models; however, for one student neither method was effective.

Source: Shukla-Mehta, Miller, and Callahan, 2010, p. 30.

Note. MBL = Multiple Baseline design.

Table 4.4 Studies where video self-modelling was the primary intervention

Study	*Design*	*Participants*	*Target Skills*	*Setting*	*Intervention Components*	*Outcome*
Bellini, Akullian, and Hopf, 2007	MBL across students	Two children, 4.4 and 5.2 years	Unprompted social engagement with peer	School	A two-min video of children displaying target behaviour; prompts for attending but not for eliciting target responses	Highly variable behaviour pattern despite an overall increase in target responses; social engagement maintained after VSM was withdrawn
Buggey, 2005	MBL across students or behaviour	five children (across three studies), five to 11 years	Social initiations, response to questions, and problem behaviour	School	A three-min videotape using role-play scripts for self and peers; praise embedded in the video but not during the viewing	Target responses improved for all, but the response rate for two students decreased during the maintenance phase. Problem behaviour for all students decreased.
Buggey et al., 1999	MBL across students	Three children, eight to 11 years	Verbal responses to questions of an adult	Home	Prompts for attending to video; children could watch the three- to five-min video as many times as they wished	Overall increase in appropriate responding were noted; however, gains were noted during baseline, and responses decreased during maintenance.
Wert and Neisworth, 2003	MBL across participants	Four children, three to six years	Spontaneous requesting	School and home	A five-min video with embedded adult prompts that children watched at home on five school days	Spontaneous requesting increased and maintained for three of four children; maintenance was not evaluated for one child.

Source: Shukla-Mehta, Miller, and Callahan, 2010, p. 31.

Note. MBL = Multiple Baseline design.

Studies in which only a point-of-view video-modelling intervention was used

Point-of-view video-modelling involves videotaping from the participant's perspective elements of the environment or task that they are learning. Out of the 26 studies that Shukla-Mehta, Miller, and Callahan examined in their literature review, two used point-of-view video-modelling as the only intervention (Hine & Wolery, 2006; Schreibman, Whalen, & Stahmer, 2000) (See Table 4.5). Point-of-view video-modelling resulted in increased toy-play skills, which were maintained and generalised across toys and play settings (Hine & Wolery, 2006). This form of video-modelling was also found to decrease behaviours described as severe problem behaviours (e.g., crying, screaming, dropping on the floor) regardless of the environment as well as during new transitional situations (Schreibman, Whalen, & Stahmer, 2000).

In 2014, Fragale published a literature review in which they examined studies about the impact that video-modelling had on the play skills and behaviours of autistic children. They examined 22 studies, which were divided into two categories; solitary play, and social play. Based on the studies collected, Fragale (2014, p. 174) concluded that:

> The results suggest that video modeling is an effective intervention, corresponding with the positive findings reported in other reviews on video modeling … Of the 22 reviewed studies, use of video modeling was effective for 82% of participants in increasing scripted play actions and vocalizations.

Fragale's study only reported play behaviour as a dependent variable. If video-modelling provided any other benefits or issues, they were not considered. In addition, there were no studies that had participants aged 12 years or older. Whether or not older autistic children and adults can obtain benefits from video-modelling was unexplored.

Another technique that researchers have used to measure the efficacy of video-modelling is to compare it to other types of strategies used to support autistics. Wang, Cui, and Parrila (2011) compared the effectiveness of peer-mediated activities and video-modelling by evaluating studies about each of these approaches. They compared four studies about video-modelling and nine studies about peer-mediated activities. For their meta-analysis, they used hierarchical linear modelling (HLM) to examine the single-case studies collected about these two approaches to teach social skills to autistic children. After applying HLM they concluded that:

> Both approaches were found to be effective. In order to benefit more from the intervention, it is recommended that social skills training, especially the video-modeling intervention, should be provided to children with ASD as soon as they are identified.

4.4.2 Evaluation of video-modelling strategies

Rating: Silver – Usually promising

Our assessment of the studies contained in Shukla-Mehta, Miller, and Callahan's (2010) literature review about the benefits that video-modelling can give autistics

Table 4.5 Studies where point-of-view video-modelling was the primary intervention

Study	*Design*	*Participants*	*Target Skills*	*Setting*	*Intervention Components*	*Outcome*
Hine and Wolery, 2006	Multiple-probe design across two behaviours and across two participants	Two children, 2.5 and 3.6 years	Toy-play skills	University based preschool	Point-of-view modelling that showed adult's hands performing actions with target materials	Point-of-view modelling was effective in teaching toy-play actions for both children. Target behaviour was maintained and generalised across materials and activity settings.
Schreibman, Whalen, and Stahmer, 2000	MBL Multiple Baseline across participants	Three children, three to six years	Severe problem behaviour (e.g., crying, screaming, dropping on the floor)	Home and community	Transition routine as a child would see it when progressing from one setting to another; video showed only the settings	Video instruction led to decreases in problem behaviour with generalisation to new transition situations.

Source: Shukla-Mehta, Miller, and Callahan, 2010, p. 32.

Note. MBL = Multiple Baseline design.

revealed two concerns. First, the studies reviewed did not all conclude that the tasks mastered after participating in video-modelling programs could be generalised across multiple settings, with some children unable to maintain skills. Second, all of the studies that Shukla-Mehta, Miller, and Callahan examined had based their results on samples of autistic children. Consequently, they noted that there was a scarcity of research about the benefits that video-modelling can provide autistic adults. To confirm this point, we searched for studies about this topic on Google Scholar, PubMed, SpringerLink, SAGE, and Taylor and Francis, and reached the same conclusion, namely that there was minimal research about the utility of video-modelling for autistic adults. Since not all lessons taught through video-modelling can be generalised and since it is unknown what benefits autistic adults can obtain from this technological approach, we have rated video-modelling as 'Silver – Usually promising'.

4.4.3 Directions for research in the future about video-modelling strategies

Despite Fragale (2014) and Shukla-Mehta, Miller, and Callahan (2010) examining a large number of studies, there are still two areas where additional research can be conducted in the future. These areas are conducting more research to discover the most beneficial video-based approach and conducting more research about the benefits that autistic adults can obtain from video-modelling.

An inspection of the studies examined by Shukla-Mehta, Miller, and Callahan showed that point-of-view video-modelling and video self-modelling have the potential to help autistics improve their social and communication abilities. However, they only examined four studies about the utility of video self-modelling for autistics (Bellini, Akullian, & Hopf, 2007; Buggey, 2005; Buggey et al., 1999; Wert & Neisworth, 2003) and two studies about the potential benefits autistics have obtained from point-of-view video-modelling (Hine & Wolery, 2006; Schreibman, Whalen, & Stahmer, 2000). Due to the paucity of literature, it is not possible to confidently conclude that point-of-view video-modelling and video self-modelling are beneficial for autistics. Thus, to improve our understanding about the utility of these video-modelling strategies for autistics more research should be conducted about their efficacy.

An examination of the studies reviewed by Shukla-Mehta, Miller, and Callahan showed that there were no studies about the benefits that video-modelling gave autistic adults. This is despite the researchers not placing any caveats on the age ranges of the participants in the studies that they reviewed. In an attempt to find literature that Shukla-Mehta, Miller, and Callahan did not examine, we searched for available peer-reviewed literature about the benefits that autistic adults have obtained from different types of video-based instructions (i.e., video-modelling, video self-modelling, and point-of-view video-modelling). Based on an appraisal of the published literature there were many gaps in the research. For example, the potential of such strategies to teach autistic adults daily living skills, such as cooking, or age-appropriate sexual behaviours within a relationship remain unexplored areas. In the interest of finding strategies that can potentially help adult autistics, along with improving our knowledge about support strategies for autistics, it would be advantageous to study the outcomes of using video-based instructions to teach new skills to autistic adults.

4.4.4 Autistic views about video-modelling strategies

Have you experienced video modelling as a support?

Out of 206 respondents who completed the online survey, 61 (29.61%) answered the question 'Have you experienced video modelling as a support?' Most (n = 54, 88.52%) stated that they had never experienced video-modelling as a support, and seven (11.48%) noted that they had used this form of support.

Respondents' ratings of the efficacy of video-modelling

We have not rated autistic respondents' ratings of video-modelling due to the low number of respondents having used video-modelling. This may be due to the respondents being adult and video-modelling becoming more common after they left school, which is the most common setting for the use of video-modelling. Of the respondents (7) who did use video-modelling, two (3.85%) respondents said it was 'not helpful', two (3.85%) stated that they found it 'a bit helpful', and three (5.77%) noted that they found it 'helpful sometimes but not other times'. This reflects the literature which noted that video-modelling was not universally helpful for autistics.

Respondents' comments about video-modelling

Five respondents provided a comment to the question 'What is your experience with video modelling?' Two respondents believed that it was an effective form of teaching for them because it presented typical situations that sometimes could be watched multiple times.

> "It depends on context. I actually find watching TV shows or movies with audio descriptions turned on more useful because they are more natural and contextual modelling."
>
> "I find imitation helpful so I like video modelling. I can also watch multiple times with no pressure to learn quickly."

However, two respondents were ambivalent about the efficacy of video-modelling for autistics. The first comment relates to videos rather than video-modelling.

> "Online videos were the only info I could find. Some help, some not. Not much info around strategies for managing life."
>
> "seems to work for some and not others, also self-modelling seems to be more powerful than peer-modelling."

The autistic educational consultant and researcher noted that in their opinion, video-modelling expectations is helpful in autism, because many autistics relate better to watching something on video as the real-life distractions aren't present.

> "Also you can stop it and rewind and replay as much as you need. We've used it help autistics to understand things people were instructing, taking out the person and showing instead."

The responses collected indicated that some believed video-modelling was beneficial while others did not hold this view. Considering there are contradictory views about the efficacy of video-modelling, it is important that its usage should be tested by an individual before using as a consistent strategy.

4.5 Conclusion

This chapter examined the findings in literature reviews about the benefits that autistics can obtain from robots, portable electronic devices, and different forms of video-modelling. It was found that portable devices can help autistics communicate with others and may help them improve their academic skills. Programs that included robots were also found to help autistic children learn social skills and other age-appropriate skills. Finally, video-modelling was found to help autistics learn important lessons. All assistive technologies in this chapter were rated as 'Silver – Usually promising'. At the end of each section the views of several autistics about the benefits of technology were presented. Their insights showed that some autistics benefited from technology while others did not.

References

Alzrayer, N., Banda, D. R., & Koul, R. K. (2014). Use of iPad/iPods with individuals with autism and other developmental disabilities: A meta-analysis of communication interventions. *Review Journal of Autism and Developmental Disorders*, 1(3), 179–191. doi:10.1007/s40489-014-0018-5.

Bellini, S., Akullian, J., & Hopf, A. (2007). Increasing social engagement in young children with autism spectrum disorders using video self-modeling. *School Psychology Review*, 36(1), 80–90.

Buggey, T. (2005). Video Self-modeling applications with students with autism spectrum disorder in a small private school setting. *Focus on Autism and Other Developmental Disabilities*, 20(1), 52–63. doi:10.1177/10883576050200010501.

Buggey, T., Toombs, K., Gardener, P., & Cervetti, M. (1999). Training responding behaviors in students with autism: Using videotaped self-modeling. *Journal of Positive Behavior Interventions*, 1(4), 205–214. doi:10.1177/109830079900100403.

Charlop, M. H., & Milstein, J. P. (1989). Teaching autistic children conversational speech using video modeling. *Journal of Applied Behavior Analysis*, 22(3), 275–285. doi:10.1901/jaba.1989.22-275.

Charlop-Christy, M. H., & Daneshvar, S. (2003). Using video modeling to teach perspective taking to children with autism. *Journal of Positive Behavior Interventions*, 5(1), 12–21. doi:10.1177/10983007030050010101.

Charlop-Christy, M. H., Le, L., & Freeman, K. A. (2000). A comparison of video modeling with in vivo modeling for teaching children with autism. *Journal of Autism and Developmental Disorders*, 30(6), 537–552. doi:10.1023/A:1005635326276.

D'Ateno, P., Mangiapanello, K., & Taylor, B. (2003). Using video modeling to teach complex play sequences to a preschooler with Autism. *Journal of Positive Behavior Interventions*, 5(1), 5–11doi:10.1177/10983007030050010801.

de Vries, M., Prins, P. J., Schmand, B. A., & Geurts, H. M. (2015). Working memory and cognitive flexibility-training for children with an autism spectrum disorder: A randomized controlled trial. *Journal of Child Psychology and Psychiatry*, 56(5), 566–576. doi:10.1111/jcpp.12324.

Diehl, J. J., Schmitt, L. M., Villano, M., & Crowell, C. R. (2012). The clinical use of robots for individuals with autism spectrum disorders: A critical review. *Research in Autism Spectrum Disorders*, 6(1), 249–262. doi:10.1016/j.rasd.2011.05.006.

DiPietro, J., Kelemen, A., Liang, Y., & Sik-Lanyi, C. (2019). Computer-and robot-assisted therapies to aid social and intellectual functioning of children with autism spectrum disorder. *Medicina*, 55(8), 440. doi:10.3390/medicina55080440.

Fragale, C. L. (2014). Video modeling interventions to improve play skills of children with autism spectrum disorders: A systematic literature review. *Review Journal of Autism and Developmental Disorders*, 1(3), 165–178. doi:10.1007/s40489-014-0019-4.

Gena, A., Couloura, S., & Kymissis, E. (2005). Modifying the affective behavior of preschoolers with autism using *in-vivo* or video modeling and reinforcement contingencies. *Journal of Autism and Developmental Disorders*, 35(5), 545–556. doi:10.1007/s10803-005-0014-9.

Hart, J. E., & Whalon, K. J. (2012). Using video self-modeling via iPads to increase academic responding of an adolescent with autism spectrum disorder and intellectual disability. *Education and Training in Autism and Developmental Disabilities*, 47, 438–446.

Hersh, M. (2015). Overcoming barriers and increasing independence–service robots for elderly and disabled people. *International Journal of Advanced Robotic Systems*, 12(8), 1–33. doi:10.5772/59230.

Hine, J. F., & Wolery, M. (2006). Using point-of-view video modeling to teach play to preschoolers with autism. *Topics in Early Childhood Special Education*, 26(2), 83–93. doi:10.1177/02711214060260020301.

Huskens, B., Palmen, A., Van der Werff, M., Lourens, T., & Barakova, E. (2015). Improving collaborative play between children with autism spectrum disorders and their siblings: The effectiveness of a robot-mediated intervention based on Lego® therapy. *Journal of Autism and Developmental Disorders*, 45(11), 3746–3755. doi:10.1007/s10803-014-2326-0.

Jowett, E. L., Moore, D. W., & Anderson, A. (2012). Using an iPad-based video modelling package to teach numeracy skills to a child with an autism spectrum disorder. *Developmental Neurorehabilitation*, 15(4), 304–312. doi:10.3109/17518423.2012.682168.

Kagohara, D. M., Sigafoos, J., Achmadi, D., O'Reilly, M. F., & Lancioni, G. (2012). Teaching children with autism spectrum disorders to check the spelling of words. *Research in Autism Spectrum Disorders*, 6, 304–310. doi:10.1016/j.rasd.2011.05.012.

Kagohara, D. M., van der Meer, L., Ramdoss, S., O'Reilly, M. F., Lancioni, G. E., Davis, T. N., … & Green, V. A. (2013). Using iPods® and iPads® in teaching programs for individuals with developmental disabilities: A systematic review. *Research in Developmental Disabilities*, 34(1), 147–156. doi:10.1016/j.ridd.2012.07.027.

Kroeger, K. A., Schultz, J. R., & Newsom, C. (2007). A comparison of two group-delivered social skills programs for young children with autism. *Journal of Autism and Developmental Disorders*, 37(5), 808–817. doi:10.1007/s10803-006-0207-x.

Larwin, K. H., & Aspiranti, K. B. (2019). Measuring the academic outcomes of iPads for students with autism: A meta-analysis. *Review Journal of Autism and Developmental Disorders*, 6 (2), 233–241. doi:10.1007/s40489-019-00165-y.

Ledbetter-Cho, K., O'Reilly, M., Lang, R., Watkins, L., & Lim, N. (2018). Meta-analysis of tablet-mediated interventions for teaching academic skills to individuals with autism. *Journal of Autism and Developmental Disorders*, 48(9), 3021–3036. doi:10.1007/s10803-018-3573-2.

Lorah, E. R., Parnell, A., Whitby, P. S., & Hantula, D. (2015). A systematic review of tablet computers and portable media players as speech generating devices for individuals with autism spectrum disorder. *Journal of Autism and Developmental Disorders*, 45(12), 3792–3804. doi:10.1007/s10803-014-2314-4.

MacDonald, R., Clark, M., Garrigan, E., & Vangala, M. (2005). Using video modeling to teach pretend play to children with autism. *Behavioral Interventions*, 20(4), 225–238. doi:10.1002/bin.197.

Mayes, S. D., & Calhoun, S. L. (2007). Learning, attention, writing, and processing speed in typical children and children with ADHD, autism, anxiety, depression, and oppositional-defiant disorder. *Child Neuropsychology*, 13(6), 469–493. doi:10.1080/09297040601112773.

Nikopoulos, C. K., & Keenan, M. (2004). Effects of video modelling on training and generalisation of social initiation and reciprocal play by children with autism. *European Journal of Behaviour Analysis*, 5(1), 1–13. doi:10.1080/15021149.2004.11434227.

Nikopoulos, C. K., & Keenan, M. (2007). Using video modeling to teach complex social sequences to children with autism. *Journal of Autism and Developmental Disorders*, 37(4), 678–693. doi:10.1007/s10803-006-0195-x.

Paterson, C. R., & Arco, L. (2007). Using video modeling for generalizing toy play in children with autism. *Behavior Modification*, 31(5), 660–681. doi:10.1177/0145445507301651.

Pennisi, P., Tonacci, A., Tartarisco, G., Billeci, L., Ruta, L., Gangemi, S., & Pioggia, G. (2016). Autism and social robotics: A systematic review. *Autism Research*, 9(2), 165–183. doi:10.1002/aur.1527.

Reichow, B., Volkmar, F. R., & Cicchetti, D. V. (2008). Development of the evaluative method for evaluating and determining evidence based practices in autism. *Journal of Autism and Developmental Disorders*, 38(7), 1311–1319. doi:10.1007/s10803-007-0517-74.

Saadatzi, M. N., Pennington, R. C., Welch, K. C., & Graham, J. H. (2018). Small-group technology-assisted instruction: Virtual teacher and robot peer for individuals with autism spectrum disorder. *Journal of Autism and Developmental Disorders*, 48(11), 3816–3830. doi:10.1007/s10803-018-3654-2.

Schreibman, L., Whalen, C., & Stahmer, A. C. (2000). The use of video priming to reduce disruptive transition behavior in children with autism. *Journal of Positive Behavior Interventions*, 2(1), 3–11. doi:10.1177/109830070000200102.

Sharkey, A. (2014). Robots and human dignity: A consideration of the effects of robot care on the dignity of older people. *Ethics and Information Technology*, 16(1), 63–75. doi:10.1007/s10676–10014–9338–9335.

Sherer, M., Pierce, K. L., Paredes, S., Kisacky, K. L., Ingersoll, B., & Schreibman, L. (2001). Enhancing conversation skills in children with autism via video technology: Which is better, "self" or "other" as a model? *Behavior Modification*, 25(1), 140–158. doi:10.1177/0145445501251008.

Shukla-Mehta, S., Miller, T., & Callahan, K. J. (2010). Evaluating the effectiveness of video instruction on social and communication skills training for children with autism spectrum disorders: A review of the literature. *Focus on Autism and Other Developmental Disabilities*, 25 (1), 23–36. doi:10.1177/1088357609352901.

Sigafoos, J., Lancioni, G. E., O'Reilly, M. F., Achmadi, D., Stevens, M., Roche, L., … & Marschik, P. B. (2013). Teaching two boys with autism spectrum disorders to request the continuation of toy play using an iPad®-based speech-generating device. *Research in Autism Spectrum Disorders*, 7(8), 923–930. doi:10.1016/j.rasd.2013.04.002.

Smith, B. R., Spooner, F., & Wood, C. L. (2013). Using embedded computer-assisted explicit instruction to teach science to students with autism spectrum disorder. *Research in Autism Spectrum Disorders*, 7(3), 433–443. doi:10.1016/j.rasd.2012.10.010.

Sparrow, R., & Sparrow, L. (2006). In the hands of machines? The future of aged care. *Minds and Machines*, 16(2), 141–161. doi:10.1007/s11023–11006–9030–9036.

Strasberger, S. K., & Ferreri, S. J. (2014). The effects of peer assisted communication application training on the communicative and social behaviors of children with autism. *Journal of Developmental and Physical Disabilities*, 26(5), 513–526. doi:10.1007/s10882-013-9358-9.

Taylor, B. A., Levin, L., & Jasper, S. (1999). Increasing play-related statements in children with autism toward their siblings: Effects of video modeling. *Journal of Developmental Disabilities*, 11(3), 253–264. doi:10.1023/A:1021800716392.

van der Meer, L., Kagohara, D., Achmadi, D., Green, V. A., Herrington, C., Sigafoos, J., … & Rispoli, M. (2011). Teaching functional use of an iPod-based speech-generating device to

individuals with developmental disabilities. *Journal of Special Education Technology*, 26(3), 1–11. doi:10.1177/016264341102600301.
van der Meer, L., Kagohara, D., Roche, L., Sutherland, D., Balandin, S., Green, V. A., … & Sigafoos, J. (2013). Teaching multi-step requesting and social communication to two children with autism spectrum disorders with three AAC options. *Augmentative and Alternative Communication*, 29(3), 222–234. doi:10.3109/07434618.2013.815801.
Walker, V. L., & Snell, M. E. (2013). Effects of augmentative and alternative communication on challenging behavior: A meta-analysis. *Augmentative and Alternative Communication*, 29(2), 117–131. doi:10.3109/07434618.2013.785020.
Wang, S. Y., Cui, Y., & Parrila, R. (2011). Examining the effectiveness of peer-mediated and video-modeling social skills interventions for children with autism spectrum disorders: A meta-analysis in single-case research using HLM. *Research in Autism Spectrum Disorders*, 5 (1), 562–569. doi:10.1016/j.rasd.2010.06.023.
Wert, B. Y., & Neisworth, J. T. (2003). Effects of video self-modeling on spontaneous requesting in children with autism. *Journal of Positive Behavior Interventions*, 5(1), 30–34. doi:10.1177/10983007030050010501.
Xin, J. F., Sheppard, M. E., & Brown, M. (2017). Brief report: Using iPads for self-monitoring of students with autism. *Journal of Autism and Developmental Disorders*, 47(5), 1559–1567. doi:10.1007/s10803-017-3055-y.
Yakubova, G., Hughes, E. M., & Hornberger, E. (2015). Video-based intervention in teaching fraction problem-solving to students with autism spectrum disorder. *Journal of Autism and Developmental Disorders*, 45(9), 2865–2875. doi:10.1007/s10803-015-2449-y.

Chapter 5

Therapeutic supports involving animals

5.1 Introduction

This chapter presents the literature about the efficacy of animal-assisted programs for autistics. It begins with an overview of the literature about the therapeutic value of dogs for autistics, followed by our evaluation of this as well as our recommendations for where more research can be conducted. The insights from autistics who completed our survey about the benefits they obtained after interacting with dogs completes this section. The same sequence of topics is then used for equine assisted therapies. This chapter concludes with insights from autistics who completed our survey about the efficacy of interacting with animals in general.

5.2 Dog therapy

5.2.1 Dogs as supports or therapy

Berry and colleagues (2013) examined six studies about the social and behavioural impacts demonstrated by autistic children after briefly interacting with therapy dogs as well as the impact of introducing dogs to families raising autistic children. They discovered that many of the studies that they examined based their results on small sample sizes. Due to the small number of participants, the results presented may not be widely applicable. Based on the literature reviewed they concluded:

> … intervention strategies, based on exploiting the emotional aspects of the relationship with a dog, can overcome the inability of children affected by ASD to relate and interact with others …
>
> (Berry et al., 2013, p. 77).

Recently, Hill and colleagues (2019) applied the single-case experimental design scale and the *Downs and Black checklist* for non-randomised control to 13 studies about the social benefits that autistic children obtained from therapy dogs. They concluded that the results reported by the studies they examined should be treated with caution since the studies contained many methodological shortcomings, including small sample sizes, inconsistent usage of terminology, lack of participant blinding, and a minimal use of research protocols. While these limitations may hamper the reliability of the results, they concluded that:

> Overall results from this review indicate interaction with a therapy dog that can have a positive impact on the social behaviours of children on the autism spectrum, in particular, improving verbal communication, non-verbal communication, desired social behaviours, as well as reducing undesired social behaviours.
>
> (Hill et al., 2019, pp. 23–24).

In summary, interacting with dogs has been found to give autistics many benefits, including reductions in social isolation (Berry et al., 2013), and improvements with verbal and non-verbal communication (Hill et al., 2019). However, despite these benefits, Berry et al. and Hill et al. suggested that these benefits are uncertain since the studies they examined contained many methodological limitations.

5.2.2 Evaluation of support programs that use dogs

Rating: Silver – Usually promising

The results reported in the studies examined by Berry et al. (2013) and Hill et al. (2019) have shown that interacting with dogs can give some autistics some benefits. Although such outcomes are promising they are largely speculative since existing findings are based on studies that have common methodological weaknesses, including small sample sizes and an inconsistent use of terms. Until more methodologically rigorous research has been published it is not possible to definitively claim that most autistics will obtain benefits after interacting with dogs. Due to this uncertainty, support programs for autistics that include the usage of dogs have been rated as 'Silver – Usually promising'.

5.2.3 Directions for research in the future about support programs that use dogs

Based on the current state of research there are three areas where more research can be conducted on the therapeutic benefits that autistics can obtain from dogs. First, Hill et al. (2019) and Berry et al. (2013) explained that most of the studies that they reviewed contained methodological weaknesses, such as small sample sizes and an inconsistent usage of terms. In the future, researchers should address these limitations so that we can have a more consistent understanding about the potential therapeutic benefits that dogs can give autistics. Second, there is a scarcity of longitudinal research on the level of maintenance of benefits autistics obtained from dogs over time. Consequently, it is not possible to claim with confidence that support programs that contain dogs can provide autistics with long-term benefits. In the future, researchers should address this limitation by conducting follow-up research, which compares and contrasts the outcomes from short-term therapeutic interactions with long-term sustained therapeutic interactions between autistics and dogs. Third, most of the studies examined by Berry et al. have explored the benefits that autistic children have obtained from interacting with dogs. Consequently, the benefits that adult autistics have obtained from canine interactions remains unknown since there is a paucity of studies. In the interests of improving our knowledge studies that measure the benefits autistic adults obtain from dogs should be conducted.

5.2.4 Autistic views about using dogs as supports or therapeutic interventions

Have you personally had/used an assistance or therapy dog?

Most respondents (n = 41, 69.49%) selected the option 'No' when answering the question 'Have you personally had/used an assistance or therapy dog?' This was followed by eight (13.56%) respondents who stated that they had used a therapy dog at their school, work, or a group that they attended.

Respondents' ratings of the efficacy of using an assistance or therapy dog

Out of the 206 respondents who completed our online survey, 48 (23.30%) rated the efficacy of using an assistance or therapy dog. Most selected the option 'enjoyed, found useful and was able to be more confident or confident even without the dog' (n = 11, 22.92%), followed by four (8.33%) who selected the option 'enjoyed and found useful'. Since most respondents selected one of these options, the efficacy of therapy dogs for autistics as perceived by autistics was calculated as 4.2 stars. This can be seen as a stronger endorsement than the literature.

Respondents' comments about using an assistance or therapy dog

When asked 'How was your experience of a therapy or assistance dog?' 19 respondents provided a comment. Our examination of these comments illustrated a belief that interacting with a dog calmed them down.

> "She is a constant source of reliably positive interaction. She interrupts negative stims and provides compression stimuli to calm me down. She alerts to my heart rate and building anxiety. She is a miracle."
>
> "I've never had a proper therapy dog, but our family dog was very helpful-cuddling her was calming ..."
>
> "I cannot imagine my life now without my therapy dog. She has enabled me to feel more confident, manage my anxiety, get out more and her fur is a soothing stim."
>
> "I brought my therapy dog to school and he would curl up with students who were distressed until they calmed down, which made me more confident."

Additionally, two respondents explained that they would like a therapy dog.

> "I would love a therapy dog, but they are extremely expensive here, and only trained for autistic children, not adults."
>
> "I'm going to get my own assistant dog next year. I am very excited because I believe once I have a dog I will be able to access more environments. Also I hope I will have less meltdowns because the dog will help me know when I'm getting stressed and even if I do have a meltdown at least I will have a mate with me and then other people in public won't be scared of me when I'm behaving autistic because the dog will advocate for me being autistic when currently most people don't believe me unless they know me personally because I'm good at passing."

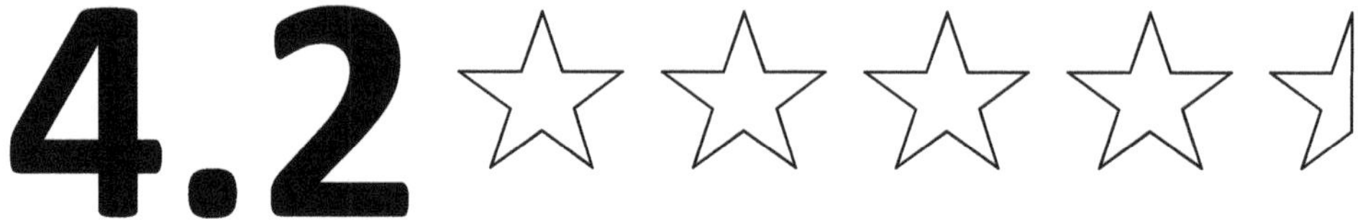

Figure 5.1 4.2 stars

While most respondents claimed that a therapy dog helped them, there were some who did not share this view. Due to these opposing views, it is important to take into consideration the views of autistics about therapy dogs before they are given such an animal. Despite some autistic respondents clearly describing the benefits of therapy dogs, one individual succinctly stated, 'It was horrific'. However, they did not provide any elaboration as to why their experience of therapy dogs was 'horrific'. It is probable that they dislike or have a phobia of dogs, which highlights the need to make sure that before such an animal is used in therapy the autistic client needs to feel comfortable around dogs.

5.3 Equine therapy

5.3.1 Equine therapy

Conducting activities with horses, such as riding, feeding, or brushing the animal's hair, is 'Equine therapy'. At the time of writing this book we located three literature reviews of the therapeutic benefits that equine activities brought to autistics (Mapes & Rosén, 2016; Srinivasan, Cavagnino, & Bhat, 2018; Tan & Simmonds, 2019). Mapes and Rosén (2016) reviewed 12 studies about this topic (See Table 5.1).

Mapes and Rosén (2016) found that most of the studies that they examined shared two common methodological weaknesses. First, just over 50% of the studies they examined did not contain a control or wait group. Since studies did not use such groups it was not possible to measure the efficacy of equine therapy for autistics, versus changes that would have occurred anyway over that period of time. Second, eight out of the 12 studies they examined had small sample sizes that in turn reduced the diversity of the autistic population represented. Despite these limitations, Mapes and Rosén (2016, p. 384) concluded that:

> The majority of the research surrounding EAT [Equine Assisted Therapy] for children with ASD yielded significant results ranging from increasing physical and social functioning, communication, sensory motivation, self-regulation, adaptive skills, motor skills, as well as decreasing aberrant behavior and severity of symptoms, and improved volition.

In 2018, Srinivasan, Cavagnino, and Bhat examined 15 studies about the social, communication, and behavioural benefits that autistics obtained from horses. They also examined the methodological quality of the studies collected. Based on their analysis they concluded:

> Our review suggested that equine therapy has beneficial effects on behavioral and to some extent on social communication skills in ASD. The evidence for positive effects of equine therapy on perceptual-motor, cognitive, and functional skills is currently limited." (Srinivasan, Cavagnino, & Bhat, 2018, p. 156).

Recently, Trzmiel et al. (2019) conducted a literature review to examine the effectiveness of equine-assisted activities and therapies (EAAT) for autistics. They searched for articles that were hosted on PUBMED, Cochrane Library, Web of Science, ClinicalTrials.gov, and PEDro. For the study to be included in their analysis, it had to have been published in English, after 1999, in a journal with a review process, contain a control group or present comparative pre- and post-therapy resulted in participants, and have a clear inclusion and exclusion criteria. They then used the *Quality Assessment Tools for Quantitative Studies* to assess the methodological quality of the included studies. They examined 15 studies that collectively assessed the impact of EAAT on 390 participants. They found that after EAAT sessions autistics exhibited an increase in socialisation, engagement, and shorter reaction time in problem-solving situations. Despite these potential benefits, Trzmiel et al. (2019, p. 111) urged caution, stating that:

> it is impossible to draw universal conclusions due to the considerable discrepancies in therapeutic protocols and measurement instruments of the … studies. Further, longitudinal trials, with standardized EAAT protocols and representative large sample groups are necessary. Also, it is crucial to establish homogeneous tools to measure therapeutic progress and outcomes, especially with regard to social functioning.

Also, during 2019 Tan and Simmonds published a literature review in which they examined 16 studies that explored the benefits that interacting with horses gave autistic children and adolescents. They reported that autistic children and adolescents obtained many benefits, including significant improvements with communication, coping and daily living skills, social participation, empathy, expressive language skills, motor planning skills, and self-regulation. Additionally, they also exhibited reductions in maladaptive and hyperactive behaviours, irritability, and off-task behaviours (See Table 5.2).

5.3.2 Evaluation of equine therapy programs

Rating: Silver – Usually promising

Based on the studies that we reviewed, equine therapy can provide many benefits to autistics, such as increased social skills, physical functioning, adaptive skills, motor skills, and self-regulation, as well as decreased aberrant behaviour (Mapes & Rosén, 2016). Despite these benefits, there was no research which explored if there were any unintended negative outcomes or impacts for individual autistics participating in equine therapy; for example, the possibility that some individuals may have a fear or anxiety about being around such a large animal. Additionally, there is insufficient research to conclude that the benefits that autistics obtain from equine therapy can be sustained once equine therapy has ended or if the benefits obtained can be generalised to multiple settings. This is because, according to Mapes and Rosén (2016), most studies about this topic either contained small sample sizes or were single-case studies and

Table 5.1 Summary of studies examined by Mapes and Rosén (2016)

Study	*Strengths*	*Weaknesses*	*Conclusion*
Bass et al., 2009	• Pre- Post-test Design with Random Assignment and high internal validity • Control group • Standardised Questionnaires with high internal consistency • Structured lesson plan	• Relatively Small sample size • Low external validity • Did not indicate if benefits were maintained	Effective for increasing social motivation, sensory seeking, sensory integration, directed attention, sensory sensitivity and reduction in sedentary behaviour, inattention/distractibility
Gabriels et al., 2012	• Control group • Multiple sources of data • Pre- Post-test Design with high internal validity	• Low external validity due to small sample size • Possible Rater bias • Results were not corrected • No examination of long-term effects • Lacked standardised THR intervention protocol	Effective for self-regulation behaviours (irritability, lethargy, stereotypical behaviour, hyperactivity) expressive language, motor skills, and adaptive learning skills
García-Gómez et al., 2014	• Control group • BASC collects data of children in different contexts	• "Quasi-Control" Test-Retest Design, no random assignment, poor internal validity • Small sample size, lowering external validity • No indication that benefits were maintained	Effective for reducing aggressiveness
Holm et al., 2014	• Single-Subject ABA Design • Examined behavioural changes magnitude correspondence with dose of THR • Multiple sources of data in multiple settings • Standardised measures	• Small sample size, lowering external validity • Parents were not masked to the general purpose of study • No control group	Effective for decreased target behaviours nominated by parents such as clapping, chewing, snapping, spontaneous verbal communication, and pounding surfaces
Jenkins and Reed, 2013	• Single-Subject Multiple Baseline Across Participants Design • Control group	• Low external validity due to small sample size and single-case design • Only evidence for efficacy is anecdotal • Failure to replicate • Used self-report forms	Not effective for response to others' initiations, or spontaneous initiations. Not effective for off-task behaviour, compliance, or problem behaviour

Study	*Strengths*	*Weaknesses*	*Conclusion*
Kern et al., 2011	• Pre- Post-test Design with Follow-Up • Standardised measures	• No control group	Effective for interactive competencies, reduction in severity of symptoms, improvements on Mood and Tone subscale of questionnaire, and improved quality of life
Lanning et al., 2014	• Control Group • Control Group was a Social Circle • High reliability of measures • Information indicating what point behaviour change occurred • Appropriate statistical analysis to address issues related to small sample size	• Longitudinal Quasi-Experimental Design with Repeated Measures, no random assignment, low internal validity • Small sample size • No knowledge of prior experiences to equines for parent reports • Varied lesson plans based on individual	Effective for improvements in physical, emotional, and social functioning
Nelson et al., 2011	• Single-Subject ABAB Reversal Design, good internal validity • Direct observation of three boys allowed for detailed explanations for each participant	• Small sample size due to Single-Subject design, low external validity	Effective for increasing social behaviour and decreasing aberrant behaviour
Taylor et al., 2009	• Appropriate use of PVQ	• No control • Small sample size	Effective for increasing volition over time
Van den Hout and Bragonje, 2010	• Prospective Single-Blinded Clinical Trial, high internal validity • Large sample size, high external validity • Included analysis of magnitude • Included differences in terms of severity of ASD • Scales had strong psychometric properties • Included examination of concurrent therapies	• Only the parent-rated measure was significant • No control group • Majority of participants participating in a concurrent therapy	Demonstrated minor improvements in communication, and large improvements in sociability, and sensory/cognitive awareness

(*continued*)

Table 5.1 *(coninued)*

Study	*Strengths*	*Weaknesses*	*Conclusion*
Ward et al., 2013	• Interrupted Time Series Design examined if behavioural changes were maintained and reinstated	• Single-Group Quasi-Experimental and Interrupted Time Series Design, no random assignment, low internal validity • Relatively small sample size • Did not include a control group	Effective for improved social interaction, sensory processing, and decreasing severity of symptoms. The effects were not sustained during breaks, but were reestablished once treatment began
Weber and Westmoquette, 2010	• Great amount of information for further generation of hypotheses • Gather information about behaviour in different environments	• Qualitative Design (semi-structured interviews) • No proof of cause and effect; no direction comparison between differential reinforcement of alternative behaviour with and without equine • Limitations of interviews • No standardised measurements	Interviewees reported improvements in physical and psychological developments such as developments in communication, motivation, awareness, interest in surroundings, self-confidence, and reduction in fears or phobias

Source: Mapes and Rosén, 2016, pp. 379–380.

Table 5.2 Summary of studies examined by Tan and Simmonds (2019)

Authors and year	*Sample (size, IQ/level of functioning)*	*Age range (mean) and gender*	*Outcomes of EAAT*	*Length of EAAT (session time in minutes)/ study design*
Ajzenman, Standeven, and Shurtleff, 2013	$N = 6$	5–12 years	Significant improvement in communication, coping and daily activity and social participation	12 weeks (45)/quasi-experimental
Anderson and Meints, 2016	$N = 15$	5–16 years ($M = 10$) 11 males, four females	Some decrease in maladaptive behaviours and increase in empathy No significant change in communication, socialisation and overall maladaptive behaviours.	Five weeks (180)/quasi-experimental
Bass, Duchowny, and Llabre, 2009	$N = 34$ Experimental $n = 19$ Control, waitlisted $n = 15$	Experimental 5–10 years ($M = 6.95$) 17 males, two females Control 4–10 years ($M = 7.73$) 12 males, three females	Significant treatment effects in overall social responsiveness profiles for experimental group, no significant change for control	12 weeks (60)/randomised controlled trial
Borgi et al., 2016	$N = 28$ Intervention $n = 15$ Control, no treatment $n = 13$	6–12 years ($M = 8.6$) Males only	Significant improvement in social functioning and quicker planning time in intervention group, but not controls	25 weeks (60–70)/randomised controlled trial
Gabriels et al., 2012	$N = 42$ Intervention $n = 26$ Waitlist $n = 16$	6–16 years ($M = 8.7$) 36 males, six females	Significant improvements on measures of irritability, lethargy, stereotypic behaviour, hyperactivity, expressive language skills, motor planning skills, and self-regulation in experimental group compared to controls	Ten weeks (60)/quasi-experimental

(*continued*)

Table 5.2 (*coninued*)

Authors and year	*Sample (size, IQ/level of functioning)*	*Age range (mean) and gender*	*Outcomes of EAAT*	*Length of EAAT (session time in minutes)/ study design*
Gabriels et al., 2015	$N = 116$ Experimental $n = 58$ Mean IQ = 86.7 Control $n = 58$ Mean IQ = 86.1	6–16 years ($M = 10.2$) Experimental: $M = 10.5$ 49 males, nine females Control: $M = 10.0$ 52 males, six females	Significant improvement in experimental group compared to control in irritability, hyperactivity, social communication, total words spoken, number of new words spoken; borderline significant for social cognition	Ten weeks (45)/randomised control trial
García-Gómez et al., 2014	$N = 16$ Experimental $n = 8$ Control $n = 8$	7–14 years 13 males, three females	Significant improvement in aggressive behaviours only in experimental group. Significant improvement on only two quality of life indicators (interpersonal relations and social inclusion) in experimental group only	12 weeks (45)[b]/quasi-experimental
Ghorban et al., 2013	$N = 6$	6–12 years ($M = 8.5$) one male, five females	Significant improvement in understand emotions and perspective-taking, initiating and maintaining interaction, and overall social skills score No change only in response to interaction	Four weeks (45)[b]/quasi-experimental
Harris and Williams, 2017	$N = 26$ One third of participants had "limited language"; majority were "mainly non-verbal"	6.08–9.33 years ($M = 7.5$) 22 males, four females Experimental: $M = 8.2$ Control: $M = 7$	Significant reduction in severity of ASD symptoms and hyperactivity for intervention group only No significant changes to energy levels, irritability, stereotypy, inappropriate speech	Seven weeks (45)/quasi-experimental
Holm et al., 2014	$N = 3$	6–8 years Males only	Significant improvement in some target behaviours, which varied across participants Positive changes in multiple target behaviours carried over to home and community context	12 weeks (45)[b]/single-subject

Table 5.2 (*coninued*)

Authors and year	*Sample (size, IQ/level of functioning)*	*Age range (mean) and gender*	*Outcomes of EAAT*	*Length of EAAT (session time in minutes)/ study design*
Jenkins and Reed, 2013	$N = 7$ Experimental: $n = 4$ Control: $n = 3$	6–14 years ($M = 9.5$) Six males, one female	No significant effect on dependent variables in both groups.	Nine weeks (60)/single-subject
Kern et al., 2011	$N = 24$	Age range not provided ($M = 7.8$) 18 males, six females	Significant decrease in CARS score (reduction of severity of ASD symptoms), significant overall increase in parent-rated quality of life, significant improvement in sensory auditory processing No significant change in parent-child interaction quality, overall sensory profile	24 weeks (60)/quasi-experimental
Lanning et al., 2014	$N = 25$ Experimental $n = 13$ Comparison $n = 12$	Experimental: 4–15 years ($M = 7.5$) nine males, four females Control: 5–14 years ($M = 9.8$) 12 males	Significant improvement in quality of life domains for both groups: Physical, psychological and emotional functioning Significantly more improvement in physical and psychosocial functioning domains for experimental group compared to comparison	12 weeks (60)/quasi-experimental
Llambias et al., 2016	$N = 7$	4–7 years ($M = 5.1$) Four males, three females	Significant improvement in task engagement across all participants	9–12 weeks (45–60)/single-subject
Memishevikj and Hodzhikj, 2010	$N = 4$ $n = 2$: Mild intellectual disability (IQ = 50–70) $n = 2$: Severe intellectual disability (IQ = 20–35)	8–10 years two males, two females	In two with mild ID: Significant improvement in speech, socialisation, cognitive and overall Autism Treatment Evaluation Checklist score. No or minimal change for health/behaviour domain In two with severe ID: No or minimal improvement overall. Decrease in behaviour rating from pre- to post-test	Ten weeks (30)/single-subject

(*continued*)

Table 5.2 (*coninued*)

Authors and year	*Sample (size, IQ/level of functioning)*	*Age range (mean) and gender*	*Outcomes of EAAT*	*Length of EAAT (session time in minutes)/ study design*
Petty et al., 2017	$N = 67$ Mean IQ = 87.84 Experimental: $n = 31$ Control: $n = 36$	6–16 years ($M = 10.45$) Experimental: $M = 10.95$ 27 males, four females Control: $M = 10.01$ 33 males, three females	Significant improvement in social interactions with family pet in experimental group only	Ten weeks (120)/randomised controlled trial
Taylor et al., 2009	$N = 3$	4–6 years old	Overall improved motivation to engage in daily activities	16 weeks (45)/single-subject
Ward et al., 2013	$N = 21$	Age range not provided ($M = 8.1$) 15 males, six females	Significant improvement in social interaction and overall autism index.	30 weeks (60)/quasi-experimental

Key: The term 'significant' indicates that statistical significance was reported by the study.
[a] Programs that qualify for the definition 'therapy'.
[b] Frequency of more than once a week.
Source: Tan and Simmonds, 2019, pp. 328–330.

that most studies did not include any follow-up periods to see if the benefits obtained during equine therapy were maintained long-term. Although equine therapy can offer some autistics benefits it is not possible to claim with confidence that these benefits can be sustained or generalised to multiple settings. Due to these limitations, we have rated equine therapy as 'Silver – Usually promising'.

5.3.3 Directions for research in the future about equine therapy programs

Despite there being many studies about the benefits that equine therapy can give autistics, as well as personal accounts from autistics about the benefits of horses (Grandin, 2019), there are still four areas where more research in the future could be conducted.

First, Mapes and Rosén (2016) found that just over 50% of the studies that they examined did not contain a control or wait list group. Consequently, it was not possible to compare the benefits a group of autistics obtained from equine therapy to a group of autistics who did not participate in this therapy. In the future, researchers should incorporate into their study's design a control group so that the benefits that equine therapy can give autistics can be contrasted against a group of autistics who did not participate in equine therapy.

Second, Mapes and Rosén examined eight out of 12 studies that based their findings on small sample sizes (Bass, Duchowny, & Llabre, 2009; García-Gómez et al., 2014; Holm et al., 2014; Lanning et al., 2014; Nelson et al., 2011; Taylor et al., 2009; Ward et al., 2013). Due to small sample sizes, it was not possible to guarantee that the results apply to the whole autistic community. In the future, researchers should conduct studies that have larger sample sizes so that the results collected can be more applicable to the autistic community.

Third, most studies about this topic have based their results on samples of autistic children. Consequently, there is not much research that has measured the benefits that autistic adults could obtain after interacting with horses. In the interests of increasing our knowledge about the potential benefits from equine interactions, in the future researchers could examine if autistic adults obtain any benefits from equine therapy.

Fourth, most researchers have examined if horse riding activities provide immediate benefits to autistics. Consequently, there is not much research about the long-term benefits that autistics have obtained from horse riding. In the future, researchers should incorporate into their studies follow-up assessments to examine if the benefits autistics obtain from horse riding are maintained long-term. Such research will increase our understanding about the long-term impacts autistics obtain from equine therapy. It will also help autistics, and those who support them, to make an informed choice about if other treatment options might be required once equine therapy has ended.

5.3.4 Autistic views about equine therapy

Have you personally experienced equine therapy (horse riding as a therapy for autism)?

Out of the 206 respondents who completed our online survey, 58 (28.15%) answered the question 'Have you personally experienced equine therapy (horse riding as a therapy for autism)?' Most (n = 50, 86.21%) selected the option 'No', three (5.17%) noted that they had used equine therapy more than ten times, three (5.17%) stated that they had used it between two and ten times, and two (3.45%) stated that they had participated in one equine therapy session.

Respondents' ratings of the efficacy of equine therapy

Since less than ten respondents rated the efficacy of equine therapy its efficacy for autistics was not rated.

Respondents' comments about equine therapy

Nine respondents answered the question 'How was your experience of an equine therapy (horse riding as a therapy for autism)?' Our examination of these comments showed that three believed horses were a beneficial form of therapy.

> "I volunteer for a group that does equine therapy and not only do I get to ride very occasionally but there are also lots of autistic kids and it really seems to help their confidence, communication, mood, and build other skills."
>
> "I've ridden before, but not as a therapy (I was obsessed with horses!). But I really enjoyed riding and being around horses is definitely calming."
>
> "My aunt owned horses and my family had me work with them through childhood until they couldn't afford it. It wasn't formal therapy but it was extremely helpful."
>
> In contrast, two respondents claimed that they did not like equine therapy.
>
> "It didn't help. I like horses. I like being around horses. But it didn't help. (they wouldn't let me ride them)."
>
> "This was a no go. I'm terrified of horses after being thrown from one when I was younger (pre-autism diagnosis and not meant for therapeutic purposes)."

Some respondents believed equine therapy was beneficial while others clearly articulated the opposite view. Therefore, before autistics participate in an equine therapy program they should be asked if they want to ride horses and/or participate in equine therapy. If they have not ever seen a horse, it would be useful for them to observe a horse from afar before being asked if they would like to participate in equine therapy.

5.4 Autistic views about using other animal species

Respondents' experiences of other animal assisted therapies

Most respondents (n = 45, 77.59%) stated that they have not used an animal assisted therapy. However, seven (12.07%) responded that they had used a variety of animal assisted therapies, four (6.90%) stated that they had experienced one animal assisted therapy, and two (3.45%) stated that they had one animal assisted therapy experience.

Respondents' ratings of the efficacy of another animal assisted therapies

Most respondents (n = 37, 75.51%) declined to rate the efficacy of another animal assisted therapy. However, six (12.24%) reported that they 'enjoyed, found useful and was able to be more confident or confident' after interacting with animals. This was followed by five (10.20%) who stated that they found interacting with other animals enjoyable and useful. Due to most respondents selecting favourable ratings, the efficacy of animal assisted therapies for autistics as perceived by autistics was calculated as 4.3 stars.

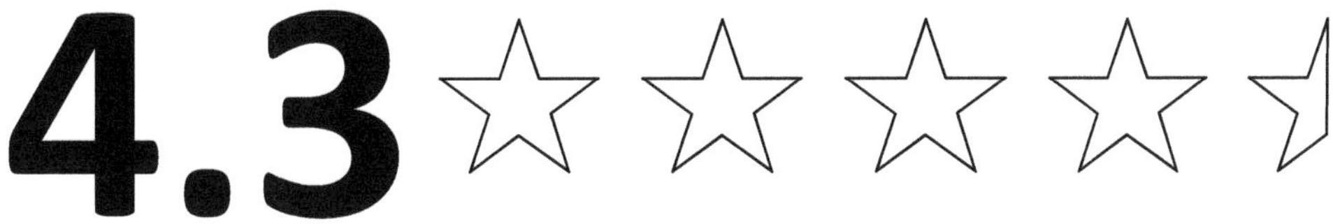

Figure 5.2 4.3 stars

Respondents' comments about other animal assisted therapies

Eight respondents provided comments when asked 'How was your experience of an animal assisted therapy as a therapy for autism?' An examination of these comments showed that animals provided 'calming' and 'anxiety reducing effects'.

> "Cats I find them calming and a nice obsession. Lots of people want to talk cats, info dump heaven. :-) Alpacas. My wife raises them and on an informal basis we have disabled groups visit the farm. Children who clearly have signs of autism will interact with alpacas. The ones my wife raised are very curious and very gentle."
>
> "All about reducing anxiety and improving sensory touch with me."
>
> "Again, not a therapy as such but I do find being around animals calming and I volunteered at the SPCA for a few years for that reason, plus we had lots of pets when I was little."

Interviewing an adult autistic educational consultant and researcher, they talked about their love for animals and the role of animals in their life.

> "Animals are accepting, they don't put on airs and graces, it is easier to relate to them, to their spirit, which I don't experience with people. I used to want puppies when I grew up, not babies!"

Many respondents explained the benefits animals provided. In contrast, no respondents expressed the view that they were ineffective. Although there were no negative views collected, this is not evidence in and of itself that all autistics find interacting with animals beneficial. Therefore, before giving autistics the opportunity to interact with animals it is important that they be asked if they wish to be a participant in an animal therapy program.

5.5 Conclusion

This chapter examined the literature about the therapeutic benefits that two animal species can give autistics; dogs and horses. Based on the literature reviewed, dog programs and equine therapy were rated as 'Silver – Usually promising'. Throughout this chapter, the views of autistics that were collected via the online survey were presented. These views illustrated that many autistics report that they do obtain benefits after interacting with animals, such as developing a sense of calmness.

References

Ajzenman, H. F., Standeven, J. W., & Shurtleff, T. L. (2013). Effect of hippotherapy on motor control, adaptive behaviors, and participation in children with autism spectrum disorder: A pilot study. *American Journal of Occupational Therapy*, 67(6), 653–663. doi:10.5014/ajot.2013.008383.

Anderson, S., & Meints, K. (2016). Brief report: The effects of equine-assisted activities on the social functioning in children and adolescents with autism spectrum disorder. *Journal of Autism and Developmental Disorders*, 46(10), 3344–3352. doi:10.1007/s10803-016-2869-3.

Bass, M. M., Duchowny, C. A., & Llabre, M. M. (2009). The effect of therapeutic horseback riding on social functioning in children with autism. *Journal of Autism and Developmental Disorders*, 39(9), 1261–1267. doi:10.1007/s10803-009-0734-3.

Berry, A., Borgi, M., Francia, N., Alleva, E., & Cirulli, F. (2013). Use of assistance and therapy dogs for children with autism spectrum disorders: A critical review of the current evidence. *The Journal of Alternative and Complementary Medicine*, 19(2), 73–80. doi:10.1089/acm.2011.0835.

Borgi, M., Loliva, D., Cerino, S., Chiarotti, F., Venerosi, A., Bramini, M., ... & Bisacco, F. (2016). Effectiveness of a standardized equine-assisted therapy program for children with autism spectrum disorder. *Journal of Autism and Developmental Disorders*, 46(1), 1–9. doi:10.1007/s10803-015-2530-6.

Gabriels, R. L., Agnew, J. A., Holt, K. D., Shoffner, A., Zhaoxing, P., Ruzzano, S., ... & Mesibov, G. (2012). Pilot study measuring the effects of therapeutic horseback riding on school-age children and adolescents with autism spectrum disorders. *Research in Autism Spectrum Disorders*, 6(2), 578–588. doi:10.1016/j.rasd.2011.09.007.

Gabriels, R. L., Pan, Z., Dechant, B., Agnew, J. A., Brim, N., & Mesibov, G. (2015). Randomized controlled trial of therapeutic horseback riding in children and adolescents with autism spectrum disorder. *Journal of the American Academy of Child & Adolescent Psychiatry*, 54(7), 541–549. doi:10.1016/j.jaac.2015.04.007.

García-Gómez, A., Risco, M. L., Rubio, J. C., Guerrero, E., & García-Peña, I. M. (2014). Effects of a program of adapted therapeutic horse-riding in a group of autism spectrum disorder children. *Electronic Journal of Research in Educational Psychology*, 12(1), 107–128.

Ghorban, H., Sedigheh, R. D., Marzieh, G., & Yaghoob, G. (2013). Effectiveness of therapeutic horseback riding on social skills of children with autism spectrum disorder in Shiraz, Iran. *Journal of Education and Learning*, 2(3), 79–84.

Grandin, T. (2019). Case Study: How horses helped a teenager with autism make friends and learn how to work. *International Journal of Environmental Research and Public Health*, 16(13), 2325. doi:10.3390/ijerph16132325.

Harris, A., & Williams, J. M. (2017). The impact of a horse riding intervention on the social functioning of children with autism spectrum disorder. *International Journal of Environmental Research and Public Health*, 14(7), 776. doi:10.3390/ijerph14070776.

Hill, J., Ziviani, J., Driscoll, C., & Cawdell-Smith, J. (2019). Can canine-assisted interventions affect the social behaviours of children on the autism spectrum? A Systematic Review. *Review Journal of Autism and Developmental Disorders*, 6(1), 13–25. doi:10.1007/s40489-018-0151-7.

Holm, M. B., Baird, J. M., Kim, Y. J., Rajora, K. B., D'Silva, D., Podolinsky, L., ... & Minshew, N. (2014). Therapeutic horseback riding outcomes of parent-identified goals for children with autism spectrum disorder: An ABA' multiple case design examining dosing and generalization to the home and community. *Journal of Autism and Developmental Disorders*, 44(4), 937–947. doi:10.1007/s10803-013-1949-x.

Jenkins, S. R., & Reed, F. D. (2013). An experimental analysis of the effects of therapeutic horseback riding on the behavior of children with autism. *Research in Autism Spectrum Disorders*, 7(6), 721–740. doi:10.1016/j.rasd.2013.02.008.

Kern, J. K., Fletcher, C. L., Garver, C. R., Mehta, J. A., Grannemann, B. D., Knox, K. R., ... & Trivedi, M. H. (2011). Prospective trial of equine-assisted activities in autism spectrum disorder. *Alternative Therapies in Health & Medicine*, 17(3), 14–20.

Lanning, B. A., Baier, M. E. M., Ivey-Hatz, J., Krenek, N., & Tubbs, J. D. (2014). Effects of equine assisted activities on autism spectrum disorder. *Journal of Autism and Developmental Disorders*, 44(8), 1897–1907. doi:10.1007/s10803-014-2062-5.

Llambias, C., Magill-Evans, J., Smith, V., & Warren, S. (2016). Equine-assisted occupational therapy: Increasing engagement for children with autism spectrum disorder. *American Journal of Occupational Therapy*, 70(6), 1–9. doi:10.5014/ajot.2016.020701.

Mapes, A. R., & Rosén, L. A. (2016). Equine-assisted therapy for children with autism spectrum disorder: A comprehensive literature review. *Review Journal of Autism and Developmental Disorders*, 3(4), 377–386. doi:10.1007/s40489-016-0090-0.

Memishevikj, H., & Hodzhikj, S. (2010). The effects of equine-assisted therapy in improving the psycho-social functioning of children with autism. *Journal of Special Education and Rehabilitation*, 11(3–4),57–67.

Nelson, K., Axtell, J., Derby, K. M., Moug, R., Berrera, S., & McLaughlin, T. F. (2011). A preliminary analysis of therapeutic horseback riding. *International Journal of Social Sciences and Education*, 1(4), 644–656.

Petty, J. D., Pan, Z., Dechant, B., & Gabriels, R. L. (2017). Therapeutic horseback riding crossover effects of attachment behaviors with family pets in a sample of children with autism spectrum disorder. *International Journal of Environmental Research and Public Health*, 14(3), 256. doi:10.3390/ijerph14030256.

Srinivasan, S. M., Cavagnino, D. T., & Bhat, A. N. (2018). Effects of equine therapy on individuals with autism spectrum disorder: A systematic review. *Review Journal of Autism and Developmental Disorders*, 5(2), 156–175. doi:10.1007/s40489-018-0130-z.

Tan, V. X. L., & Simmonds, J. G. (2019). Equine-assisted interventions for psychosocial functioning in children and adolescents with autism spectrum disorder: A literature review. *Review Journal of Autism and Developmental Disorders*, 6(3), 325–337. doi:10.1007/s40489-018-0143-7.

Taylor, R. R., Kielhofner, G., Smith, C., Butler, S., Cahill, S. M., Ciukaj, M. D., & Gehman, M. (2009). Volitional change in children with autism: A single-case design study of the impact of hippotherapy on motivation. *Occupational Therapy in Mental Health*, 25(2), 192–200. doi:10.1080/01642120902859287.

Trzmiel, T., Purandare, B., Michalak, M., Zasadzka, E., & Pawlaczyk, M. (2019). Equine assisted activities and therapies in children with autism spectrum disorder: A systematic review and a meta-analysis. *Complementary Therapies in Medicine*, 42, 104–113. doi:10.1016/j.ctim.2018.11.004.

Van den Hout, C. M. A., & Bragonje, S. (2010). *The effect of equine assisted therapy in children with autism spectrum disorders.* Unpublished Master's Thesis. Amsterdam:Vrije Universiteit Faculty of Human Movement Sciences.

Ward, S. C., Whalon, K., Rusnak, K., Wendell, K., & Paschall, N. (2013). The association between therapeutic horseback riding and the social communication and sensory reactions of children with autism. *Journal of Autism and Developmental Disorders*, 43(9), 2190–2198. doi:10.1007/s10803-013-1773-3.

Weber, Y., & Westmoquette, K. (2010). Equine-assisted therapy as a treatment for children with autism spectrum disorders—a qualitative study. *Karolinska Institutet*, 6–19.

Chapter 6

Sensory-based strategies

6.1 Introduction

This chapter reviews the literature on typical sensory-based strategies that can be used to support autistics. It begins with an examination of the literature about the possible benefits that weighted clothes and blankets might give autistics. It then rates the efficacy of these sensory-based strategies as well as presenting several directions for research in the future. Afterwards, this chapter presents insights and experiences from a group of autistics about weighted blankets and weighted clothes. It then examines the literature about the therapeutic benefits that aromatherapy massage, acupuncture, holding therapy, and Sensory Integration Therapy (SIT) for autistics. It then concludes with a series of views from autistic adults about sensory-based strategies.

6.2 Weighted blankets and vests

6.2.1 Weighted blankets

Many autistics experience insomnia and to address such difficulties, some autistics use weighted blankets (Allik, Larsson, & Smedje, 2006; Mannion & Leader, 2014; Richdale & Schreck, 2009). Gee et al. (2016) explored the effectiveness of weighted blankets in helping autistic children manage their sleep disturbances. Two male autistic children with sensory over-responsivity difficulties participated in a study with three phases. During the first phase seven days of baseline data was collected via an online survey, that was completed each day by the child's caregivers. For the second phase, which lasted 14 days, the children used weighted blankets. The child's caregivers received the weighted blanket along with oral and written instructions about how it was to be used, as well as precautions about its usage. During this phase, the child's caregivers completed an online survey daily that contained the same questions from the baseline survey (i.e., how much time it took for the child to fall asleep the previous night, how many times the previous night had the child awoken, the total duration of sleep the child had the previous night, and the child's mood upon waking in the morning). During the third and final phase, which lasted seven days, the autistic boys did not use their weighted blankets. During this phase the 'long-term' effects of the weighted blanket intervention was evaluated by the child's caregivers who continued to complete the online survey each day. Based on the results collected, Gee et al. concluded that:

> the findings indicate that an improvement in sleep duration and time to fall asleep may be improved with the use of a weighted blanket. However, the mood of the child upon waking the next morning does not appear to be influenced by the use of the weighted blanket. (2016, p. 180).

While Gee et al.'s study provides some support for the usage of weighted blankets for autistic children, their results need to be cautiously adopted. First, they only examined the consequences of using weighted blankets with two autistic boys. Since there were only two participants in their study the conclusions obtained cannot be generalised and applied to the broader population of autistics. Furthermore, some autistics prefer firm touch whilst others prefer light touch, so it is likely that weighted blankets would not be universally enjoyed by autistics. Since their research had such a small participant pool, Gee et al. did not cover the effects on individuals who do not naturally prefer weighted blankets. Second, the second boy in their study had difficulty breathing because of an ear infection. This medical condition meant that it was not possible to accurately determine the effectiveness of the weighted blanket program on their sleep quality.

6.2.2 Weighted vests

Weighted vests have been used to potentially help autistic children manage instances of sensory-overload. According to Olson and Moulton (2004, p. 53) weighted vests are typically "10% of a person's body weight evenly distributed around the vest". It has been proposed that wearing a weighted vest can give people deep pressure stimulation, which can have a calming effect (VandenBerg, 2001).

Studies have measured the proportion of the autistic population that have used weighted vests. Green et al. (2006) found that 12.8% of parents used weighted vests on their children with autism at the time of completing their survey and 25.7% had used weighted blankets in the past. Olson and Moulton (2004) distributed a 43-item questionnaire to 514 members of the American Occupational Therapy Association. They received 349 (68%) responses and of these most (82%) indicated that they have recommended the use of weighted vests to help autistic children manage their sensory overload. Several respondents also claimed that such vests increased the child's attention to tasks and reduced stereotypic behaviours. However, some respondents believed that more research about the benefits that weighted vests can give autistic children needs to be conducted.

There are several literature reviews in which studies about the efficacy of weighted vests for autistic children have been examined (Morrison, 2007; Stephenson & Carter, 2009; Taylor et al., 2017). Morrison (2007) examined five studies about this topic and concluded:

> Although there seems to be a consensus among occupational therapists that regularly use weighted vests that the vests are beneficial, the evidence to support their effectiveness with students on the autism spectrum is limited. (Morrison, 2007, p. 326).

Stephenson and Carter (2009) examined five peer-reviewed studies, one non-peer reviewed article, and one poster presentation about the benefits that weighted vests gave autistic children and children with other disabilities (See Table 6.1). They found that

Table 6.1 Summaries of studies reviewed by Stephenson and Carter (2009)

Study	*Participants and behaviour*	*Design*	*Vest characteristics*	*Reported outcome*
Deris et al., 2006 (ERIC document)	Four-year-old boy with ASD. Attention to task and self-stimulation	Alternating treatment design comparing no vest, to pressure vest and weighted vest	Weight – 3 lbs (approx 10% of body weight). Worn for 30 min intervals every 2 hours throughout day. Assessed after having worn vest for at least 15 min	No clinically significant effect on self-stimulation or attention to task
Barton, Reichow, and Wolery, 2007 (Poster)	Four-year-old boy with autism (Tommy) Four-year-old boy with developmental-delay and autism-like behaviours (Bert)	Alternating treatment design comparing weighted vest, vest without weights and no vest (observers were blinded when vest was weighted). Engagement, non-engagement, stereotypic behaviour and problem behaviour were measured during morning table-time activities (painting, gluing, colouring and cutting)	No details of weight. Tommy wore irregularly and Bert wore for part of each school day	No difference in engagement across conditions Tommy's problem behaviours increased while wearing the vest, but stereotypic behaviours decreased
Carter, 2005 (Refereed article)	Four-year-old boy with autism Self-injurious behaviour (hitting head or back of hand)	Alternating treatment functional analysis of SIB (attention, demand, alone and play conditions) when infection was present/absent and when vest was present/absent	Weight – 3 lb (7.5% of body weight) Worn during 5 min assessment sessions	SIB was more likely to be present when student had a sinus infection, high rates across all conditions showed it was maintained by automatic reinforcement Presence or absence of vest had no effect

(*continued*)

Table 6.1 (*coninued*)

Study	*Participants and behaviour*	*Design*	*Vest characteristics*	*Reported outcome*
Fertel-Daly, Bedell, and Hinojosa, 2001 (Refereed article)	Two years seven-month girl with PDD Two years ten-month boy with PDD Three years one-month boy with PDD Two years nine-month girl with PDD Two years ten-month boy with autism All had some self-stimulatory behaviour and problems attending to task	Observation of behaviour during a 5-min fine motor activity	Weight of 1 lb in all vests. Worn for 2 hours and observations made after the vest was worn for 1.5 hours	Participant 1 showed most attention, fewest distractions in the vest condition, and least self-stimulatory behaviour in baseline Participant 2 showed most attention and least distraction in the vest condition and most self-stimulatory behaviour in the withdrawal condition Participant 3 showed most attention and least distractions and stereotypy in the vest condition Participant 4 showed most attention in the vest condition, least distraction in the vest condition and least stereotypy in the withdrawal condition Participant 5 showed most attention in the vest condition, least distraction and least stereotypy in the vest condition These judgments were made on means
Kane et al., 2004, 2005 (Refereed article)	Eight-year-old boy (Jerry) with autism Ten-year-old girl (Elsie) with autism 11-year-old girl (Eileen) with autism Eight-year-old boy (Norman) PDD-NOS All with stereotypic behaviours	ABC design involving baseline (no vest); weighted vest and vest without weights (treatments were counter-balanced across the four participants)	Weight – 5% of individual's body weight Placed on child 1 min before the 10 min observation session	Jerry's attention to task increased slightly with the no-weight vest, and stereotypy also decreased during this condition. Stereotypy was highest during the weighted-vest condition Elsie's stereotypy occurred during 100% of intervals in all conditions. Attention to task was best in baseline Norman had high levels of stereotypy in all conditions, and attention to task was highest in baseline Eileen engaged in stereotypy for 2.5% of intervals in baseline and not at all in either vest condition. Attention to task was highest in baseline

Study	*Participants and behaviour*	*Design*	*Vest characteristics*	*Reported outcome*
Myles et al., 2004 (Refereed article)	Student 1, boy, five years seven months, autism, developmental age 20 months, non-verbal Student 2, boy, three years six months, autism, non-verbal Student 3, boy, four years 11 months, autism, developmental age 22 months, some verbal skills	ABAB designs. Comparing on task behaviour (first and second students) and duration of self-stimulation (third student) during school activities. Observations were made in 5 min individual sessions and group sessions of unspecified length for Student 1 and group activities of 15 min for Students 2 and 3	Weight – 10% of child's boy weight for Student 1 and 5% for Students 2 and 3 Vests worn for duration of activities for student 1 (5 min) and Student 2 (15 min). For Student 3 vest was worn for 30 min BEFORE activity and removed for the activity itself (15 min)	Student 1 – no clinically significant changes Student 2 – mean increase of on task time from 9% to 34% (based on graphic data) Student 3 – mean time spent in self-stimulation decreased from 19% to 6%
VandenBerg, 2001 (Refereed article)	Student 1, girl, six years ten months, speech and language impairment, ADHD Student 2, girl, six years and six months speech and language impairment, ADHD Student 3, boy, six years and nine months ADHD Student 4, boy, five years and nine months, ADHD Excessive movement, overreaction to extraneous stimuli, inability to complete tasks, difficulties with fine-motor tasks	AB design. Measured "on-task" behaviour during a wide range of fine-motor activities. A phase, without vest and B phase with vest. Also wore vests at other times 15 min observations	Weight – 5% of child's body weight Vests put on 5 min before the observation interval and removed after 20–30 min	Student 1–25% mean increase in time on task while wearing vest Student 2, 3, 4-Mean increase of 17–18% time on task

Source: Stephenson & Carter, 2009, pp. 107–108.

four studies concluded that weighted vests were not an effective intervention, one reported mixed results, and two concluded that they produced positive outcomes. Stephenson and Carter concluded that:

> Weighted vests are reportedly a widely employed intervention. While it should be acknowledged there is only a limited body of research, on balance, indications are that weighted vests are ineffective … until such time as well-conducted studies can provide replicated evidence to the contrary, weighted vests cannot be recommended for clinical applications. (2009, pp. 112–113).

A recent systematic literature review about the utility of weighted vests for autistics was published in 2017 by Taylor and colleagues. They examined 32 studies and found that these studies were conducted in different settings and were aimed at addressing different target behaviours. They also found that all studies were conducted in the participants' classroom. Eight studies were conducted in a public elementary school, three were conducted in university-affiliated early childhood centres, and two studies were conducted in early childhood special education classrooms. Taylor et al. concluded that based on the studies examined the use of weighted vests with autistic children is not an effective evidence-based practice.

6.2.3 Evaluation of weighted blankets and weighted vests

Weighted blankets

Rating: Insufficient information to make a recommendation

We did not locate a sufficient amount of research to decide about the efficacy of weighted blankets for autistics.

Weighted vests

Rating: Bronze – Safe but ineffective (IF USED CORRECTLY – can be dangerous if too heavy or tight)

Stephenson and Carter (2009), Morrison (2007), and Taylor et al. (2017) all concluded that weighted vests did not provide autistics with any benefits. Additionally, the literature these studies reviewed did not note that weighted vests could be dangerous for autistics if they were not used as intended. Thus, provided the correct weight is used we have rated weighted vests as 'Bronze – Safe but ineffective'.

6.2.4 Directions for research in the future about weighted blankets and weighted vests

Currently, there is a paucity of literature evaluating the therapeutic benefits of weighted blankets and weighted vests for autistics. Due to this dearth of literature, particularly for weighted blankets, there are many opportunities for research in the future to be conducted into this topic. Most of the literature that has evaluated the possible therapeutic benefits that weighted vests and blankets may give autistics are based on samples of autistic children. One consequence is that we do not know if autistic adults could obtain therapeutic benefits. To fill this gap in our understanding studies should explore what therapeutic benefits autistic adults feel they do or do not obtain from weighted blankets and clothes.

Most of the research about the benefits of weighted vests and blankets for autistics have not used a control group, nor have they examined individual preference for firm or light pressure prior to assigning the use of weighted blanket or clothes. Such research designs have made it difficult to accurately ascertain the impact of these items for individual autistics with differing preferences around pressure and touch. To fill this gap in our knowledge, studies should incorporate into their research design a control group and obtain information about individual preferences about pressure and touch prior to, and during, the intervention. Similarly, studies could compare the outcomes of a group of autistics that used weighted blanket or vests and a group of autistics that used another type of support. Such comparisons can ascertain if weighted vests and blankets are more effective than other types of support. An area for future research could be the use of clothes that provide deep pressure, such as compression leggings and vests, as these may be safer and more accessible and acceptable than weighted clothes for some children and adults.

6.2.5 Autistic views about weighted blankets and vests

Have you personally used weighted blankets and/or weighted vests?

When asked 'Have you personally used weighted blankets and/or weighted vests?' 57 respondents provided an answer. Most (n = 30, 52.63%) stated that they have only used weighted blankets, one (1.75%) noted that they have only used weighted vests, and three (5.26%) revealed that they have used both weighted vests and weighted blankets. Additionally, 23 (40.35%) stated that they have not used a weighted vest or a weighted blanket.

Respondents' ratings of the efficacy of using weighted blankets

Out of the 206 respondents who completed our online survey, 53 (25.72%) rated the efficacy of weighted blankets. Most selected favourable ratings, with 10 (18.87%) selecting 'enjoyed, found useful and was able to be more confident or confident after using' and 17 (32.08%) selecting 'enjoyed and found useful'. Since most selected a positive result, the efficacy of weighted blankets for autistics as perceived by autistics was calculated as 3.9 stars.

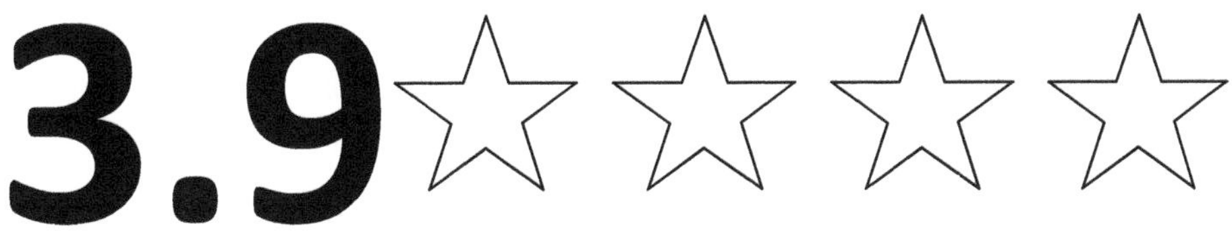

Figure 6.1 3.9 stars

Respondents' comments about using weighted blankets

When asked 'How was your experience of using weighted blankets?' 22 respondents who completed our online survey provided their insights. In our judgement, three respondents did not find them useful, whilst eight detailed their benefits and ten provided an answer that did not answer the question.

Of those who endorsed the usage of weighted blankets or who experienced the benefits of such items, four explained that weighted blankets helped them stay calm and fall asleep.

> "If I don't have a weighted blanket, I need lots of pillows. I like to feel supported on all sides. My weighted blanket was a game changer. I get to sleep much faster with it."
>
> "Always calms me down. Hard to travel with though."
>
> "The weight is really good to release stress and help me sleep."
>
> "I enjoy the deep pressure so much I now have an additional weighted blanket to use two blankets for particularly bad sensory overload and also have weighted eye patches and also a weighted neck blanket."

Although four respondents believed weighted blankets provided a calming effect, three articulated the opposite view.

> "Love the feel of it. Very soothing. But doesn't improve sleep or anxiety for me."
>
> "I'm the complete opposite – sleep with no blankets – really touch sensitive."
>
> "I hate weighted blankets, and much prefer very light blankets and clothing."

Aside from explaining if weighted blankets were beneficial or not, four explained that they did not have the financial means to afford this item.

> "Can't currently afford one of my own but from my experience of using one can assume it would be of great help to have because they make me feel more calm."
>
> "I would like to try a weighted blanket as I know I find deep pressure calming, but they are very expensive so I don't have one yet."
>
> "I use heavyweight cotton blankets as I haven't yet been able to afford a weighted blanket."
>
> "But I really like the idea of a weighted blanket because I like tight hugs and my bed sheets to be really tight, they're just expensive."

The comments collected showed that some respondents liked using weighted blankets while others did not. Due to the diversity of views and experiences collected, autistics should be asked if they would like to use a weighted blanket before such an item is purchased. Furthermore, if they are unsure then it might be advantageous to hire and try a weighted blanket first, ensuring that a SAFE weight is selected. An occupational therapist should be able to help with selecting a safe weight level for an individual.

Respondents' ratings of the efficacy of using weighted vests

The efficacy of weighted vests for autistics was not rated since less than ten respondents rated its efficacy.

Respondents' comments about weighted vests

Three respondents provided a comment when asked 'How was your experience using weighted vests?' We discovered that two respondents did not like weighted vests.

> "I don't like pressure on my chest for too long, vests tend to make me more anxious because I can't always get them off fast enough."
>
> "Normally very uncomfortable and I won't touch let alone use."

While one respondent expressed the opposite view.

> "I like weight so I can sleep at night, but I don't like the feel of being trapped under a full blanket so this is a good compromise."

Asking an adult autistic researcher that strongly advocates for their own use of a squeeze jacket, they discussed how personal sensory preferences can impact each individual so it can be hard to research the use of sensory clothing. They like their squeeze jacket because it can be controlled by the wearer.

> "When I wear my squeeze jacket it's like I have armour on and I am protected. I gave one away to one of the students that I worked with and he wouldn't give it back, he said it changed his life. He loved the pressure and enabled him to stay grounded and confident, and he could wear it under his school shirt and no-one knew, so no-one ridiculed him."

Like weighted blankets, respondents expressed both an endorsement and a reluctance to the use of weighted vests. Therefore, an autistic should be asked if they would like to use such an item. Like weighted blankets, if they cannot provide an answer then it might be advantageous to hire and try a weighted vest first.

6.3 Aromatherapy massage

6.3.1 Aromatherapy massage

There are a few studies about the possible therapeutic benefits which aromatherapy massage may provide autistics (Solomons, 2005; Williams, 2006). Williams (2006) examined if aromatherapy massage improved the sleep quality of children with autism. Their sample contained 12 children with autism and learning difficulties (two females, ten males), who were aged between 12 years and two months to 15 years and seven months. For three nights these children were given aromatherapy massage and for 14 nights they were not given aromatherapy massage. These children were checked every 30 minutes throughout the night to measure the time it took for them to fall asleep as well as the number of awakenings and the sleep duration. The results collected showed that there were no differences in any sleep measurements between the nights when they received aromatherapy massage and the nights when this massage therapy was not used. Williams concluded that for children with autism aromatherapy massage with lavender oil does not improve their quality of sleep.

6.3.2 Evaluation of aromatherapy massage

Rating: Insufficient amount of literature to rate the support's efficacy

We did not locate a sufficient amount of research to rate the efficacy of aromatherapy massage for autistics.

6.3.3 Directions for research in the future about aromatherapy massage

Since few researchers have measured the potential benefits of aromatherapy massage for autistics, there are two areas where research could be conducted in the future. First, most of the research about this topic has examined the benefits that autistic children have obtained from aromatherapy massage. Consequently, studies should examine if autistic adults can obtain any benefits from this massage and if so what areas of life they feel may have improved. Second, it is acknowledged that some autistics have olfactory and/or touch sensitivities (Tavassoli & Baron-Cohen, 2012a; Tonacci et al., 2017). In the future, research should explore the impacts that the fragrances and level of pressure used in aromatherapy massage can have on autistics. It is possible that some autistics will find such olfactory or touch sensations uncomfortable, which could subsequently hamper treatment success.

6.3.4 Autistic views about aromatherapy massage

Have you personally used aromatherapy and/or aromatherapy massage to manage anything related to your autism?

Out of the 206 respondents who completed our online survey, 57 (27.66%) answered the question 'Have you personally used aromatherapy and/or aromatherapy massage to manage anything related to your autism?' Most selected the option 'No' (N= 30, 52.63%), whilst 12 (21.05%) stated that they had used aromatherapy, one (1.75%) stated that they had used aromatherapy massage, and 14 (24.56%) stated that they had used both aromatherapy and aromatherapy massage.

Respondents' ratings of the efficacy of aromatherapy massage

Most respondents who rated the efficacy of aromatherapy massage reported that they either found it enjoyable and useful (n = 8, 16%) or enjoyable, useful, and were able to be more confident after having aromatherapy massage (n = 2, 4%). However, three (6%) did not enjoy or find aromatherapy massage useful. Based on the distribution of responses, the efficacy of aromatherapy massage for autistics as perceived by autistics was calculated as 3.3 stars.

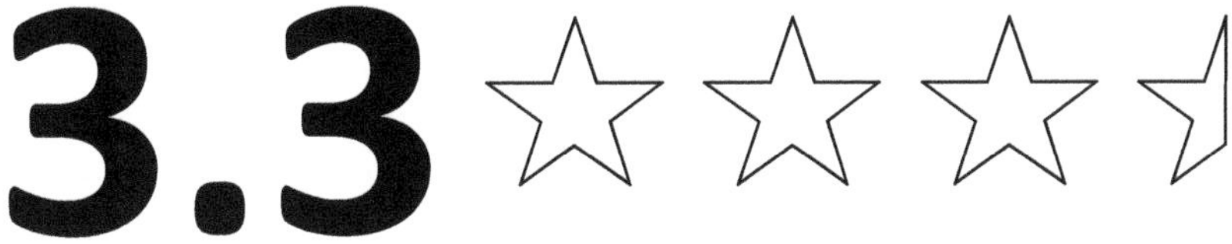

Figure 6.2 3.3 stars

Respondents' comments about aromatherapy massage

Six respondents provided a comment when asked 'How was your experience of aromatherapy massage as an autism therapy?' One respondent found it useful, stating 'Helps with relaxation', while two expressed the opposite view, stating 'massage makes me ill and overwhelmed' and 'Sensory nightmare!' These opposing views illustrate the range of sensory preferences and highlights that it is important that autistics be provided with the opportunity to decline this support if they believe it will cause more problems than it aims to solve.

Interviewing some autistic adults, they talked about the need to know and trust the person doing the massage, that it couldn't be just anyone. The use of essential oils is again a strong preference, with some autistics loving particular smells, but feeling revolted by some smells that therapists recommend.

6.4 Acupuncture

6.4.1 Acupuncture

We identified four literature reviews about the therapeutic benefits of acupuncture for autistics (Cheuk, Wong, & Chen, 2011; Lee et al., 2012, 2018; Liu et al., 2019). In 2011, Cheuk, Wong, and Chen attempted to determine if acupuncture improved an autistic's communication, cognition, overall functioning, and quality of life. They examined ten studies that collectively examined 390 autistic children. The acupuncture programs that they reviewed ranged in duration from four weeks to nine months. The studies were conducted in Hong Kong, Egypt, and mainland China. They found that four studies reported that acupuncture produced some adverse consequences, namely bleeding, crying due to fear of pain, irritability, sleep disturbances, and increased hyperactivity. They also found that there were a number of methodological problems inherent within the examined studies, namely small sample sizes, studies containing only children, and brief follow-up periods that meant that the long-term benefits were not measured. Based on the results collected, they concluded:

> Current evidence does not support the use of acupuncture for treatment of ASD. There is no conclusive evidence that acupuncture is effective for treatment of ASD in children and no RCTs have been carried out with adults. Further high quality trials of larger size and longer follow-up are needed. (Cheuk, Wong, & Chen, 2011, p. 2).

In 2012, Lee et al. searched for studies which were hosted on 15 electronic databases from their inception until June 2011. The aim of their study was to assess the effectiveness of acupuncture as a support for autistics. Based on the 11 studies that they examined, they concluded:

> ... the results of our systematic review provided limited evidence of acupuncture's effectiveness on treating ASD ... The total number of studies included in the analysis, their total sample sizes and their methodological quality, however, were too low to draw firm conclusions ... (Lee et al., 2012, pp. 1681–1682).

In 2018, Lee and colleagues searched through 13 databases for studies published up until December 2016 about the safety and effectiveness of acupuncture for autistic children. Based on the 27 randomised controlled trials that they reviewed, Lee et al. (2018, p. 19) concluded that:

> The results of this systematic review indicated that acupuncture may improve the overall symptoms of ASD. The reported adverse events associated with acupuncture were mild and acceptable. However, due to heterogeneities among the trials and the low methodological quality of some of the studies, additional rigorous, well-designed RCTs [Randomised Controlled Trials] with larger sample sizes should be performed to confirm these results.

While their study has added to our understanding of the efficacy of acupuncture for autistics it does have several limitations. First, many studies had performance bias because it was difficult to mask the acupuncture treatment. Second, 74% of the studies examined were conducted in China, where acupuncture is viewed as a positive and helpful treatment for a wide range of conditions. It is possible that studies conducted in other parts of the world could have contradicted the results collected as they may not have had the same Chinese cultural influences. In addition, they did not explain what the 'mild and acceptable' reported adverse effects were. It may be that these are not acceptable to some or even most autistics. Thus, when evaluating any possible benefits, these adverse effects will need to be weighed up against the possible benefits.

Recently, Liu et al. (2019) published a systematic review and meta-analysis of studies about the benefits of scalp acupuncture for autistic children. They searched through six databases and examined 14 trials that were conducted from 1980 through to September 2018. They concluded that for some autistic children scalp acupuncture might be beneficial in terms of reducing their anxiety. However, they did not report on side effects, which are likely to be similar to acupuncture on other body parts, such as fear of pain or discomfort. These may be unacceptable and distressing to some or even most autistics.

6.4.2 Evaluation of acupuncture

Rating: Bronze – Safe but ineffective (Tin for autistics with needle phobias or bleeding disorders)

The notion that acupuncture can help autistics was mostly unsupported by the literature reviews examined in the last section (Cheuk, Wong, & Chen, 2011; Lee et al., 2012). However, all literature reviews did conclude that the evidence about the efficacy of acupuncture for autistics contained several methodological flaws that could compromise the results. If practiced correctly, acupuncture can be safe. Yet the current literature does not support the notion that it can help autistics beyond what it might offer non-autistics. Provided acupuncture is performed correctly, and the autistic has no apprehension about receiving acupuncture, we have rated it as 'Bronze – Safe but ineffective'.

6.4.3 Directions for research in the future about acupuncture

Due to a paucity of literature, additional research on acupuncture would help to clarify if it gives autistics any benefits. Lee et al. (2012, 2018) reported that most of the studies about the efficacy of acupuncture for autistics have been conducted in China. Although valuable, such studies might have been influenced by the value Chinese society gives acupuncture. To counteract any potential cultural influences, studies about this topic should be conducted in other countries and cultures. In addition, most of the findings about the efficacy of acupuncture for autistics are based on samples of autistic children. Consequently, it is unclear if autistic adults might obtain the same benefits from acupuncture, or if they would find possible adverse effects unacceptable and not be willing to trial acupuncture. To fill this gap in our knowledge, studies should test acupuncture programs on autistic adults to see if they obtain any benefits from such programs. Finally, acupuncture can be applied to different areas of the body. In the interests of furthering our knowledge studies should examine which areas of an autistic's body are the most receptive to acupuncture. It could be, for instance, that cranial acupuncture is more effective for autistics than acupuncture applied to other areas of the human body.

6.4.4 Autistic views about acupuncture

Have you personally used acupuncture to manage anything related to your autism?

Out of 206 respondents who completed our online survey, 56 (27.18%) answered the question 'Have you personally used acupuncture to manage anything related to your autism?' Most selected the option 'No' (n = 41, 73.21%), 11 (19.64%) selected the option 'have used acupuncture but not for anything related to my autism', and four (7.14%) used acupuncture exclusively to help them manage their autism.

Respondents' ratings of the efficacy of acupuncture

Since there are less than ten responses, the efficacy of acupuncture for autistics was not rated.

Respondents' comments about acupuncture

Eight respondents provided a comment to the question 'How was your experience of acupuncture as an autism therapy?' However, many of their comments were related to the use of acupuncture to manage physical symptoms. Several examples were:

> 'Dry-needling by a physiotherapist for neck spasms. It was very effective.'
>
> "I sought acupuncture when I was a young adult (pre Autistic diagnosis) when I was experiencing feeling tired all the time. At the time I did not notice any positive benefits though."
>
> "It was like putting a dam across a raging river it worked to stop the pain for a while but then the pain came rushing back."

Few respondents found acupuncture beneficial in any way, so it is important that autistics be provided with the opportunity to decline this support if they believe it will cause more problems than it aims to solve, especially if they have a needle phobia. Following initial sessions, autistics should be asked if they would like to receive acupuncture. Acupuncture should not be undertaken by autistics with bleeding disorders, such as haemophilia, or those on blood thinners.

6.5 Holding therapy

6.5.1 Holding therapy

Holding therapy was developed to theoretically help autistic children become more socially and emotionally connected to others. One common type of holding therapy is performed by parents under the supervision of their therapist and it involves them placing their child's head in their lap and then making eye contact. This form of holding therapy was developed by Martha Welch and Jirina Prekopova and has been described in the following way:

> The child is held in a position that allows the parent to make direct eye contact while controlling the child's attempts to protest, to struggle, and to escape. The technique anticipates and indeed facilitates confrontation so that problems can be resolved … As the child's emotions are aroused, the child struggles to turn away. The mother expresses verbally her feelings – concerns, frustrations, hope, anger, as well as affection and love – to the child. She uses her strength and tenacity to intensify contact and prevent withdrawal. The struggle becomes desperate for both, and then, if the mother perseveres throughout the child's rejection, it dissolves into tender intimacy with intense eye contact, exploratory touching, usually of the mother's face, and gentle conversation highly gratifying to both mother and child. (Welch, 1988, p. 27).

Our review of the literature yielded multiple studies which do not support the usage of holding therapy for autistics (Lilienfeld, 2007; Mercer, 2013, Pignotti & Mercer, 2007). Mercer (2013) published a systematic literature review about holding therapy for autistics. Based on the eight studies that they collected and analysed, Mercer concluded that the few empirical studies that have claimed that holding therapy is an effective strategy for autistic children have not been replicated. In addition, all studies that they examined had a high rate of bias because they used non-blinded parental assessments to measure outcomes. Mercer concluded that the evidence about the effectiveness of holding therapy is insufficient and that this therapy should not be recommended as a strategy to help autistics.

Aside from academic literature, there are also many professional organisations that have condemned the usage of holding therapy. For example, in the United States such organisations include the American Psychological Association, the American Psychiatric Association, and the National Association of Social Workers (Mercer, 2014). Furthermore, the American Professional Society on Abuse of Children assembled a task force that examined the benefits and risks associated with holding therapy. They recommended that this therapy and other similar methods should not be used (Chaffin et al., 2006). Furthermore, in the United Kingdom the British Association for Adoptions and Fostering has rejected the usage of holding therapy (Mercer, 2014).

6.5.2 Evaluation of holding therapy

Rating: Tin – Extremely unsafe and potentially life threatening

Based on the volume of literature that has claimed that holding therapy is ineffective (Lilienfeld, 2007; Mercer, 2013; Pignotti & Mercer, 2007), along with it contributing to the deaths of children (Mercer, Sarner, & Rosa, 2003), and that many professional organisations have condemned its usage (Mercer, 2014) we have rated it as 'Tin – Extremely unsafe and potentially life threatening'. Under no circumstances should it be used as a method to help autistics since there is a high probability that it will cause psychological and/or physical injury or death. No research should be conducted in the future to determine the efficacy of holding therapy for autistics, as this would be unethical.

6.5.3 Autistic views about holding therapy

Have you personally experienced holding therapy?

Out of the 206 respondents who completed our online survey, 56 (27.18%) answered the question 'Have you personally experienced holding therapy?' Of those who answered this question, 50 (89.29%) stated 'No' and six (10.71%) stated 'Yes'.

Respondents' ratings of holding therapy

Since there were less than ten responses, the efficacy of holding therapy for autistics has not been rated.

Respondents' comments about holding therapy

Six respondents provided a comment when asked 'How was your experience of holding therapy?' Our analysis of these comments illustrated the psychological and physical distress that holding therapy can result in distress and harm.

> "Couldn't cope with the emotional intensity of physical contact."
> "I do not like being touched unless I ask for it."
> "touch sensitive ... HATE it."
> "Very early years of my life. Vague memories of it. Primary the stress that came from it."

While these four respondents gave statements demonstrating that they did not like holding therapy, there were no comments that were positive about holding therapy. Since the literature claims that holding therapy is dangerous and ineffective, and the autistic experience is negative, under no circumstances should autistics participate in holding therapy.

One autistic adult psychologist had worked in a clinic where holding therapy was used. They talked about how distressing this was and how the other therapists ridiculed them for this attitude. They refused to take part in the holding therapy and reported that the clinic has since been closed down.

6.6 Sensory Integration Therapy (SIT)

6.6.1 Sensory Integration Therapy (SIT)

One common characteristic of the autism spectrum is sensory sensitivities to different sensations, such as taste (Tavassoli & Baron-Cohen, 2012b). One of the earliest documented reports of sensory sensitivities exhibited by autistics was published in 1943 by Kanner. He described children with autism who had a sensory fascination with light as well as over-sensitivity to sounds (Kanner, 1943). Due to sensory sensitivities, some autistics can experience sensory difficulties, including sensory over-stimulation. Sensory Integration Therapy (SIT) has been proposed to help autistics manage their sensory difficulties. SIT was first conceived in 1972 by Ayers, who claimed that it is a:

> neurological process that organizes sensation from one's own body and from the environment and makes it possible to use the body effectively within the environment. (Ayers, 1979, p. 11).

Some of those who have used SIT have claimed that it can produce many benefits, including enhancing a person's ability to utilise objects in educational and social environments (Wilbarger & Wilbarger, 1991). It has also been claimed that SIT can reduce instances of challenging behaviours (i.e., self-injury) (Bright, Bittick, & Fleeman, 1981) and can improve one's cognitive capabilities, such as their ability to read and use language (Ayres, 1979; Devlin, Leader, & Healy, 2009; Magrun et al., 1981).

The utility of SIT for autistics has been explored from the perspective of professionals and parents raising autistic children. In Watling et al.'s (1999) study, 82% of occupational therapists surveyed reported that they have used SIT or other sensory approaches when treating children with autism. Smith and Antolovich (2000) surveyed parents raising children with autism about their use and perceptions of supplemental treatments. They found that 56% of respondents had at some point used SIT. Finally, Green et al. (2006) found that 38.2% of parents raising autistic children revealed that their child was receiving SIT at the time of completing their survey. Furthermore, 33.2% of respondents disclosed that their child had received SIT in the past.

There are several literature reviews in which studies explaining the benefits that SIT can give autistics have been explored (Case-Smith, Weaver, & Fristad, 2015; Lang et al., 2012; Leong, Carter, & Stephenson, 2015). Case-Smith, Weaver, and Fristad (2015) examined research published between 2000 to 2012 about two types of sensory interventions for autistic children who had concurrent sensory processing problems; SIT and sensory-based interventions. Based on their eligibility criteria and the databases searched, they identified five studies that examined the impact of SIT for autistic children and 14 studies that examined the impact of sensory-based interventions for autistic children. They concluded that within some clearly defined goals their systematic review:

> found that SIT [Sensory Integration Therapy] for children with ASD and sensory processing problems demonstrates positive effects on the child's individualized goals; however, additional studies are needed to confirm these results. (Case-Smith, Weaver, & Fristad, 2015, p. 145).

The other two literature reviews identified concluded that SIT does not provide any benefits to autistics (Lang et al., 2012; Leong, Carter, & Stephenson, 2015). Lang et al. (2012) identified, analysed, and summarised research about the usage of SIT programs for autistic children. The search procedures and the application of the predetermined eligibility criteria resulted in the identification and inclusion of 25 studies. They found that three studies concluded that SIT was effective, eight reported mixed results, and 14 claimed that it had no benefits for autistics. However, some of the studies, including the three that reported positive benefits, had serious methodological flaws. Based on these results, Lang et al. concluded that SIT had no positive benefits for autistics. The conclusions reported by Lang et al. have also been echoed by Leong, Carter, and Stephenson (2015). In their systematic review of single case design studies about SIT for individuals with disabilities, they found that:

> Overall the studies do not provide convincing evidence for the efficacy of sensory integration therapy. Given the findings of the present review and other recent analyses it is advised that the use of SIT be limited to experimental contexts. (Leong, Carter, & Stephenson, 2015, p. 334).

6.6.2 Evaluation of Sensory Integration Therapy (SIT)

Rating: Bronze – Safe but ineffective

Most of the literature has concluded that while SIT is safe, autistics do not obtain any benefits from it. Thus, we have rated SIT for autistics as 'Bronze – Safe but ineffective'. Furthermore, since SIT does not provide any benefits there is no point conducting further research into SIT as a support for autistics in the future.

6.6.3 Autistic views about Sensory Integration Therapy (SIT)

Have you personally used Sensory Integration therapy (SIT) and/or Auditory Integration therapy (AIT) to manage anything related to your autism?

Out of the 56 respondents who answered this question, two (3.57%) stated that they had used both approaches and one (1.7%) stated that they had only used SIT. The remaining participants stated that they have not used either approach.

Respondents' ratings of Sensory Integration Therapy (SIT)

No respondents commented on their experiences of SIT, therefore the efficacy of SIT for autistics has not been rated.

6.7 Conclusion

This chapter reviewed the literature about the benefits that autistics might obtain from strategies that support their sensory needs. Out of the six strategies examined, three (i. e., weighted vests, acupuncture, and SIT) were rated as 'Bronze – Safe but ineffective'. In contrast, holding therapy was given the lowest possible rating, 'Tin – Extremely unsafe and potentially life threatening', since the research has showed that it can cause death. Finally, aromatherapy and weighted blankets were not rated because there was an insufficient amount of information to determine their efficacy. The literature reviewed has also shown that there are still many areas where additional research can be conducted. For example, most of the literature in this chapter has evaluated the benefits that autistic children can obtain from sensory-based approaches. As a consequence, there is a lack of published literature about the benefits that such strategies can give autistic adults. In the interests of increasing our knowledge, it is important that more research about sensory-based strategies be conducted with autistic adults, exploring what they find useful. Insights and experiences from autistics about the efficacy of the sensory supports were varied, meaning that while some autistics benefited from particular sensory supports others did not.

References

Allik, H., Larsson, J. O., & Smedje, H. (2006). Insomnia in school-age children with Asperger syndrome or high-functioning autism. *BMC Psychiatry*, 6(1), 18. doi:10.1186/1471-244X-6-18.

Ayres, A. J. (1979). *Sensory integration and the child.* Los Angeles: Western Psychological Services.

Barton, E.E., Reichow, B., & Wolery, M. (2007, May). Double blind placebo evaluation on the engagement of young children with autism. Poster session presented at the International Meeting for Autism Research, Seattle Washington.

Bright, T., Bittick, K., & Fleeman, B. (1981). Reduction of self-injurious behavior using sensory-integrative techniques. *American Journal of Occupational Therapy*, 35, 167–172.

Carter, S. L. (2005). An empirical analysis of the effects of a possible sinus infection and weighted vest on functional analysis out comes of self-injury exhibited by a child with autism. *Journal of Early and Intensive Behavior Interventions*, 2(4), 252–258. doi:10.1037/h0100318.

Case-Smith, J., Weaver, L. L., & Fristad, M. A. (2015). A systematic review of sensory processing interventions for children with autism spectrum disorders. *Autism*, 19(2), 133–148. doi:10.1177/1362361313517762.

Chaffin, M., Hanson, R., Saunders, B. E., Nichols, T., Barnett, D., Zeanah, C., … & Miller-Perrin, C. (2006). Report of the APSAC task force on attachment therapy, reactive attachment disorder, and attachment problems. *Child Maltreatment*, 11(1), 76–89. doi:10.1177/1077559505283699.

Cheuk, D. K., Wong, V., & Chen, W. X. (2011). Acupuncture for autism spectrum disorders (ASD). *Cochrane Database of Systematic Reviews*, 2011(9), 1–89. doi:10.1002/14651858.CD007849.pub2.

Deris, A. R., Hagelman, E. M., Schilling, K., & DiCarlo, C. F. (2006). *Using a weighted or pressure vest for a child with autistic spectrum disorder.* ERIC Clearinghouse.

Devlin, S., Leader, G., & Healy, O. (2009). Comparison of behavioral intervention and sensory-integration therapy in the treatment of self-injurious behavior. *Research in Autism Spectrum Disorders*, 3(1), 223–231. doi:10.1016/j.rasd.2008.06.004.

Fertel-Daly, D., Bedell, G., & Hinojosa, J. (2001). Effects of a weighted vest on attention to task and self-stimulatory behaviors in preschoolers with pervasive developmental disorders. *American Journal of Occupational Therapy*, 55(6), 629–640. doi:10.5014/ajot.55.6.629.

Gee, B. M., Peterson, T. G., Buck, A., & Lloyd, K. (2016). Improving sleep quality using weighted blankets among young children with an autism spectrum disorder. *International Journal of Therapy and Rehabilitation*, 23(4), 173–181. doi:10.12968/ijtr.2016.23.4.173.

Green, V. A., Pituch, K. A., Itchon, J., Choi, A., O'Reilly, M., & Sigafoos, J. (2006). Internet survey of treatments used by parents of children with autism. *Research in Developmental Disabilities*, 27(1), 70–84. doi:10.1016/j.ridd.2004.12.002.

Kane, A., Luiselli, J. K., Dearborn, S., & Young, N. (2004–2005). Wearing a weighted vest as an intervention for children with autism/pervasive developmental disorder. *The Scientific Review of Mental Health Practice*, 3(2), 19–24.

Kanner, L. (1943). Autistic disturbances of affective contact. *Nervous Child*, 2(3), 217–250.

Lang, R., O'Reilly, M., Healy, O., Rispoli, M., Lydon, H., Streusand, W., … & Didden, R. (2012). Sensory integration therapy for autism spectrum disorders: A systematic review. *Research in Autism Spectrum Disorders*, 6(3), 1004–1018. doi:10.1016/j.rasd.2012.01.006.

Lee, B., Lee, J., Cheon, J. H., Sung, H. K., Cho, S. H., & Chang, G. T. (2018). The efficacy and safety of acupuncture for the treatment of children with autism spectrum disorder: A systematic review and meta-analysis. *Evidence-Based Complementary and Alternative Medicine*, 1–21, doi:10.1155/2018/1057539.

Lee, M. S., Choi, T. Y., Shin, B. C., & Ernst, E. (2012). Acupuncture for children with autism spectrum disorders: A systematic review of randomized clinical trials. *Journal of Autism and Developmental Disorders*, 42(8), 1671–1683. doi:10.1007/s10803-011-1409-4.

Leong, H. M., Carter, M., & Stephenson, J. (2015). Systematic review of sensory integration therapy for individuals with disabilities: Single case design studies. *Research in Developmental Disabilities*, 47, 334–351. doi:10.1016/j.ridd.2015.09.022.

Lilienfeld, S. O. (2007). Psychological treatments that cause harm. *Perspectives on Psychological Science*, 2(1), 53–70.

Liu, C., Li, T., Wang, Z., Zhou, R., & Zhuang, L. (2019). Scalp acupuncture treatment for children's autism spectrum disorders: A systematic review and meta-analysis. *Medicine*, 98(13). doi:10.1097/MD.0000000000014880.

Magrun, W. M., Ottenbacher, K., McCue, S., & Keefe, R. (1981). Effects of vestibular stimulation on spontaneous use of verbal language in developmentally delayed children. *American Journal of Occupational Therapy*, 35, 101–104.

Mannion, A., & Leader, G. (2014). Sleep problems in autism spectrum disorder: A literature review. *Review Journal of Autism and Developmental Disorders*, 1(2), 101–109. doi:10.1007/s40489-013-0009-y.

Mercer, J. (2013). Holding therapy: A harmful mental health intervention. *Focus on Alternative and Complementary Therapies*, 18(2), 70–76. doi:10.1111/fct.12024.

Mercer, J. (2014). International concerns about holding therapy. *Research on Social Work Practice*, 24(2), 188–191. doi:10.1177/1049731513497518.

Mercer, J., Sarner, L., & Rosa, L. (2003). *Attachment therapy on trial*. Westport, CT: Praeger.

Morrison, E. E. (2007). A review of research on the use of weighted vests with children on the autism spectrum. *Education*, 127(3), 323–327.

Myles, B. S., Simpson, R. L., Carlson, J., Laurant, M., Gentry, A. M., & Cook, K. T. (2004). Examining the effects of the use of weighted vests for addressing behaviors of children with autism spectrum disorders. *Journal of the International Association of Special Education*, 5(1), 47–62.

Olson, L. J., & Moulton, H. J. (2004). Use of weighted vests in pediatric occupational therapy practice. *Physical & Occupational Therapy in Pediatrics*, 24(3), 45–60. doi:10.1300/J006v24n03_04.

Pignotti, M., & Mercer, J. (2007). Holding therapy and dyadic developmental psychotherapy are not supported and acceptable social work interventions: A Systematic Research Synthesis Revisited. *Research on Social Work Practice*, 17(4), 513–519. doi:10.1177/1049731506297046.

Richdale, A. L., & Schreck, K. A. (2009). Sleep problems in autism spectrum disorders: prevalence, nature, & possible biopsychosocial aetiologies. *Sleep Medicine Reviews*, 13(6), 403–411. doi:10.1016/j.smrv.2009.02.003.

Smith, T., & Antolovich, M. (2000). Parental perceptions of supplemental interventions received by young children with autism in intensive behavior analytic treatment. *Behavioral Interventions*, 15(2), 83–97.

Solomons, S. (2005). Using aromatherapy massage to increase shared attention behaviours in children with autistic spectrum disorders and severe learning difficulties. *British Journal of Special Education*, 32(3), 127–137. doi:10.1111/j.0952-3383.2005.00385.x.

Stephenson, J., & Carter, M. (2009). The use of weighted vests with children with autism spectrum disorders and other disabilities. *Journal of Autism and Developmental Disorders*, 39(1), 105. doi:10.1007/s10803-008-0605-3.

Tavassoli, T., & Baron-Cohen, S. (2012a). Olfactory detection thresholds and adaptation in adults with autism spectrum condition. *Journal of Autism and Developmental Disorders*, 42(6), 905–909. doi:10.1007/s10803-011-1321-y.

Tavassoli, T., & Baron-Cohen, S. (2012b). Taste identification in adults with autism spectrum conditions. *Journal of Autism and Developmental Disorders*, 42(7), 1419–1424. doi:10.1007/s10803-011-1377-8.

Taylor, C. J., Spriggs, A. D., Ault, M. J., Flanagan, S., & Sartini, E. C. (2017). A systematic review of weighted vests with individuals with autism spectrum disorder. *Research in Autism Spectrum Disorders*, 37, 49–60. doi:10.1016/j.rasd.2017.03.003.

Tonacci, A., Billeci, L., Tartarisco, G., Ruta, L., Muratori, F., Pioggia, G., & Gangemi, S. (2017). Olfaction in autism spectrum disorders: A systematic review. *Child Neuropsychology*, 23(1), 1–25. doi:10.1080/09297049.2015.1081678.

VandenBerg, N. L. (2001). The use of a weighted vest to increase on-task behavior in children with attention difficulties. *The American Journal of Occupational Therapy*, 55(6), 621–628.

Watling, R., Deitz, J., Kanny, E. M., & McLaughlin, J. F. (1999). Current practice of occupational therapy for children with autism. *The American Journal of Occupational Therapy*, 53(5), 498–505.

Welch, M. (1988). *Holding time: How to eliminate conflict, temper tantrums, and sibling rivalry and raise happy, loving, successful children*. New York: Simon & Schuster.

Wilbarger, P., & Wilbarger, J. (1991). *Sensory defensiveness in children aged 2–12: An intervention guide for parents and caregivers*. Denver, CO: Avanti Educational Programs.

Williams, T. I. (2006). Evaluating effects of aromatherapy massage on sleep in children with autism: A pilot study. *Evidence-Based Complementary and Alternative Medicine*, 3(3), 373–377. doi:10.1093/ecam/nel017.

Chapter 7

Dietary programs

7.1 Introduction

This chapter examines the findings in the literature about the efficacy of ketogenic and gluten-free and/or casein-free (GFCF) diets for autistics. It begins with a succinct explanation of these diets, followed by a presentation of the findings in the literature about possible therapeutic benefits that these diets might provide autistics. It then rates their efficacy and recommends a series of opportunities in which more research could be conducted in the future. This chapter concludes with a collection of insights and experiences about dietary programs from a sample of autistics.

7.2 What are ketogenic, gluten free, and casein free diets?

7.2.1 What are ketogenic diets?

In 1921, Russell Morse Wilder (24 November 1885–16 December 1595) conceived ketogenic diets. A typical ketogenic diet is comprised of 8% protein, 2% carbohydrate, and 90% fat. Wilder created this diet to help treat epilepsy. However, after the development of anticonvulsant drugs, such as phenytoin and sodium valproate, the usage of ketogenic diets started to diminish. However, they continued to be used to treat epilepsy when anticonvulsant drugs were ineffective. Since their discovery, ketogenic diets have been used for patients with cancer (Klement, 2019; Schwartz et al., 2018; Sremanakova, Sowerbutts, & Burden, 2018), Alzheimer's disease (Broom, Shaw, & Rucklidge, 2018; Taylor et al., 2018), Type II diabetes (Cox et al., 2019), and Type I diabetes (Leow et al., 2018).

7.2.2 What are gluten-free and casein-free diets?

In 1881, Samuel Gee (13 September 1839–3 August 1911), a paediatric physician practicing in London, published *The Coeliac Affection*; one of our earliest clinical descriptions of coeliac disease. He suggested that this disease could affect any person at any age and proposed that it could be cured if the patient consumed gluten-free and/or casein-free (GFCF) foods (Losowsky, 2008). Casein-free foods do not contain the protein casein, which is in all milk-based products, such as cheese, yogurt, and milk. Often they are used in combination with a gluten-free diet, which is a diet in which a person does not consume any wheat, barley, rye, oats, or any foods that contain gluten.

7.3 Dietary programs and the autism spectrum

7.3.1 Ketogenic diets

Our search retrieved one meta-analysis, published by Castro et al. (2015), which examined studies about the efficacy of ketogenic diets for autistics. Castro et al. examined three studies about the efficacy of ketogenic diets on animals that 'exhibited autistic characteristics' (Ahn et al., 2014; Mantis et al., 2009; Ruskin et al., 2013). They also examined five studies about the therapeutic benefits that autistics obtained from ketogenic diets (Evangeliou et al., 2003; Frye, Sreenivasula & Adams, 2011; Herbert & Buckley, 2013; Jurecka et al., 2014; Spilioti et al., 2013).

The five studies that Castro et al. (2015) examined shared several methodological flaws. First, some of these studies did not specify if the participants were also using medications whilst using a ketogenic diet. By not taking into consideration medication usage, it was not possible to attribute any improvements to the ketogenic diet itself, the possible medication that the participants were using, or a combination of both of these factors. Second, the studies examined by Castro et al. did not specify the length of the dietary program or details about the foods consumed in the ketogenic diet. Due to this lack of detail, it was not possible to replicate the studies examined in order to validate their findings. Subsequently, Castro et al. (2015, p. 31) concluded:

> The limited number of reports of improvements after treatment with the KD [ketogenic diets] is insufficient to attest to the practicability of the KD as a treatment for ASD.

7.3.2 Evaluation of ketogenic diets

Rating: Insufficient information to make a recommendation

Since there were less than five studies about the benefits of ketogenic diets for autistics, we were not able to rate the efficacy of this support.

7.3.3 Gluten-free and casein-free (GFCF) diets

A search through the literature about supports for autistics revealed several studies about the efficacy of GFCF diets for autistics. This section presents the findings of several meta-analysis studies and literature reviews about the therapeutic benefits that GFCF diets can give autistics.

Arguably, Elder and colleagues (2015) published one of the most comprehensive meta-analysis studies about GFCF diets for autistics. They searched for studies that were hosted on five databases; PubMed, Web of Knowledge, EBSCO, ProQuest, and WorldCat. They only examined peer-review English-language articles that were published between January 2005 to February 2015. They examined 11 systematic literature reviews or meta-analysis, seven group experimental studies, five case reports, and four group observational studies.

Elder et al. examined 11 literature reviews or meta-analysis studies (See Table 7.1). They found that most of the reviews that they examined concluded that there was an insufficient amount of information to conclude that GFCF diets helped autistics. For

Table 7.1 Literature reviews/meta-analysis studies examined by Elder et al. (2015)

Study	*Age of participants*	*Number and types of studies included*	*Author's conclusions regarding GFCF diet in ASD*
Christison and Ivany, 2006	Authors did not report ages included in search. Participant ages in included studies: 3–22 years.	$N = 7$ six uncontrolled clinical trials one single-blind RCT	Inadequate evidence to clearly support or refute use of GFCF for ASD symptom alleviation. Outcome assessments should include measurement of nonverbal cognition.
Elder, 2008	Author did not report ages included in search or review.	N = unreported $n = 3$ three studies regarding effectiveness of GFCF diet in treatment of ASD one systematic review two RCTs	Great need for additional research exists on order to address remaining questions from both researchers and families; great needs exist for patients with ASD and their families.
Millward et al., 2008	Children, adolescents and adults included in search. Participant ages in included studies: 2–16 years.	$N = 2$ one single-blind RCT one double-blind RCT	Authors cannot recommend gluten and/or casein exclusion diets as standard treatment of individuals with ASD. Larger well-controlled trials are needed.
Mulloy et al., 2010	Authors did not report ages included in search. Participant ages in included studies: 2–7 years.	N = 14 studies two case observational studies four group observational studies two single-subject experimental studies six group experimental studies	Evidence is limited and weak in supporting use of GFCF diets for treatment of ASD. GFCF diets should only be used when behavioural changes appear to be associated with diet changes and/or in the presence of confirmed allergy to gluten and/or casein.
Mulloy et al., 2011	Participant ages in included study: four years to ten years 11 months.	$N = 1$ one single-blind RCT	Researchers maintain their position as published in 2010; no new conclusions in light of the newly published study reviewed in this addendum to the systematic review conducted by Mulloy et al., 2010.

(*continued*)

Table 7.1 (*coninued*)

Study	*Age of participants*	*Number and types of studies included*	*Author's conclusions regarding GFCF diet in ASD*
Buie, 2013	Author did not report ages included in search or review	N = unreported n = 4 clinical trials of GFCF diet in treatment of ASD	Insufficient evidence to support GF diet as treatment for ASD. Gluten sensitivity can present with a variety of symptoms. Identification of a subgroup of characteristic presentation may help predict response to dietary interventions. Additional considerations are needed as to what may constitute response to interventions (e.g. better sleep, improved task performance) in individuals with ASD.
Dosman et al., 2013	Authors did not report ages included in search or review.	Authors did not report total number or types of articles reviewed. n = 7 testing effect of GFCF diet in treatment of ASD two systematic reviews three single-blind RCTs two double-blind RCTs	Inconclusive evidence regarding GFCF diet effectiveness due to methodological limitations. Studies suggest existence of a subgroup of responders to GFCF diet.
Hurwitz, 2013	Age of participants included in search: < 18 years. Participant ages in included studies: 2–16 years.	N = 5 one open RCT two single-blind RCTs two double-blind RCTs	Effect of GFCF diet on behaviour of children with ASD is inconclusive; GFCF diet does not significantly change functioning or behaviour.
Whiteley et al., 2013	Authors did not report ages included in search or review.	Author did not report total number or types of articles reviewed. n = 12 regarding effectiveness of GFCF diet in treatment of ASD one survey three open clinical trials three single-blind RCTs two double-blind RCTs four systematic reviews	Experimental studies suggest improved symptoms and improved development for some individuals with ASD. Dietary studies do not yet adequately measure GFCF diet effects having clinical significance (as opposed to statistical significance) such as effects that, if exist, positively increase quality of life and overall daily functioning.

Study	*Age of participants*	*Number and types of studies included*	*Author's conclusions regarding GFCF diet in ASD*
Zhang, Mayton, and Wheeler, 2013	Authors did not report ages included in search or review.	$N = 23$ seven group comparison studies two single subject designs seven AB designs seven studies did not identify research design	Evidence insufficient to draw firm conclusions as to efficacy of GFCF diets for individuals with ASD.
Marí-Bauset et al., 2014a	All ages included in the search. Participant ages in included studies: two years – adults.	$N = 32$ total $n = 24$ regarding effectiveness of GFCF diet in treatment of ASD three observational case reports/case series two experimental case reports one experimental cohort study one open-label study two open-label experimental studies two open-label cohort studies one open-label experimental cohort study one open-label double-blind controlled cohort study one open-label randomised experimental study one double-blind randomised experimental cohort study one retrospective double-blind randomised trial two single-blind RCTs three double-blind RCTs three systematic reviews	Evidence is limited and weak in supporting use of GFCF diets for treatment of ASD. Authors advise against introduction of gluten-free and/or casein-free diets unless gluten and/or casein intolerance or allergy has been diagnosed. Future research can target identification of a diet-related phenotype and/or discovery of a marker for responsiveness to GFCF dietary intervention.

Source: Elder et al., 2015, pp. 91–93.

example, they cited Mulloy et al. (2010, 2011) and Zhang, Mayton, and Wheeler (2013) who reached this conclusion. However, both studies also suggested that such diets might be beneficial for autistics ***if*** their behavioural challenges were caused by an intolerance or allergy to gluten and/or casein.

Elder et al. examined seven group experimental studies (See Table 7.2). Of these, five only focused on a GFCF diet (Elder et al., 2006; Hyman et al., 2010; Johnson et al., 2011; Seung et al., 2007; Whiteley et al., 2010) and two used three different experimental groups (i.e., casein-free diet group, gluten-free diet group, and GFCF diet group) to compare the effectiveness of gluten-free, casein-free, and GFCF diets for autistics (Mageshwari & Minitha, 2006; Nazni, Wesely, & Nishadevi, 2008). The length of the dietary program ranged from six weeks (Elder et al., 2006; Seung et al., 2007) to 24 months (Whiteley et al., 2010). Elder et al. found that three studies reported that the behavioural, sleep, activity, attention, and verbal communication outcomes of autistic children did not improve whilst they were on a GFCF diet (Hyman et al., 2010; Johnson et al., 2011; Seung et al., 2007). Additionally, one study found GFCF diets did not improve the objectively measured behaviour of autistic children aged between two to 16 years, despite there being positive parental claims to the contrary (Elder et al., 2006). Interestingly, three studies using parental ratings of behaviour showed that GFCF diets did produce significant improvements between pre- and post-intervention behavioural ratings (Mageshwari & Minitha, 2006; Nazni, Wesely, & Nishadevi, 2008; Whiteley et al., 2010). It is possible that using objective measures of behaviour would have shown that GFCF diets did not produce positive behavioural changes in these participants. However, Mageshwari and Minitha (2006) suggested that gluten-free, casein-free, and GFCF diets can improve behavioural challenges and reduce hyperactivity and digestion problems. Based on the results, it appears that GFCF diets can reduce disruptive behaviours that are caused by digestive problems. However, this conclusion is speculative since none of the studies that they examined explored the dietary intolerances prior to intervention, nor the possible role of dietary intolerances or allergies on disruptive behaviour.

In their review of research, Elder et al. (2015) examined five case studies. All five case studies were about the efficacy of GFCF diets on autistic children, with the youngest being 42 months old (Hsu et al., 2009) and the oldest being 12 years old (Irvin, 2006). Some studies indicated that GFCF diets might be promising for autistic children. For example, after starting a GFCF diet the female participant in Herbert and Buckley's (2013) case study demonstrated immediate improvements in language, a gradual reduction in tantrum severity, and a reduction in gastrointestinal symptoms. Furthermore, during the course of the GFCF diet this child's autistic symptoms reduced to a point where they did not exhibit autistic symptoms as evaluated on the *Childhood Autism Rating Scale* (CARS). Reductions in autistic symptomology is not synonymous with curing autism, rather these reductions show a greater ability to function in an adaptive way. In another study, the five-year-old male participant in Genuis and Bouchard's (2010) case study was placed on a gluten-restricted diet with nutritional supplementation (i.e., Omega 3 and 6 fatty acids, and folic acid). After three months on this diet, their functioning improved to the point where they were enrolled in a typical classroom without an individualised learning program. It is unknown if their improved outcomes were attributed to the removal of a food allergy, or if they consumed supplements that supported their improved outcomes, or if there were other

Table 7.2 Case studies examined by Elder et al. (2015)

Study	*Age and diagnosis*	*Previous/ additional therapies*	*Behavioural/ developmental symptoms preceding intervention*	*Gastrointestinal/ physiologic symptoms preceding intervention*	*Intervention*	*Behavioural outcome*	*Gastrointestinal outcome*
Irvin, 2006	12 year-old male ASD and intellectual disability	GCCF diet for one year prior to initial trial.	Extreme self-injury, physical aggression, property destruction, and self-restraint	None reported	Single case ABAB quasi-experimental design A1: one year GFCF diet B1: 12 days regular diet A2: ten days GFCF diet B2: 30 months regular diet	No change in problem behaviours. Behaviours measured during attention, demand, and play conditions.	None reported.
Hsu et al., 2009	42 month-old male ASD and CHARGE syndrome	Speech, occupational, physical, and sensory integration therapy	Delayed motor, language, concept, social comprehension, and general development. 3rd percentile height and weight.	Postprandial vomiting and long-term constipation	GFCF diet	Improved eye contact after 2.5 months. Improved physiological biometry and interpersonal relations after five months. Improved development within 11 months.	Improved appetite, and reduced postprandial vomiting and constipation within 2.5 months.
Gannage, 2010	Three year-old male Regressive autism at 18 months old	Previous therapies – Supplements: probiotics, essential fatty acids, B vitamins. Additional therapies – Behavioural therapies	Language loss, self-stimulatory behaviour, hyperactivity.	Abnormal stool colour and consistency	CAM interventions: Dietary: GFCF diet Medication: anti-fungal and anti-viral medications. Heavy metal toxicity treatment: chelation therapy, dimercapto-succinic acid, alpha-lipoic acid, zinc, selenium, vitamin C, methylsulfonly-methane, taurine, and vitamin E Nutrition supplementation: glutathione, carosine.	At three years following CAM interventions, which included GFCF diet, child had greatly improved language, toilet training, increased play interaction, lowered hyperactivity. At age 11, functions as a neurotypical child without symptoms of ASD.	Improved stool consistency, three months after implementation of GFCF diet.

(continued)

Study	*Age and diagnosis*	*Previous/ additional therapies*	*Behavioural/ developmental symptoms preceding intervention*	*Gastrointestinal/ physiologic symptoms preceding intervention*	*Intervention*	*Behavioural outcome*	*Gastrointestinal outcome*
Genuis and Bouchard, 2010	Five year-old male Regressive autism diagnosed at three years old; language disorder, positive screen for coeliac disease at five years old	Speech language therapy, intensive educational programing	Developmental delay, language and communication impairment, difficulty sleeping, depressed mood, disproportionate anger, inappropriate emotions, inability to tolerate bright lights	Abdominal bloating/pain, belching, nausea, vomiting, diarrhea; chronic upper respiratory infections, chronic congestion.	Gluten restricted diet with nutritional supplementation (omega 3 and omega 6 fatty acids, folic acid)	After three months of initiating gluten restricted diet, the child's functioning improved enough to enable enrollment in a typical classroom without an aide; the individualised learning program was no longer needed three months post initiation of gluten restricted diet.	Gastrointestinal symptoms were relieved within one month of initiating gluten restricted diet.
Herbert and Buckley, 2013	Five year-old female Regressive autism at four years old; seizure onset at puberty (12 years old)	Speech and physical therapy	Escalating tantrums, no eye contact, lack of social awareness, hypersensitivity to sensory stimulation, hypotonia, stereotypies	Foul smelling orange diarrhoea, abdominal distension, daily morning moaning; asthma, recurrent otitis media, recurrent sinusitis	Parents implemented GFCF diet when the child was five years old. Recurrent illness treated with intravenous immunoglobulins; asthma with nutritional supplements and pharmacological supports. Treatment for inflammatory bowel disease. Seizures at 12 years; non-responsive to pharmacological therapy, ketogenic GFCF diet implemented.	Language improvements immediately after implementation of GFCF diet. Gradual improvement in auditory sensitivity; gradual reduced tantrum severity. Autism symptoms reduced over time to non-autistic range on Childhood Autism Rating Scale. Seizures were significantly improved several weeks after GFCF-ketogenic diet was implemented.	Following implementation of GFCF diet, gastrointestinal symptoms improved but did not resolve.

Source: Elder et al., 2015, pp. 96–97.

strategies that addressed their behavioural support needs. However, not all case studies showed that autistic children achieved beneficial outcomes whilst being on a GFCF diet. For example, the 12-year-old male participant in Irvin's (2006) case study showed no change in behaviours that others found challenging whilst on a GFCF diet. In conclusion, while some single case studies showed that GFCF diets can help autistic children (Genuis & Bouchard, 2010; Herbert & Buckley, 2013; Hsu et al., 2009) this finding was not universal (Irvin, 2006) and it may be, as mentioned earlier, that where GFCF diets address dietary intolerance or allergies, then and only then are they beneficial for relieving gastrointestinal symptoms such as those in Table 7.2.

Elder et al. (2015) examined four group observational studies. The study with the largest sample was published by Pennesi and Klein (2012) (n = 387), while the study with the smallest sample was published by Patel and Curtis (2007) (n = 10). Three reported positive benefits (Patel & Curtis, 2007; Pedersen et al., 2014; Pennesi & Klein, 2012), while Harris and Card (2012) found that eating foods not containing gluten and casein did not alleviate gastrointestinal symptoms or disruptive behaviours.

Compared to other literature reviews, Elder et al.'s (2015) study is unique because they analysed a methodologically diverse range of studies (i.e., systematic literature reviews, group experimental studies, case reports, and group observational studies). Despite examining a large number of studies, their meta-analysis had several limitations. For example, they did not examine what type of participant characteristics (i.e., food intolerance or allergy, age, gender, level and type of support needs) could have influenced the efficacy of GFCF diets. In spite of such limitations, based on the evidence that they examined, Elder et al. (2015, p. 99) concluded that:

> until such evidence is available, clinicians should advise those wishing to implement the GFCF diet that it is not likely to be a "miraculous cure" as some claim. As such, clinicians should use caution and consider a number of factors, such as the individual's overall nutritional status as well as potential added family burden related to cost and time commitments, when advising regarding implementation of the GFCF diet for individuals with ASD.

Earlier, Mulloy and colleagues (2010) examined 14 studies about possible therapeutic benefits that GFCF diets can have for autistics. Seven reported positive results, four reported negative results, two reported mixed results, and one did not evaluate the efficacy of GFCF diets. They found that all the studies that reported positive effects had problems with measurement validity, such as basing the results on surveys developed by the researcher or basing results on the subjective perceptions of teachers, parents, and physicians who were not blind to treatment conditions. Despite these limitations, Mulloy et al. (2010, p. 328) stated:

> In view of the lack of empirical support identified through this systematic review, the authors conclude that the research does not support the use of GFCF diets in the treatment of ASD … Unless conclusive evidence is found in support of GFCF diets, the authors recommend that restrictive diets should be implemented only when a food allergy or intolerance is detected.

Unlike other literature reviews about the efficacy of GFCF diets for autistics, Marí-Bauset et al. (2014a) used a rating system to examine the methodological quality of the 32 studies they collected. They identified several methodological limitations including studies that based their results on small sample sizes, studies that did not use a control group or clear definitions of inclusion criteria, and studies that based their results on anecdotal information. Despite these limitations, they concluded that:

> On the basis of this review, we conclude that the evidence to support gluten-free, casein-free diets is limited and weak … Hence, we advise against resorting to elimination diets in an attempt to treat autism spectrum disorders. Specifically, until there is conclusive evidence of the benefits of gluten-free, casein-free diets in autism spectrum disorders, **they should only be introduced after the diagnosis of an intolerance or allergy to allergens in the food that would be eliminated in such a diet.** (Marí-Bauset et al., 2014a, p. 1725).

Zhang, Mayton, and Wheeler (2013) examined 32 studies about the benefits that GFCF diets gave autistics. While they only examined English-language studies, they found little scientific evidence to conclude that such diets were effective in helping autistics:

> Results of this synthesis indicated that the efficacy of GFCF diet interventions for individuals with ASD is inconclusive, and the field needs better controlled studies to provide the scientific evidence base for the intervention. (Zhang, Mayton, & Wheeler, 2013, p. 276).

Recently, Piwowarczyk and colleagues (2018) examined six randomised controlled trials (RCTs) and found that the studies examined had low methodological quality, namely a lack of large sample sizes and brief GFCF dietary periods. Based on these methodological problems they concluded:

> The current systematic review was designed to resolve uncertainty regarding the role of a GFCF diet in children with ASD. … The limited available evidence suggests that there is no consistent evidence to support the use of a GFCF diet in children with ASD. (Piwowarczyk et al., 2018, pp. 439–440).

Most of the literature has examined either the effects of ketogenic diets or GFCF diets on autistics. However, El-Rashidy and colleagues (2017) compared the efficacy of both of these diets for autistics. They divided 45 children who had a diagnosis of autism spectrum disorder from the *Fifth Edition of the Diagnostic and Statistical Manual of Mental Disorders* into three groups. The first group received a ketogenic diet (n = 15), the second group received a GFCF diet (n = 15), and the third group was a control group that received a nutritionally balanced diet (n = 15). Before and six months after starting their dietary programs, all participants completed the CARS, *Autism Treatment Evaluation Test* (ATEC), and neurological examinations and anthropometric measures. In comparison to the control group, both the ketogenic and GFCF groups showed significant improvements in ATEC and CARS scores. However, those in the ketogenic diet group exhibited better cognition and sociability outcomes than those in the GFCF diet group. Despite these results, El-Rashidy et al. cautioned that their study contained a small number of participants in each group and that studies in the future should have larger sample sizes so that the results obtained could be more representative. Furthermore, they did not screen the participants for food intolerances or allergies. Thus, some on a ketogenic or GFCF diet might have shown improvements because they were no longer eating foods that caused gastrointestinal stress.

7.3.4 Evaluation of gluten-free and casein-free (GFCF) diets

Rating: Bronze – Safe but ineffective (in the short-term, unknown safety in the long-term)

Most of the research that we located and examined concluded that GFCF diets are safe but that they do not provide any benefits to autistics, except in situations when they have an intolerance or allergy to gluten and/or casein. Thus, we have rated GFCF diets for autistics as 'Bronze – Safe but ineffective'. However, obviously for individuals who are allergic to gluten and/or casein, they require the relevant diets, which will be gluten and/or casein free.

7.4 Directions for research in the future about dietary programs for autistics

Despite there being a large amount of literature examining possible therapeutic benefits that GFCF and ketogenic diets give autistics, there remains areas where more research in the future could be conducted.

7.4.1 Sensory sensitivities to taste and the texture of food

There is research that has suggested that some autistics have sensory sensitivities to taste and the texture of food and that such sensitivities can influence their selection of foods (Bandini et al., 2017; Curtin et al., 2015; Kuschner et al., 2015; Marí-Bauset et al., 2014b). However, we found that researchers who have examined the benefits that GFCF and ketogenic dietary programs can provide autistics have failed to take into consideration how such sensory sensitivities can affect an autistic's dietary choices or how this may have an impact on their behaviours. In the future, it would be useful for research to examine how an autistic's sensory sensitivities to food can influence their dietary choices and decisions. For autistic children, such studies can base their results on both data that is objective (e.g., parental reports as to what their child did or did not eat) and subjective (e.g., an autistic child explaining what they do and do not like to eat and why). For autistic adults, objective data might be difficult to obtain, especially considering if they live alone. However, this living arrangement does not prevent subjective data from being collected. Most autistic adults are capable of explaining how their sensory sensitivities to the texture and taste of food can have an impact on their dietary choices and this may provide illuminating insights into why some autistics seem to have highly restricted diets by choice whilst others eat a much wider range of foods. Obtaining such information can equip nutritionists and other healthcare professionals with an understanding of how to determine suitable alternative food options that they can recommend to their autistic patients when they express a sensory discomfort with a particular meal.

7.4.2 Researching additional benefits

Currently, most of the literature about dietary interventions for autistics have focused on the role that such interventions play in modifying autistic characteristics (e.g., increasing communication and social behaviours) or improving desirable behaviours (e.g., increasing concentration levels and reducing disruptive behaviours). The role that such diets can play in assisting autistics with managing weight is one area of research that has not been comprehensively examined. Studies have shown that autistics have greater rates of eating disorders (Huke et al., 2013) and higher rates of being overweight or obese than non-autistics (Broder-Fingert et al., 2014; de Vinck-Baroody et al., 2015; Healy, Aigner, & Haegele, 2018; Matheson & Douglas, 2017; McCoy, Jakicic, & Gibbs, 2016). Being obese or overweight or having an eating disorder are all contributing causational factors of health complications, such as the development of heart disease (Piché et al., 2018). Due to these potential health complications, it would seem prudent to conduct more research into how to help autistics manage food choices and eating healthily so that they can avoid potential health consequences.

7.4.3 Combined supports

We recommend that in the future studies about dietary programs for autistics should take into consideration other forms of supports that can help maximise desired outcomes. For example, a ketogenic diet might help autistics manage seizures and lose weight. However, the probability of this outcome might be increased if those on this diet also used an additional support, such as participating in a physical exercise program. Supplementary supports can also be used to achieve other desirable outcomes that dietary activities alone cannot achieve. For example, a gluten-free diet can help alleviate the intestinal discomfort that some autistics with an intolerance for gluten experience. While this discomfort can be mitigated by a gluten-free diet such a dietary intervention cannot help them perfect their social skills. Perhaps a suitable combination of supports could be a gluten-free diet to help them reduce their intestinal disruption so that they can participate in peer-mentoring activities that can help them refine their social skills. Currently, the viability and effectiveness of combining dietary activities with other supports are unknown since most of the literature has only examined the therapeutic benefits of dietary activities in isolation.

7.4.4 Longitudinal research

Most of the studies in the literature reviews that we evaluated did not use follow-up procedures to examine the potential long-term benefits that autistics obtained from ketogenic and GFCF diets. The lack of longitudinal research has meant that very little is known about whether or not autistics and/or their families have the capacity and/or resources to continue dietary activities after the study has concluded. It could be that there are long-term factors that can influence the continuation of a dietary program, such as a sense of complacency emerging or the novelty of the diet fading. Until more longitudinal research is conducted, the long-term viability and benefits of GFCF and ketogenic diets for autistics remains unknown.

7.4.5 Studies about autistic adults using diets

Most of the studies examined in the literature reviews about the efficacy of GFCF and ketogenic diets for autistics have based their results on samples of autistic children. For example, all five studies about the efficacy of ketogenic diets for autistics that Castro et al. (2015) examined based their results on samples of autistic children. In the interests of examining if such dietary programs can help autistic adults more research about this topic should be conducted with autistic adults.

7.4.6 Other dietary programs

Most of the literature about dietary programs for autistics have focused on the efficacy of ketogenic and GFCF diets. However, there are other diets that have not received much research; for instance, Vegetarian or Vegan diets, the Paleo diet, GAPS diet, and the Raw food diet. It is possible that such diets will be beneficial for autistics. Alternatively, such diets might produce detrimental outcomes, such as restricting essential nutrients that are used for the development and maintenance of health. Until more research is conducted, the potential benefits and drawbacks of any type of diets for autistics, other than ketogenic of GFCF diets, will remain a source of speculation.

7.5 Autistic perspectives about dietary programs

Have you ever used a specific type of diet to manage any symptoms related to your autism?

Of the 206 respondents who completed our online survey, 54 (26.21%) answered the question 'Have you ever used a specific type of diet to manage any symptoms related to your autism?' Of those who answered this question, most respondents selected the option 'No, I eat pretty much whatever I want' (n = 20, 37.04%), followed by respondents stating 'No, but I have a restricted diet of preferred foods' (n = 16, 29.63%), and 'Gluten free (GF) diet' (n = 14, 25.93%).

Respondents' ratings of the efficacy of particular diets

Most respondents selected options that explained that particular diets were undesirable and/or ineffective; 'did not enjoy or find useful' (n = 7, 13.46%), 'enjoyed but did not find useful' (n = 3, 5.77%), and 'did not enjoy but found useful' (n = 10, 19.23%). However, six respondents (11.54%) selected the option 'Enjoyed, found useful and found that my wellbeing and mood were improved'. Based on the distribution of responses, the efficacy of particular diets for autistics as perceived by autistics was calculated as 2.8 stars.

Figure 7.1 2.8 stars

Respondents' comments about particular diets

During the course of completing our online survey, 24 respondents provided a comment to the question 'How did you find using a particular diet to help you manage symptoms related to your autism?' Our examination of the collected responses found that two respondents explained that gluten-free diets helped them reduced their 'brain fog'.

> "I tried gluten-free briefly. I found my mind was slightly clearer (less brain-fog) but it wasn't enough of an improvement to justify maintaining the very difficult gluten free diet. I always eat a pretty limited diet of familiar foods because it's just my preference, it's easy and predictable. I eat a vegetarian diet partly for ethical reasons, and partly because I find it easier to make decisions about what to eat if my options are limited (e.g. at a restaurant there are usually only a few veggie options, so I can actually make a decision instead of getting overwhelmed with dozens of options from the full menu)."
>
> "I can't have gluten because it makes my brain foggy, everything overwhelms me and I get very depressed."

Interviewing a coeliac autistic, they noted that they had not been diagnosed as coeliac until they were 50 years old.

> "I had classic symptoms of coeliac disease for more than a decade before I was diagnosed, because I'd had tummy troubles all my life, I don't think I was taken seriously. Anxiety would go straight to my tummy, and I think they thought I was just being anxious. It was terrible, the Dr kept saying there had to be a reason I was so unwell. I changed GPs and asked for the coeliac disease blood test, and then they did the genetic testing too and the endoscopy and found I was coeliac and had a lot of damage by then. So for me a gluten free diet is amazing, I have healthy bowels, I'm not anaemic anymore, I feel so much more comfortable and healthy and well."

The lack of responses to this question could be because the question was too ambiguous or that not many respondents have used special diets and therefore were not in a position to provide an adequate comment. Regardless of these potential limitations, the small number of experiences showed that in certain circumstances special diets might be beneficial.

7.6 Conclusion

This chapter examined literature reviews and meta-analysis studies that examined studies about the benefits that autistics have obtained from ketogenic and GFCF diets. It presented the findings of one literature review about ketogenic diets for autistics (Castro et al., 2015). In comparison, multiple literature reviews that have examined studies about the possible benefits that autistics have obtained from GFCF diets were explained (Elder et al., 2015; Hyman et al., 2010; Johnson et al., 2011; Seung et al., 2007; Whiteley et al., 2010). Most of the literature reviews examined concluded that autistics did not obtain any therapeutic benefits from GFCF diets. Hence, GFCF diets were rated as 'Bronze – Safe but ineffective'. However, it should be noted that autistics with coeliac disease must adhere to gluten free diets to prevent serious health complications. In contrast, the efficacy of ketogenic diets for autistics were not rated due to a lack of literature. This chapter concluded with a series of views from autistic participants who completed our survey about their insights and experiences of dietary programs.

References

Ahn, Y., Narous, M., Tobias, R., Rho, J. M., & Mychasiuk, R. (2014). The ketogenic diet modifies social and metabolic alterations identified in the prenatal valproic acid model of autism spectrum disorder. *Developmental Neuroscience*, 36(5), 371–380. doi:10.1159/000362645.

Bandini, L. G., Curtin, C., Phillips, S., Anderson, S. E., Maslin, M., & Must, A. (2017). Changes in food selectivity in children with autism spectrum disorder. *Journal of Autism and Developmental Disorders*, 47(2), 439–446. doi:10.1007/s10803-016-2963-6.

Broder-Fingert, S., Brazauskas, K., Lindgren, K., Iannuzzi, D., & Van Cleave, J. (2014). Prevalence of overweight and obesity in a large clinical sample of children with autism. *Academic Pediatrics*, 14(4), 408–414. doi:10.1016/j.acap.2014.04.004.

Broom, G. M., Shaw, I. C., & Rucklidge, J. J. (2018). The ketogenic diet as a potential treatment and prevention strategy for Alzheimer's disease. *Nutrition*, 60, 118–121. doi:10.1016/j.nut.2018.10.003.

Buie, T. (2013). The relationship of autism and gluten. *Clinical Therapeutics*, 35(5), 578–583. doi:10.1016/j.clinthera.2013.04.011.

Castro, K., Faccioli, L. S., Baronio, D., Gottfried, C., Perry, I. S., & dos Santos Riesgo, R. (2015). Effect of a ketogenic diet on autism spectrum disorder: A systematic review. *Research in Autism Spectrum Disorders*, 20, 31–38. doi:10.1016/j.rasd.2015.08.005.

Christison, G. W., & Ivany, K. (2006). Elimination diets in autism spectrum disorders: Any wheat amidst the chaff? *Journal of Developmental & Behavioral Pediatrics*, 27(2), S162–S171.

Cox, N., Gibas, S., Salisbury, M., Gomer, J., & Gibas, K. (2019). Ketogenic diets may reverse Type II diabetes and ameliorate clinical depression: A case study. *Diabetes & Metabolic Syndrome: Clinical Research & Reviews*, 13(2), 1475–1479. doi:10.1016/j.dsx.2019.01.055.

Curtin, C., Hubbard, K., Anderson, S. E., Mick, E., Must, A., & Bandini, L. G. (2015). Food selectivity, mealtime behavior problems, spousal stress, and family food choices in children with and without autism spectrum disorder. *Journal of Autism and Developmental Disorders*, 45(10), 3308–3315. doi:10.1007/s10803-015-2490-x.

de Vinck-Baroody, O., Shui, A., Macklin, E. A., Hyman, S. L., Leventhal, J. M., & Weitzman, C. (2015). Overweight and obesity in a sample of children with autism spectrum disorder. *Academic Pediatrics*, 15(4), 396–404. doi:10.1016/j.acap.2015.03.008.

Dosman, C., Adams, D., Wudel, B., Vogels, L., Turner, J., & Vohra, S. (2013). Complementary, holistic, and integrative medicine: Autism spectrum disorder and gluten-and casein-free diet. *Pediatrics in Review*, 34(10), e36–e41. doi:10.1542/pir.34-10-e36.

Elder, J. H. (2008). The gluten-free, casein-free diet in autism: An overview with clinical implications. *Nutrition in Clinical Practice*, 23(6), 583–588. doi:10.1177/0884533608326061.

Elder, J. H., Kreider, C. M., Schaefer, N. M., & de Laosa, M. B. (2015). A review of gluten-and casein-free diets for treatment of autism: 2005–2015. *Nutrition and Dietary Supplements*, 7, 87. doi:10.2147/NDS.S74718.

Elder, J. H., Shankar, M., Shuster, J., Theriaque, D., Burns, S., & Sherrill, L. (2006). The gluten-free, casein-free diet in autism: Results of a preliminary double blind clinical trial. *Journal of Autism and Developmental Disorders*, 36(3), 413–420. doi:10.1007/s10803-006-0079-0.

El-Rashidy, O., El-Baz, F., El-Gendy, Y., Khalaf, R., Reda, D., & Saad, K. (2017). Ketogenic diet versus gluten free casein free diet in autistic children: A case-control study. *Metabolic Brain Disease*, 32(6), 1935–1941. doi:10.1007/s11011-017-0088-z.

Evangeliou, A., Vlachonikolis, I., Mihailidou, H., Spilioti, M., Skarpalezou, A., Makaronas, N., ... & Sbyrakis, S. (2003). Application of a ketogenic diet in children with autistic behavior: Pilot study. *Journal of Child Neurology*, 18(2), 113–118. doi:10.1177/08830738030180020501.

Frye, R. E., Sreenivasula, S., & Adams, J. B. (2011). Traditional and non-traditional treatments for autism spectrum disorder with seizures: An on-line survey. *BMC Pediatrics*, 11(1), 37. doi:10.1186/1471-2431-11-37.

Gannage, J. (2010). Integrative autism treatment: Foretelling medicine's future. *Journal of Orthomolecular Medicine*, 25(4), 166–168.

Genuis, S. J., & Bouchard, T. P. (2010). Celiac disease presenting as autism. *Journal of Child Neurology*, 25(1), 114–119. doi:10.1177/0883073809336127.

Harris, C., & Card, B. (2012). A pilot study to evaluate nutritional influences on gastrointestinal symptoms and behavior patterns in children with autism spectrum disorder. *Complementary Therapies in Medicine*, 20(6), 437–440. doi:10.1016/j.ctim.2012.08.004.

Healy, S., Aigner, C. J., & Haegele, J. A. (2018). Prevalence of overweight and obesity among US youth with autism spectrum disorder. *Autism*, 23(4), 1046–1050. doi:10.1177/1362361318791817.

Herbert, M. R., & Buckley, J. A. (2013). Autism and dietary therapy: Case report and review of the literature. *Journal of Child Neurology*, 28(8), 975–982. doi:10.1177/0883073813488668.

Hsu, C. L., Lin, C. Y., Chen, C. L., Wang, C. M., & Wong, M. K. (2009). The effects of a gluten and casein-free diet in children with autism: A case report. *Chang Gung Med J*, 32(4), 459–465. doi:3204/320414p.

Huke, V., Turk, J., Saeidi, S., Kent, A., & Morgan, J. F. (2013). Autism spectrum disorders in eating disorder populations: A systematic review. *European Eating Disorders Review*, 21(5), 345–351. doi:10.1002/erv.2244.

Hurwitz, S. (2013). The gluten-free, casein-free diet and autism: Limited return on family investment. *Journal of Early Intervention*, 35(1), 3–19. doi:10.1177/1053815113484807.

Hyman, S., Stewart, P., Smith, T., Foley, J., Cain, U., Peck, R., ... & Wang, H. (2010, May). *The gluten free and casein free (GFCF) diet: A double blind, placebo controlled challenge study.* In International Meeting for Autism Research, Philadelphia, PA.

Irvin, D. (2006). Using analog assessment procedures for determining the effects of a gluten-free and casein-free diet on rate of problem behaviors for an adolescent with autism. *Behavioral Interventions*, 21(4), 281–286. doi:10.1002/bin.205.

Johnson, C. R., Handen, B. L., Zimmer, M., Sacco, K., & Turner, K. (2011). Effects of gluten free / casein free diet in young children with autism: A pilot study. *Journal of Developmental and Physical Disabilities*, 23(3), 213–225. doi:10.1007/s10882-010-9217-x.

Jurecka, A., Zikanova, M., Jurkiewicz, E., & Tylki-Szymańska, A. (2014). Attenuated adenylosuccinate lyase deficiency: A report of one case and a review of the literature. *Neuropediatrics*, 45(1), 50–55. doi:10.1055/s-0033-1337335.

Klement, R. J. (2019). The emerging role of ketogenic diets in cancer treatment. *Current Opinion in Clinical Nutrition & Metabolic Care*, 22(2), 129–134. doi:10.1097/MCO.0000000000000540.
Kuschner, E. S., Eisenberg, I. W., Orionzi, B., Simmons, W. K., Kenworthy, L., Martin, A., & Wallace, G. L. (2015). A preliminary study of self-reported food selectivity in adolescents and young adults with autism spectrum disorder. *Research in Autism Spectrum Disorders*, 15, 53–59. doi:10.1016/j.rasd.2015.04.005.
Leow, Z. Z. X., Guelfi, K. J., Davis, E. A., Jones, T. W., & Fournier, P. A. (2018). The glycaemic benefits of a very-low-carbohydrate ketogenic diet in adults with Type 1 diabetes mellitus may be opposed by increased hypoglycaemia risk and dyslipidaemia. *Diabetic Medicine*, 35(9), 1258–1263. doi:10.1111/dme.13663.
Losowsky, M. S. (2008). A history of coeliac disease. *Digestive Diseases*, 26(2), 112–120.
Mageshwari, U. S., & Minitha S. J. (2006). Impact of dietary exclusion of casein and gluten on selected autistic children. *The Indian Journal of Nutrition and Dietetics*, 43, 183–191.
Mantis, J. G., Fritz, C. L., Marsh, J., Heinrichs, S. C., & Seyfried, T. N. (2009). Improvement in motor and exploratory behavior in Rett syndrome mice with restricted ketogenic and standard diets. *Epilepsy & Behavior*, 15(2), 133–141. doi:10.1016/j.yebeh.2009.02.038.
Marí-Bauset, S., Zazpe, I., Mari-Sanchis, A., Llopis-González, A., & Morales Suárez-Varela, M. (2014a). Evidence of the gluten-free and casein-free diet in autism spectrum disorders: a systematic review. *Journal of Child Neurology*, 29(12), 1718–1727. doi:10.1177/0883073814531330.
Marí-Bauset, S., Zazpe, I., Mari-Sanchis, A., Llopis-González, A., & Morales Suárez-Varela, M. (2014b). Food selectivity in autism spectrum disorders: A systematic review. *Journal of Child Neurology*, 29(11), 1554–1561. doi:10.1177/0883073813498821.
Matheson, B. E., & Douglas, J. M. (2017). Overweight and obesity in children with autism spectrum disorder (ASD): A critical review investigating the etiology, development, and maintenance of this relationship. *Review Journal of Autism and Developmental Disorders*, 4(2), 142–156. doi:10.1007/s40489-017-0103-7.
McCoy, S. M., Jakicic, J. M., & Gibbs, B. B. (2016). Comparison of obesity, physical activity, and sedentary behaviors between adolescents with autism spectrum disorders and without. *Journal of Autism and Developmental Disorders*, 46(7), 2317–2326. doi:10.1007/s10803-016-2762-0.
Millward, C., Ferriter, M., Calver, S. J., & Connell-Jones, G. G. (2008). Gluten- and casein-free diets for autistic spectrum disorder. *Cochrane Database of Systematic Reviews*, 2008(2). doi:10.1002/14651858.CD003498.pub3.
Mulloy, A., Lang, R., O'Reilly, M., Sigafoos, J., Lancioni, G., & Rispoli, M. (2010). Gluten-free and casein-free diets in the treatment of autism spectrum disorders: A systematic review. *Research in Autism Spectrum Disorders*, 4(3), 328–339. doi:10.1016/j.rasd.2009.10.008.
Mulloy, A., Lang, R., O'Reilly, M., Sigafoos, J., Lancioni, G., & Rispoli, M. (2011). Addendum to "Gluten-free and casein-free diets in treatment of autism spectrum disorders: A systematic review". *Research in Autism Spectrum Disorders*, 5(1), 86–88. doi:10.1016/j.rasd.2010.07.004.
Nazni, P., Wesely, E., & Nishadevi, V. (2008). Impact of casein and gluten free dietary intervention on selected autistic children. *Iranian Journal of Pediatrics*, 18(3), 244–250.
Patel, K., & Curtis, L. (2007). A comprehensive approach to treating autism and attention-deficit hyperactivity disorder: A prepilot study. *Journal of Alternative and Complementary Medicine*, 13(10), 1091–1097. doi:10.1089/acm.2007.0611.
Pedersen, L., Parlar, S., Kvist, K., Whiteley, P., & Shattock, P. (2014). Data mining the ScanBrit study of a gluten-and casein-free dietary intervention for children with autism spectrum disorders: Behavioural and psychometric measures of dietary response. *Nutritional Neuroscience*, 17(5), 207–213. doi:10.1179/1476830513Y.0000000082.
Pennesi, C. M., & Klein, L. C. (2012). Effectiveness of the gluten-free, casein-free diet for children diagnosed with autism spectrum disorder: Based on parental report. *Nutritional Neuroscience*, 15(2), 85–91. doi:10.1179/1476830512Y.0000000003.

Piché, M. E., Poirier, P., Lemieux, I., & Després, J. P. (2018). Overview of epidemiology and contribution of obesity and body fat distribution to cardiovascular disease: An update. *Progress in Cardiovascular Diseases*, 61(2), 103–113. doi:10.1016/j.pcad.2018.06.004.

Piwowarczyk, A., Horvath, A., Łukasik, J., Pisula, E., & Szajewska, H. (2018). Gluten-and casein-free diet and autism spectrum disorders in children: A systematic review. *European Journal of Nutrition*, 57(2), 433–440. doi:10.1007/s00394-017-1483-2.

Ruskin, D. N., Svedova, J., Cote, J. L., Sandau, U., Rho, J. M., Kawamura Jr, M., ... & Masino, S. A. (2013). Ketogenic diet improves core symptoms of autism in BTBR mice. *PLoS One*, 8 (6), e65021. doi:10.1371/journal.pone.0065021.

Schwartz, K. A., Noel, M., Nikolai, M., & Chang, H. T. (2018). Investigating the ketogenic diet as treatment for primary aggressive brain cancer: Challenges and lessons learned. *Frontiers in Nutrition*, 5, 11. doi:10.3389/fnut.2018.00011.

Seung, H., Rogalski, Y., Shankar, M., & Elder, J. (2007). The gluten-and casein-free diet and autism: Communication outcomes from a preliminary double-blind clinical trial. *Journal of Medical Speech Language Pathology*, 15(4), 337–345.

Spilioti, M., Evangeliou, A., Tramma, D., Theodoridou, Z., Metaxas, S., Michailidi, E., ... & Tsalkidis, A. (2013). Evidence for treatable inborn errors of metabolism in a cohort of 187 Greek patients with autism spectrum disorder (ASD). *Frontiers in Human Neuroscience*, 7, 858. doi:10.3389/fnhum.2013.00858.

Sremanakova, J., Sowerbutts, A. M., & Burden, S. (2018). A systematic review of the use of ketogenic diets in adult patients with cancer. *Journal of Human Nutrition and Dietetics*, 31(6), 793–802. doi:10.1111/jhn.12587.

Taylor, M. K., Sullivan, D. K., Mahnken, J. D., Burns, J. M., & Swerdlow, R. H. (2018). Feasibility and efficacy data from a ketogenic diet intervention in Alzheimer's disease. *Alzheimer's & Dementia: Translational Research & Clinical Interventions*, 4, 28–36. doi:10.1016/j.trci.2017.11.002.

Whiteley, P., Haracopos, D., Knivsberg, A. M., Reichelt, K. L., Parlar, S., Jacobsen, J., ... & Shattock, P. (2010). The ScanBrit randomised, controlled, single-blind study of a gluten-and casein-free dietary intervention for children with autism spectrum disorders. *Nutritional Neuroscience*, 13(2), 87–100. doi:10.1179/147683010X12611460763922.

Whiteley, P., Shattock, P., Knivsberg, A. M., Seim, A., Reichelt, K. L., Todd, L., ... & Hooper, M. (2013). Gluten- and casein-free dietary intervention for autism spectrum conditions. *Frontiers in Human Neuroscience*, 6, 344. doi:10.3389/fnhum.2012.00344.

Zhang, J., Mayton, M. R., & Wheeler, J. J. (2013). Effectiveness of gluten-free and casein-free diets for individuals with autism spectrum disorders: An evidence-based research synthesis. *Education and Training in Autism and Development*, 48(2), 276–287.

Chapter 8

Physical activities

8.1 Introduction

This chapter explores the possible therapeutic benefits that autistics may obtain from physical activities. In the following order the literature about physical exercise programs, dance and movement therapy (DMT), and yoga activities are reviewed. At the end of each type of physical activity, its therapeutic value for autistics is rated along with a series of recommendations about possible directions for research in the future. At the end of this chapter a series of insights from a small sample of autistics about the efficacy of these activities is presented.

8.2 Physical exercise programs

8.2.1 Physical exercise programs

In a general sense, physical exercise has been defined as any "physical activity that is planned, structured, repetitive, and purposeful" (Griera et al., 2007, p. 1194). Such a broad definition allows for aquatic exercises (e.g., swimming) and land-based exercises (e.g., walking, jogging) to be considered as physical exercise. Physical exercise can provide everyone with benefits, regardless of their background or characteristics. For example, it can improve a person's muscle strength and coordination (Burton et al., 2015; de Labra et al., 2015). It can also improve the concentration abilities of people with Attention Deficit Hyperactivity Disorder (Den Heijer et al., 2017; Grassmann et al., 2017), as well as the mental health of people with depression (Josefsson, Lindwall, & Archer, 2014; Knapen et al., 2015). Gehricke et al. (2020) found that autistic children and adolescents typically engage in less physical activity compared to those not on the autism spectrum, although no rationale for this discrepancy was provided.

In their meta-analysis, Lang et al. (2010) examined 18 studies that measured the benefits that autistics obtained from different types of physical exercise. Most of the studies analysed involved participants running or jogging around a track or an open field (e.g., a park or a sports field at school), other types of physical exercise were; water-based exercises (e.g., swimming or aqua aerobics), stationary bike riding, treadmill walking, roller-skating, muscle toning and stretching, and walking in snowshoes. They found that physical exercise programs can help autistics improve their physical fitness, in line with the benefits of exercise for the general population (e.g., improved endurance, strength, flexibility, and aerobic fitness).

In 2012, Sowa and Meulenbroek published a meta-analysis in which they examined 16 studies on the effects of physical exercise for autistics. Most of the studies that they examined described the therapeutic benefits of jogging, followed by swimming, horseback riding, cycling, and weight training. Even though most of the collected studies based their findings on small sample sizes, they tentatively concluded that individualised physical exercise programs can improve an autistic's social skills and motor control. They also found that physical exercise can help a diverse range of autistic participants across the spectrum who had different support needs and strengths.

The literature reviews and meta-analysis studies presented thus far have examined studies about the potential benefits of physical exercise for autistics across different ages. However, we identified other literature reviews that have examined studies about the benefits which specific age cohorts of autistics can obtain from physical exercise. In 2014, Sorensen and Zarrett examined 19 studies about the benefits that autistic adolescents obtained from physical exercise. After examining these studies, they concluded that:

> The strongest empirical support for the benefits of PA [Physical activity] was identified for self-regulation, health, and motor skills, while evidence remains limited or absent for benefits related to improvements to cognitive, language, and sensorimotor functioning. (Sorensen & Zarrett, 2014, p. 344).

In 2016, Bremer, Crozier, and Lloyd published a literature review in which they evaluated studies about the influence which physical exercise had on the academic capabilities of autistic children. They found that in Rosenthal-Malek and Mitchell's (1997) study, five autistic males improved their ability to produce correct academic responses after 20 minutes of jogging. This finding was supported by Oriel et al. (2011), who reported that after 15 minutes of jogging autistic children exhibited an increase in the number of correct academic responses compared to autistic children who did not do any jogging. Finally, Nicholson et al. (2011) examined the impact that a 15-minute jogging program had on the academic performance of four nine-year-old autistic boys. They found that there was a 7.5% increase in academic tasks after the jogging session. However, although they did not offer an explanation, academic performance returned to near baseline levels four weeks after the jogging program concluded.

Bremer, Crozier, and Lloyd also examined studies that measured if physical exercise helped autistics improve their social reciprocity, communication, and behavioural skills. The physical exercise activities that they examined were horseback riding, martial arts, swimming, and a combined yoga and dance program. Out of the four studies involving horseback riding, two reported that participants exhibited increases in social responsiveness after participating in such riding sessions and the other two did not report any improvement. Movahedi et al. (2013) found that in comparison to those in the control group, participants who participated in their martial arts program exhibited significant improvements in social interactions and that these changes were maintained 30-days after the program ceased. Pan (2010) found that autistic children who participated in swimming demonstrated significant improvements in social competence and a decrease in problem behaviours. However, when compared to the measurements obtained from the control group, these benefits were not significant. Finally, Rosenblatt et al. (2011) found that yoga and dance activities resulted in significant reductions in behavioural problems among autistic participants. However, whether these benefits were a result of the yoga and dance itself remains unknown since they did not use a control group. Based on these findings, Bremer, Crozier, and Lloyd (2016, p. 899) concluded:

> Results demonstrated that exercise interventions consisting individually of jogging, horseback riding, martial arts, swimming or yoga/dance can result in improvements to numerous behavioural outcomes including stereotypic behaviours, social-emotional functioning, cognition and attention.

8.2.2 Evaluation of physical exercise programs

Gold – Extremely promising and use with confidence

There is an overwhelming amount of evidence that concludes that physical exercise programs are beneficial for most autistics, as per the general population. More specifically in relation to autism, studies have shown that aquatic exercises can reduce insomnia (Oriel et al., 2016) and *improve social skills* (Pan, 2010). As a side note, from another perspective, most aquatic occupational therapists who participated in Vonder Hulls, Walker, and Powell's (2006) study expressed opinions that aquatic exercises helped autistic children substantially increase their attention, muscle strength, balance, and initiating/maintaining joint attention. Research also shows that different types of physical exercise programs are beneficial for autistics. This means that there is a wide variety of physical activity options available to autistics. Thus, if an autistic dislikes one or more physical activities then they have the possibility of enjoying and benefiting from another physical activity program. For example, if an autistic is uncomfortable with aquatic activities, perhaps because of the water's temperature or pressure on their body, then they might find walking or weightlifting more comfortable and enjoyable. Since most of the literature has shown that physical exercise can be beneficial for autistics, we have rated physical exercise as 'Gold – Extremely promising and use with confidence'.

However, it is unknown why, or indeed if it is physical exercise (or a removal from a distracting classroom, or 1:1 interaction with a liked physical therapist/PE teacher) that can improve academic outcomes and/or social interaction skills.

8.2.3 Directions for research in the future about physical exercise programs

There are many studies that have shown that physical exercise programs can provide immediate benefits to autistics (Lang et al., 2010). However, there are not many studies that have examined if there are any specific long-term benefits that such programs can give autistics. This point was made by Sorensen and Zarrett (2014) who claimed that within their literature review there were only two studies that used follow-up assessments (Bahrami et al., 2012; Movahedi et al., 2013). It is important to examine the long-term effects of physical exercise programs to see if they have a continued impact on helping autistics manage their physical and mental health, or if any benefits are not maintained post-intervention.

The relationship between the intensity of the physical exercise and its impact on behavioural outcomes for autistics is unknown, apart from some case studies on developing body awareness (interoception) through very brief (time and intensity) physical activities over a long period of time. These case studies (Schauder et al., 2015; Shah, 2016) have indicated that developing body awareness through brief physical activities increases the ability of autistics to self-manage and self-regulate. This is a promising area of research which needs further exploration and longer-term trials. Similarly, studies in the future could incorporate measures of exercise intensity, such as maximum and average heart rate during exercise. Such measurements can be recorded by monitors, such as accelerometers or heart rate monitors, which participants can wear whilst physically exercising. Such devices have already been used to measure the stress and aggression that autistic children exhibit towards others (Goodwin et al., 2019). In future studies, such measurements would make it possible to objectively compare the benefits that different levels of physical activity and intensity can give autistics (Bremer, Crozier, & Lloyd, 2016). However, this may be impractical for children or those with sensory difficulties who may struggle to adapt to wearing monitors which exert constant physical contact and pressure.

The relationship between the amount of physical exercise and the associated benefits that autistics can receive has not been explored. It may be that frequent and longer participation in physical exercise can result in greater and long-lasting improvements in behaviour for autistics. This claim was made by Bahrami et al. (2012) and Movahedi et al. (2013) in their studies which demonstrated that autistic youths benefited from a 56-hour martial arts program which was spread over four sessions per week for a total of 14 weeks. Despite these findings, it is difficult to establish what is an ideal amount of physical exercise for optimal results for autistics. This point was stated by Bremer, Crozier, and Lloyd (2016, p. 910), who stated "we do not know whether 5 min of jogging would result in equivalent reductions in stereotypic behaviour to those evident following 15–20 min". It is simply unknown if more physical exercise can create better outcomes for autistics or if there is a ceiling effect in which the benefits obtained begin to plateau after a specific amount of physical exercise. This is not to say that decreasing stereotypic behaviour should be a desired outcome. It may also be that short exercise periods focused on interoception can have different impacts than longer periods of exercises and longer sessions as in general developing/improving interoception is beneficial as is strengthening muscles including cardiac strength from a physical health perspective. Whether this is any different for autistics in terms of how to optimise physical and/or mental health is unknown.

Similarly, another unexplored area that research could investigate is if different amounts of physical exercise can have different impacts on different behaviours. For example, one hour of intense physical exercise could reduce anxiety but might not create sustained benefits on socio-emotional behaviours, whereas developing interoception brings social-emotional skill development but may not improve physical fitness. To add to our knowledge, in the future, studies could use multiple measures to gauge the relative impact which different amounts of physical exercise can have on different behavioural outcomes.

8.3 Dance and movement therapy (DMT)

8.3.1 Dance and movement therapy (DMT)

When some think about dance, they might imagine a ballerina who has mastered their craft and who is able to choreograph their movements to the accompanying music

(Koff, 2000). However, performing competently is not the only goal of dance. It can also enable "every child, regardless of physical capabilities, to be expressive in a non-verbal manner – to explore and incorporate the physical self as a functioning part of the whole social being" (Koff, 2000, p. 27). Aside from aiding communication, dance has been used in therapy programs, which are often called dance and movement therapy (DMT) programs. DMT programs are based on the notion that "human reception, processing and response inextricably link the mind and body into a functional whole" (Fitt, 1988, p. 278). Over 2000 years ago Hippocrates conceptualised a link between mind and body. Since this time, DMT programs have been a fundamental part of healing rituals in many cultures (Chaiklin, 2009). During 1966, DMT emerged as a movement within the United States, especially after the creation of the American Dance Therapy Association, which has defined DMT as "the psychotherapeutic use of movement to further the emotional, cognitive, physical and social integration of the individual" (American Dance Therapy Association, 2009).

DMT programs can have many positive benefits for a person's physical, social, and cognitive abilities. They can improve balance, flexibility, muscular strength and tone, endurance, spatial awareness, and social skills and social relationships. From a cognitive perspective, DMT programs can help improve vocabulary development and sensory-motor systems (Scharoun et al., 2014). Despite their therapeutic potential, such programs have rarely been offered to autistics. For example, Green et al. (2006) found that 2.4% of parents sampled reported that their autistic children had used a DMT program.

A review of the available literature did not yield any literature reviews or meta-analysis studies about the efficacy of DMT programs for autistics. Consequently, the remaining part of this section will review individual studies about the efficacy of such programs for this population, beginning with case studies and then studies that have delivered such programs to groups of autistics.

Early accounts about the efficacy of DMT programs for autistics were predominantly anecdotal. Several of these anecdotal accounts were documented in Costonis's 1978 book *Therapy in Motion*. In this book, Costonis detailed her experiences of working with a five-year-old autistic girl called Patricia. Costonis measured her behaviour as she progressed through the DMT program. After four months of DMT, she exhibited major improvements in all areas of movement and behaviour, which ultimately resulted in her being transferred from a special education centre to a mainstream school. Costonis also described Boettinger's (1978) work on the implementation of a DMT program to help a four-year-old autistic girl. The DMT session lasted 30 minutes, three times per week for over eight weeks. At the conclusion of the program, the child's tolerance for physical touch and eye contact increased. These positive results led Costonis (1978) and Boettinger (1978) to suggest that components of DMT, such as moving to a rhythm, may stimulate an autistic child's unconscious ability to learn.

One of the earliest studies in which a DMT program was used with a group of autistic children was published in 2001 by Hartshorn and colleagues. A group of 38 autistic children were introduced to a 30-minute movement session twice per week for two months. The sessions included the children performing different movements with hoops, moving through an obstacle course, and dancing to the sound of a tambourine. During the first and last DMT session, specific behaviours were measured (e.g., wandering, resisting a teacher's instructions). The results collected showed that on-task behaviours increased and that behaviours perceived to be related to stress decreased. Even though there were gains, the authors reported that at the end of the DMT program the autistic children were still not able to fully engage with others.

In 2003, Torrance described the results of a DMT program that was delivered to a small group of four 16- to 18-year-old autistic males. At the time of the study, these participants were completing their schooling at a special education institution. Over the course of nine months, they completed a weekly 45-minute DMT session. Torrance noted that at the end of the DMT program the participants demonstrated increased group cohesion by way of exhibiting respect for one another, increased turn-taking, and a reduction in violent outbursts. However, it is hard to know if this was due to the DMT program itself or another aspect of their education, or simply a result of them maturing and developing over time.

One of the most contemporary studies about the efficacy of DMT for a group of autistic adults was conducted in 2015 by Koch and colleagues. They conducted a feasibility study evaluating the effects of a DMT program for 31 adults (23 males, eight females; age range = 16–47 years; mean age = 22 years) who predominantly had a diagnosis of Asperger syndrome. Of these, 16 participants were assigned to a DMT group and 15 participants were assigned to a control group. Every dance session consisted of the same four-part routine. The first part was a warm-up exercise, which lasted 10 minutes, in which the therapist identified a characteristic of each participant and asked the other group members to try and identify this characteristic. For the second part, participants were divided into pairs where one person would make a physical movement or gesture and the other person would imitate that action. Then the people in the pair would swap roles. The third part of the program, which lasted for about 20 minutes, involved participants being in a circle and then one person making a physical movement while others watched and then copied. The fourth and final part lasted about 10–15 minutes and involved participants expressing their actual feelings and opinions about the DMT session. The aim of this component was to increase body awareness (interoception/proprioception), self-awareness, empathy, social skills, and self-other awareness.

To measure the efficacy of their seven-week DMT program, Koch and colleagues asked the participants before and after their program to complete a series of questionnaires. While the findings showed that their program was beneficial for autistics, Koch et al. stressed that their results should be treated with caution since they were based on a small sample and that they only used self-reported scales instead of more objective measures, such as questionnaires completed by the participant's parents. However, the idea that reports completed by parents are of more value than the individuals' personal perspectives also highlights an important aspect of much autism research; the devaluing of autistic lived experience. If autistics and their families' value different things and interpret the idea of beneficial differently it can impact on the validity of the conclusions. Koch et al. summarised their study by stating that:

> Our pilot results suggest that DMT [Dance Movement Therapy] can be effective and feasible for the treatment of individuals with ASD, causing improvement in body awareness, self-other awareness, psychological well-being, and social skills. (2015, p. 346).

Most studies have examined the therapeutic benefits of either musical programs or DMT programs. However, there are a few studies that have examined the therapeutic benefits of a combined music and DMT program. Mateos-Moreno and Atencia-Doña's (2013) study contained 16 adults with 'severe' autism; with eight males being assigned to a control group and seven males and one female being assigned to an experimental group. Over the course of 17 weeks, each participant completed two separate one-hour sessions of dance and musical activities. Over the course of the program, eight measurements were taken (i.e., once every three weeks) from each participant. Based on the evidence collected, they found that if delivered regularly, combined DMT and musical activities could be an effective strategy to help autistics improve their physical fitness and social skills.

8.3.2 Evaluation of dance and movement therapy (DMT)

Gold – Extremely promising and use with confidence

Like physical exercise, DMT programs can provide many different benefits to autistics from different ages and backgrounds. Additionally, the duration of DMT sessions, the frequency of DMT sessions per week, the duration of the DMT program, and the activities in the DMT program can be customised to suit an autistic's abilities. Due to this flexibility and that it has the potential to provide multiple benefits to different autistics we have rated DMT has been rated as 'Gold – Extremely promising and use with confidence'. However, if an individual autistic expressed a dislike or unwilling to engage in DMT then this should be respected.

8.3.3 Directions for research in the future about dance and movement therapy (DMT)

Despite there being a growing body of literature showing that DMT programs can give autistics benefits, there are still some areas where more research in the future can be conducted. At the moment there are not many studies evaluating the long-term benefits that DMT programs might deliver to autistics. In the interests of increasing our knowledge, studies in the future should address this gap by exploring if the benefits obtained from DMT programs are maintained long-term. Such research is important because if it shows that they do not provide any long-term benefits then this will strengthen the justification for trying other supports and activities. However, if longitudinal studies show the opposite results then the usage of other supports and activities might be unnecessary. In addition, it may be useful to conduct research on purely dance programs that are focused on a particular dance style such as hip-hop, classical, folk, etc, rather than just simplistic body movements as occurs in most DMT programs. If autistics can obtain similar or other benefits from attending dance classes rather than DMT sessions, this would open up accessibility to dance as a therapeutic support to a wider range of autistics in areas where DMT programs are not provided. It is important that future research values the input of the autistic participants and records how they felt about the DMT/dance programs, and their perceptions of any benefits and any issues, both in the immediacy of the program and longer term, once the program has ceased.

8.4 Yoga activities

8.4.1 Yoga activities

Yoga is a physical activity that combines controlled breathing and body movements. It can be viewed as a mind-body form of exercise, a complementary or alternative form of medicine, or as a religious practice which can involve a person using asanas or poses, controlled breathing, and chanting. Yoga is known to develop interoception, as when taught with fidelity it is an interoceptive activity, where the person moves their body and is guided to notice how their body feels in each pose or movement. In the past few years yoga's popularity has increased and it has been demonstrated to improve the well-being of people who have Parkinson's disease (Fan & Chen, 2011; Moriello et al., 2013; Sharma et al., 2015), coronary artery disease (Pal et al., 2011), and chronic lower back pain (Tekur et al., 2012). In general, research has indicated that the benefits of doing yoga regularly are improved fitness, increases in concentration, and greater physical awareness (Ehleringer, 2010; Pal et al., 2011; Tekur et al., 2012). Recently, yoga's potential therapeutic benefits for autistics have begun to be examined (Gwynette et al., 2015). There are also anecdotal reports from therapists, who have claimed that it can improve an autistic's focus and attention, sensory processing, communication, self-regulation, and motor control (Ehleringer, 2010).

In 2015, Gwynette and colleagues reviewed four studies about the potential benefits that autistics obtained from yoga. However, they found that the research examined had low methodological quality and that there was little reliable evidence which supported the conclusion that autistics obtained any benefits from yoga. Based on this finding, they concluded:

> While there are a number of reasons why yoga could potentially benefit patients with ASD including the direct and indirect treatment pathways, there are few published reports in this area ... Before yoga can be vetted as an evidence-based treatment, more rigorous trials are needed. For example, a higher number of subjects, randomization, control groups, blinded raters, manualized interventions, and outcome measures gauging core ASD symptoms and co-morbid psychiatric symptoms would strengthen the evidence base. (Gwynette et al., 2015, p. 4).

8.4.2 Evaluation of yoga activities

Rating: Insufficient amount of literature to rate the support's efficacy

Due to the small amount of literature we were not able to rate the efficacy of yoga activities for autistics. However, if it is done correctly, with a qualified and experienced yoga instructor, it is a safe activity that is likely to produce many benefits, such as improved fitness and greater motor control.

8.4.3 Directions for research in the future about yoga activities

Due to the paucity of literature, there are many areas where more research can be conducted into the benefits that yoga might give autistics. First, research studies could include a control group so that the potential benefits of yoga activities for autistics are clearly measured. Second, more studies could be conducted to see if particular age group of autistics obtain the most benefits from yoga activities. It could be that such activities are more effective in helping autistic children to relax and develop motor coordination skills than autistic adults. Alternatively, it could be of greatest benefit for elderly autistics in helping them maintain their physical skills. As some forms of yoga activate the parasympathetic nervous system, research could investigate if these types of yoga improve quality of life and decrease anxiety for autistics with anxiety. In conjunction with these suggestions, Gwynette et al. (2015, p. 5) posed the following questions which research in the future could address.

Future research directions expressed by Gwynette and colleagues

- Is yoga effective in improving the quality of life for patients with ASD…?
- How might certain characteristics of the patients, such as severity of autism symptoms, cognitive ability, or pre-existing levels of anxiety, affect potential treatment response?
- Is a more naturalistic setting, such as in school, (or yoga class) preferred to a clinical setting?
- Are any potential gains from yoga interventions maintained over time?
- What is the minimum and optimal number of hours of yoga per week required in order to observe clinical improvement?
- What level of training should providers have in order to implement yoga interventions for patients with ASD?

Source: Gwynette et al., 2015, p. 5.

8.5 Autistic perspectives of physical exercise programs

Have you ever used any type of physical therapy or activity to manage any aspect of your autism?

Most respondents who answered the question 'Have you ever used any type of physical therapy or activity to manage any aspect of your autism?' reported that they did not engage in physical exercise (n = 24, 42.86%). However, 15 (26.79%) stated that they have engaged in 'walking and/or running', 11 (19.64%) noted that they have participated in 'dance or movement therapy', and ten (17.86%) selected the option 'yoga and/ or pilates'.

Respondents' ratings of the efficacy of using a particular physical activity or therapy to manage symptoms related to autism

Most respondents who rated the efficacy of using a particular physical activity or therapy to manage symptoms related to autism selected the response 'enjoyed, found useful and found that my wellbeing and mood were improved' (n = 16, 31.37%). This was followed by six (11.76%) who reported that they 'enjoyed and found useful' a particular physical activity, six (11.76%) who 'enjoyed but did not find useful', three (5.88%) who found it neither useful nor enjoyable. As expected following a

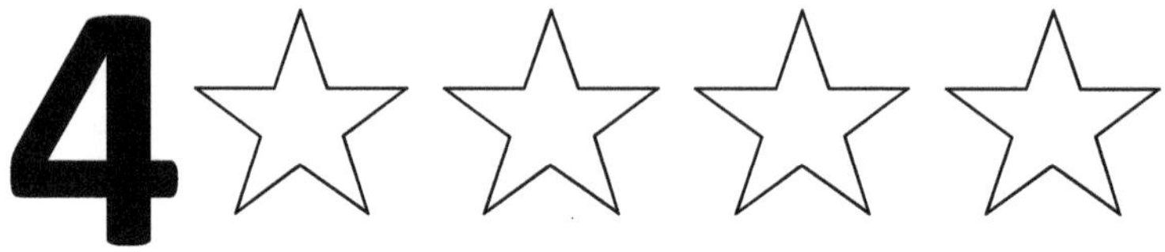

Figure 8.1 4 stars

preponderance of positive ratings, the efficacy of particular physical exercises for autistics as perceived by autistics was calculated as four stars.

Respondents' comments about using a particular physical activity or therapy to manage symptoms related to autism

When asked 'How did you find using a particular physical activity or therapy to manage symptoms related to your autism?' 19 respondents provided a comment. Our analysis of these comments showed that most believed physical exercise produced beneficial results. Of those who expressed a view that physical exercise was beneficial, six expressed a preference for walking.

> "As an adult I have found that walking every day helps me to stay physically and mentally well. If / when I experience chronic stress (which I have at various time points) I have found that by walking every day in our beautiful parkland, listening to the birds, the wind, the frogs, the trees, and breathing in the fresh air, whilst moving my body, is healing for me. It slows my 'over busy' mind down. It takes me out of my 'rumination' and quietens me down. I feel grounded, connected, whole. I would say that I practice mindfulness walking. This is my number one strategy for maintaining my mental health and wellbeing."
>
> "Dancing and walking both beneficial. I also pace as a stim, so that's not surprising. Repetitive physical actions like walking, dancing, and swinging are all very helpful."
>
> "Walking really helps regulate me when I am anxious."
>
> "Walking does help me to feel more grounded and centred."
>
> "Walking and talking. Helped clear my mind and reset myself. But it was doing this with a peer that helped."
>
> "Again, not a proper therapy but I enjoy walking as it is good thinking time and allows me to clear my mind, and I always say dancing keeps my sane – when you're in a dance class you have to be fully present, you can't be worrying about anything else."

In contrast, four believed physical exercise was stressful and did not produce any benefits. Three explained that physical exercise was stressful because of the emotional labour involved in interacting with others.

> "They had an impact on my stress and anxiety levels, and swimming especially was very calming for my nervous system, but my executive functioning issues and social anxiety make it very tough to actually engage in."
>
> "Dance and movement therapy – eventful getting me moving but emotional intensity of working 1:1 with therapist extremely hard. Hate when physical proximity too close but like doing things alongside her, following her lead."
>
> "Results great during and immediately after, but fade quickly and do not 'stick', e.g. no long-term improvement to motor skills or tactile processing. Working with a mainstream instructor (e.g. mainstream swim or yoga class) less than useless – they either completely ignore you or make you feel so incompetent/different/singled out that you leave and don't come back."

In interviewing an adult autistic with significant physical health conditions, they explained how it was very hard to sustain exercise routines unless they are based around their interests. They gave an example of a computerised component to the exercise if the person likes computers. They have done a range of physical activities and reported that.

> "any exercise reminds me of what I am capable of physically, even just swimming for a short time makes me feel great, even though I have a tendency to fear physical exercise in case it hurts. But once I do it, it connects me to my body and to the outside world. It is really good for my mental health too. I love being outside, and walking."

Since some participants explained that physical exercise was beneficial while others did not it is important that therapists take into consideration the views of their autistic clients when discussing the prospect of them engaging in physical exercise. The comments provided illustrate some of the barriers autistics feel when trying to engage in formal physical exercise, such as:

- struggling with executive functioning, which can result in arriving too late to a class to be allowed in;
- sensory difficulties which may make attending a class difficult; and
- receptive language and/or planning difficulties leading to feelings of incompetence.

8.6 Conclusion

This chapter reviewed the literature about the possible therapeutic benefits that physical activities can give autistics. It began with a review of the literature about the benefits of physical activity programs for autistics. It then examined the literature about the therapeutic benefits that DMT programs and yoga activities can give autistics. With the exception of yoga activities, which was rated as 'Insufficient information to make a recommendation, physical exercise and DMT were both rated as 'Gold – Extremely promising and use with confidence'. This chapter also examined areas where research in the future could be conducted. It stated, for example, that most studies have only explored the benefits that physical activities can give autistic children, often in the context of academic progress in school. In the future, and in the interests of furthering our knowledge in assisting autistic adults, it was argued that it would seem prudent to conduct studies about the effectiveness of physical activities for autistic adults. This chapter then concluded with a series of views and experiences from a group of autistics about the efficacy of physical activities for autistics, highlighting the benefits as well as some barriers to enjoying physical exercise activities.

References

American Dance Therapy Association. (2009). About dance/movement therapy. Retrieved from https://adta.org/faqs/.

Bahrami, F., Movahedi, A., Marandi, S. M., & Abedi, A. (2012). Kata techniques training consistently decreases stereotypy in children with autism spectrum disorder. *Research in Developmental Disabilities*, 33(4), 1183–1193. doi:10.1016/j.ridd.2012.01.018.

Boettinger, J. A. (1978). The study of the autistic child . In M. N. Costonis (Ed.), *Therapy in motion*. Urbana: University of Illinois Press.

Bremer, E., Crozier, M., & Lloyd, M. (2016). A systematic review of the behavioural outcomes following exercise interventions for children and youth with autism spectrum disorder. *Autism*, 20(8), 899–915. doi:10.1177/1362361315616002.

Burton, E., Cavalheri, V., Adams, R., Browne, C. O., Bovery-Spencer, P., Fenton, A. M., ... & Hill, K. D. (2015). Effectiveness of exercise programs to reduce falls in older people with dementia living in the community: A systematic review and meta-analysis. *Clinical Interventions in Aging*, 10, 421–434. doi:10.2147/CIA.S71691.

Chaiklin, S. (2009). We dance from the moment our feet touch the earth . In S. Chaiklin & H. Wengrower (Eds.), *The art and science of dance/movement therapy* (pp. 3–11). New York: Routledge.

Costonis, M. (Ed.). (1978). *Therapy in motion*. Chicago: University of Illinois Press.

de Labra, C., Guimaraes-Pinheiro, C., Maseda, A., Lorenzo, T., & Millán-Calenti, J. C. (2015). Effects of physical exercise interventions in frail older adults: A systematic review of randomized controlled trials. *BMC Geriatrics*, 15(1), 154. doi:10.1186/s12877-015-0155-4.

Den Heijer, A. E., Groen, Y., Tucha, L., Fuermaier, A. B., Koerts, J., Lange, K. W., ... & Tucha, O. (2017). Sweat it out? The effects of physical exercise on cognition and behavior in children and adults with ADHD: A systematic literature review. *Journal of Neural Transmission*, 124 (1), 3–26. doi:10.1007/s00702-016-1593-7.

Ehleringer, J. (2010). Yoga for children on the autism spectrum. *International Journal of Yoga Therapy*, 20(1), 131–139.

Fan, J. T., & Chen, K. M. (2011). Using silver yoga exercises to promote physical and mental health of elders with dementia in long-term care facilities. *International Psychogeriatrics*, 23(8), 1222–1230. doi:10.1017/S1041610211000287.

Fitt, S. S. (1988). *Dance Kinesiology*. New York: Schirmer Books.

Gehricke, J. G., Chan, J., Farmer, J. G., Fenning, R. M., Steinberg-Epstein, R., Misra, M., ... & Neumeyer, A. M. (2020). Physical activity rates in children and adolescents with autism spectrum disorder compared to the general population. *Research in Autism Spectrum Disorders*, 70, 101490. doi:10.1016/j.rasd.2019.101490.

Goodwin, M. S., Mazefsky, C. A., Ioannidis, S., Erdogmus, D., & Siegel, M. (2019). Predicting aggression to others in youth with autism using a wearable biosensor. *Autism Research*, 12(8), 1286–1296. doi:10.1002/aur.2151.

Grassmann, V., Alves, M. V., Santos-Galduróz, R. F., & Galduróz, J. C. F. (2017). Possible cognitive benefits of acute physical exercise in children with ADHD: A systematic review. *Journal of Attention Disorders*, 21(5), 367–371. doi:10.1177/1087054714526041.

Green, V. A., Pituch, K. A., Itchon, J., Choi, A., O'Reilly, M., & Sigafoos, J. (2006). Internet survey of treatments used by parents of children with autism. *Research in Developmental Disabilities*, 27(1), 70–84. doi:10.1016/j.ridd.2004.12.002.

Griera, J. L., Manzanares, J. M., Barbany, M., Contreras, J., Amigó, P., & Salas-Salvadó, J. (2007). Physical activity, energy balance and obesity. *Public Health Nutrition*, 10(10A), 1194–1199. doi:10.1017/S1368980007000705.

Gwynette, M. F., Warren, N. J., Warthen, J., Truleove, J. S., & Ross, C. P. (2015). Yoga as an intervention for patients with autism spectrum disorder: A review of the evidence and future directions. *Autism Open Access*, 5(3), 1–7. doi:10.4172/2165-7890.1000155.

Hartshorn, K., Olds, L., Field, T., Delage, J., Cullen, C., & Escalona, A. (2001). Creative movement therapy benefits children with autism. *Early Child Development and Care*, 166(1), 1–5. doi:10.1080/0300443011660101.

Josefsson, T., Lindwall, M., & Archer, T. (2014). Physical exercise intervention in depressive disorders: Meta-analysis and systematic review. *Scandinavian Journal of Medicine & Science in Sports*, 24(2), 259–272doi:10.1111/sms.12050.

Knapen, J., Vancampfort, D., Moriën, Y., & Marchal, Y. (2015). Exercise therapy improves both mental and physical health in patients with major depression. *Disability and Rehabilitation*, 37 (16), 1490–1495. doi:10.3109/09638288.2014.972579.

Koch, S. C., Mehl, L., Sobanski, E., Sieber, M., & Fuchs, T. (2015). Fixing the mirrors: A feasibility study of the effects of dance movement therapy on young adults with autism spectrum disorder. *Autism*, 19(3), 338–350. doi:10.1177/1362361314522353.

Koff, S. R. (2000). Toward a definition of dance education. *Childhood Education*, 77(1), 27–32. doi:10.1080/00094056.2000.10522134.

Lang, R., Koegel, L. K., Ashbaugh, K., Regester, A., Ence, W., & Smith, W. (2010). Physical exercise and individuals with autism spectrum disorders: A systematic review. *Research in Autism Spectrum Disorders*, 4(4), 565–576doi:10.1016/j.rasd.2010.01.006.

Mateos-Moreno, D., & Atencia-Doña, L. (2013). Effect of a combined dance/movement and music therapy on young adults diagnosed with severe autism. *The Arts in Psychotherapy*, 40(5), 465–472. doi:10.1016/j.aip.2013.09.004.

Moriello, G., Denio, C., Abraham, M., DeFrancesco, D., & Townsley, J. (2013). Incorporating yoga into an intense physical therapy program in someone with Parkinson's disease: A case report. *Journal of Bodywork and Movement Therapies*, 17(4), 408–417. doi:10.1016/j.jbmt.2013.01.005.

Movahedi, A., Bahrami, F., Marandi, S. M., & Abedi, A. (2013). Improvement in social dysfunction of children with autism spectrum disorder following long term Kata techniques training. *Research in Autism Spectrum Disorders*, 7(9), 1054–1061. doi:10.1016/j.rasd.2013.04.012.

Nicholson, H., Kehle, T. J., Bray, M. A., & van Heest, J. (2011). The effects of antecedent physical activity on the academic engagement of children with autism spectrum disorder. *Psychology in the Schools*, 48(2), 198–213. doi:10.1002/pits.20537.

Oriel, K. N., George, C. L., Peckus, R., & Semon, A. (2011). The effects of aerobic exercise on academic engagement in young children with autism spectrum disorder. *Pediatric Physical Therapy*, 23(2), 187–193. doi:10.1097/PEP.0b013e318218f149.

Oriel, K. N., Kanupka, J. W., DeLong, K. S., & Noel, K. (2016). The impact of aquatic exercise on sleep behaviors in children with autism spectrum disorder: A pilot study. *Focus on Autism and Other Developmental Disabilities*, 31(4), 254–261. doi:10.1177/1088357614559212.

Pal, A., Srivastava, N., Tiwari, S., Verma, N. S., Narain, V. S., Agrawal, G. G., ... & Kumar, K. (2011). Effect of yogic practices on lipid profile and body fat composition in patients of coronary artery disease. *Complementary Therapies in Medicine*, 19(3), 122–127. doi:10.1016/j.ctim.2011.05.001.

Pan, C. Y. (2010). Effects of water exercise swimming program on aquatic skills and social behaviors in children with autism spectrum disorders. *Autism*, 14(1), 9–28. doi:10.1177/1362361309339496.

Rosenblatt, L. E., Gorantla, S., Torres, J. A., Yarmush, R. S., Rao, S., Park, E. R., ... & Levine, J. B. (2011). Relaxation response–based yoga improves functioning in young children with autism: A pilot study. *The Journal of Alternative and Complementary Medicine*, 17(11), 1029–1035. doi:10.1089/acm.2010.0834.

Rosenthal-Malek, A., & Mitchell, S. (1997). Brief report: The effects of exercise on the self-stimulatory behaviors and positive responding of adolescents with autism. *Journal of Autism and Developmental Disorders*, 27(2), 193–202. doi:10.1023/A:1025848009248.

Scharoun, S. M., Reinders, N. J., Bryden, P. J., & Fletcher, P. C. (2014). Dance/movement therapy as an intervention for children with autism spectrum disorders. *American Journal of Dance Therapy*, 36(2), 209–228. doi:10.1007/s10465-014-9179-0.

Schauder, K. B., Mash, L. E., Bryant, L. K., & Cascio, C. J. (2015). Interoceptive ability and body awareness in autism spectrum disorder. *Journal of Experimental Child Psychology*, 131, 193–200. doi:10.1016/j.jecp.2014.11.002.

Shah, P. (2016). Interoception: The eighth sensory system: Practical solutions for improving self-regulation, self-awareness and social understanding of individuals with autism spectrum and related disorders. *Journal of Autism and Developmental Disorders*, 46(1), 3193–3194. doi:10.1007/s10803-016-2848-8.

Sharma, N. K., Robbins, K., Wagner, K., & Colgrove, Y. M. (2015). A randomized controlled pilot study of the therapeutic effects of yoga in people with Parkinson's disease. *International Journal of Yoga*, 8(1), 74–79. doi:10.4103/0973-6131.146070.

Sorensen, C., & Zarrett, N. (2014). Benefits of physical activity for adolescents with autism spectrum disorders: A comprehensive review. *Review Journal of Autism and Developmental Disorders*, 1(4), 344–353. doi:10.1007/s40489-014-0027-4.

Sowa, M., & Meulenbroek, R. (2012). Effects of physical exercise on autism spectrum disorders: A meta-analysis. *Research in Autism Spectrum Disorders*, 6(1), 46–57. doi:10.1016/j.rasd.2011.09.001.

Tekur, P., Nagarathna, R., Chametcha, S., Hankey, A., & Nagendra, H. R. (2012). A comprehensive yoga programs improves pain, anxiety and depression in chronic low back pain patients more than exercise: An RCT. *Complementary Therapies in Medicine*, 20(3), 107–118. doi:10.1016/j.ctim.2011.12.009.

Torrance, J. (2003). Autism, aggression, and developing a therapeutic contract. *American Journal of Dance Therapy*, 25(2), 97–109. doi:10.1023/B:AJOD.0000004757.28220.68.

Vonder Hulls, D. S., Walker, L. K., & Powell, J. M. (2006). Clinicians' perceptions of the benefits of aquatic therapy for young children with autism: A preliminary study. *Physical & Occupational Therapy in Pediatrics*, 26(1–2), 13–22. doi:10.1080/J006v26n01_03.

Chapter 9

Music and art therapy

9.1 Introduction

This chapter examines the results in the literature about the potential therapeutic benefits of music and art therapy for autistics. This chapter begins with a definition and overview of the support and then it presents the findings in the literature about its possible therapeutic benefits for autistics. A rating of the support's efficacy for autistics and an explanation for some directions for where research can be conducted in the future are then presented. Afterwards, a collection of views from a sample of autistics about their experiences and views of music and/or art for therapeutic means is then presented.

9.2 Music therapy

9.2.1 Music therapy

According to the World Federation of Music Therapy, music therapy:

> is the professional use of music and its elements as an intervention in medical, educational, and everyday environments with individuals, groups, families, or communities who seek to optimize their quality of life and improve their physical, social, communicative, emotional, intellectual, and spiritual health and wellbeing. Research, practice, education, and clinical training in music therapy are based on professional standards according to cultural, social, and political contexts. (Haase, 2012, p. 194).

Music therapy has been found to give many benefits to people of different ages and (dis)abilities. It has been found to help improve the quality of life of people with dementia (Särkämö et al., 2014), strokes (van Wijck et al., 2012), or depression (Erkkilä et al., 2011). Our review of the research about support programs for autistics revealed three literature reviews in which the authors examined studies about the efficacy of music programs of music therapy for autistics (Geretsegger et al., 2014; James et al., 2015; Shi, Lin, & Xie, 2016).

Geretsegger et al. (2014) has perhaps published one of the most comprehensive literature reviews about the possible benefits of music therapy for autistics. They examined ten studies that collectively explored the benefits that this therapy gave 165 autistic participants. The music therapy programs ranged in duration from one to seven months. Based on the diverse variety of studies analysed, Geretsegger et al. (2014, p. 3) concluded that:

> Music therapy may help children with ASD to improve their skills in important areas such as social interaction and communication. Music therapy may also contribute to increasing social adaptation skills in children with ASD and to promoting the quality of parent-child relationships ... More research with adequate design and using larger numbers of patients is needed. It is important to specifically examine how long the effects of music therapy last.

James and colleagues published a literature review about the efficacy of music therapy for autistics in 2015. They examined single-case studies and found that seven provided evidence that was conclusive. However, they found that three were deemed as having conflicting evidence (Katagiri, 2009; Lim & Draper, 2011; Pasiali, 2004). These three received this rating because they either had too many variables and possible carry-over effects (Pasiali, 2004) or an insufficient or absent inter-rated system for agreeing on the results (Katagiri, 2009; Lim & Draper, 2011). Finally, two were classified as having insufficient evidence because they used quasi-research designs to establish their conclusions (Boso et al., 2007; Kern, Wakeford, & Aldridge, 2007). Based on these findings, James et al. concluded that there is still a need for more robust, high-quality experimental research about the therapeutic benefits that music therapy can give autistics. Despite this desire, James et al. (2015, p. 39) concluded:

> Outcomes were positive for 58% of the studies and mixed for 42% of the studies. Certainty of evidence was rated as conclusive for 58% of the studies. The existing literature suggests that music therapy is a promising practice for individuals with ASD, but additional research is warranted to further establish its generality and the mechanisms responsible for behavior change.

Most of the literature about the benefits that musical activities can bring to autistics have been published in Western nations. However, some studies about this topic have been conducted in non-Western countries. Shi, Lin, and Xie (2016) searched for relevant studies conducted in China about this topic. They found that music therapy could help autistic children improve their mood, behaviour, language, sensory perception, and social skills.

9.2.2 Evaluation of music therapy

Rating: Silver – Usually promising

Based on the literature that we examined we have rated the efficacy of music therapy for autistics as *'Silver – Usually promising'* because much of the research within this area contains methodological flaws. Thus, it is not possible to conclude definitively that it can help autistics.

9.2.3 *Directions for research in the future about music therapy*

Despite there being many studies, there still remains three areas where more research can be conducted about the efficacy of music therapy for autistics. First, most of the studies examined by Geretsegger et al. (2014) and James et al. (2015) examined the benefits that autistic children have obtained from music therapy. Due to this focus, the benefits that it can provide autistic adults remains largely unknown. In the future, studies should address this gap because if the results are positive then autistic adults, their families and clinicians could consider music therapy as a potential support option. Second, James et al. highlighted that the studies about the efficacy of music therapy for autistics contain methodological flaws that could have undermined the results collected. For example, they examined two studies that had insufficient evidence because they used quasi-research designs to establish their conclusions (Boso et al., 2007; Kern, Wakeford, & Aldridge, 2007). In the future, studies should address these flaws so that we have a more robust understanding about the utility of music therapy for autistics. Third, not much longitudinal research has measured if autistics continue to use and maintain the skills developed during music therapy after the program has ended. Such research is important since it can help autistics, their families and people who support autistics decide if autistics need other supports once the music therapy program has ended.

9.2.4 *Autistic views about music therapy*

Have you personally taken part in music therapy as an autism therapy?

Out of the 206 respondents who completed our online survey, 56 (27.18%) answered the question 'Have you personally taken part in music therapy as an autism therapy?' Most respondents selected the option 'No' (n = 41, 73.21%), seven (12.50%) selected the answer 'Yes', and eight (14.29%) selected the answer 'Yes I have taken part but it was not an autism therapy'.

Respondents' ratings of the efficacy of music therapy

Most respondents (n = 4, 7.8%) selected the option 'enjoyed, found useful and was able to be more confident or confident after participating' or 'enjoyed but did not find useful'. In addition, three (5.88%) selected the option 'Enjoyed and found useful' and two (3.92%) selected the option 'Did not enjoy but found useful'. Based on the distribution of responses, the efficacy of music therapy for autistics as perceived by autistics was calculated as 3.5 stars.

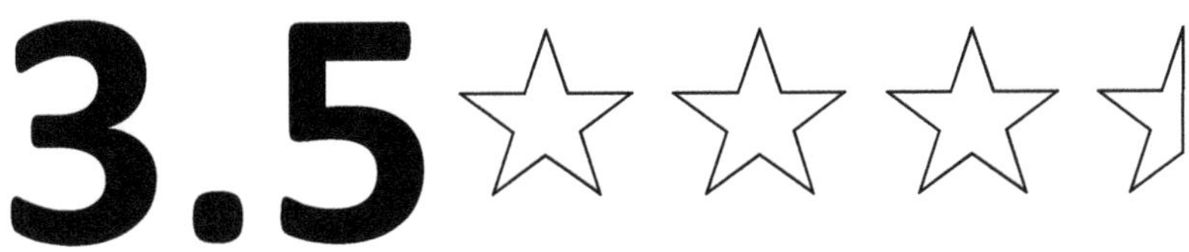

Figure 9.1 3.5 stars

Respondents' comments about music therapy

When asked 'How was your experience of music therapy?' seven respondents provided a comment. We determined that three reported favourable experiences or views of music therapy, despite never formally participating in such a therapy.

> "I have always played the piano (since age seven) as well as listening to music on a daily basis. Whilst I have not paid for "music therapy" I know that listening and playing music helps me immensely to regulate myself, express myself, feel connected, and find meaning in our world."
>
> "I use a form I taught myself and find it extremely helpful, but it's not formal."
>
> "Again due to my age it was never considered therapy but I certainly see my relationship with music as a therapy."

An autistic psychologist who has been involved in delivery music therapy, expressed how much they had enjoyed delivering this, but that.

> "it shouldn't be called music therapy, just music, it is great to see the joy on kids' faces as they engage with music, but I love music. I am not sure there was any benefit for the kids except for enjoyment, though some of the kids who didn't use speech could actually sing the songs. Sometimes, I would sing instructions to the kids instead of speaking the instructions and this was received better."

There were no comments in which respondents expressed negativity about music therapy. The paucity of comments from participants about their positive or negative experiences of music therapy could be that this therapy is not as readily accessible.

9.3 Art therapy

9.3.1 Art therapy

In an elementary sense, art therapy involves the use of artistic activities to help a client develop their social, communication, expressive, fine motor, and cognitive skills. Art therapy can be delivered individually, between the instructor and a participant, or in a group of participants with one instructor. It has traditionally been used to assist people after adverse events. For example, it has helped war veterans manage the debilitating effects of Post-Traumatic Stress Disorder (Campbell et al., 2016; Kopytin & Lebedev, 2013; Walker et al., 2016) and adults who have experienced trauma (Schouten et al., 2015) or who have substance use issues (Skeffington & Browne, 2014). The therapeutic benefits of art therapy for autistics have also been explored. Schweizer, Knorth, and Spreen (2014) examined 18 studies about the benefits that this therapy gave autistics (See Table 9.1).

They found that artistic activities have the potential to help autistics increase their tolerance of social interactions, improve social skills at home and at school, and increase verbal expressivity. Based on these findings they concluded:

> The results indicate that art therapy may add to a more flexible and relaxed attitude, a better self-image, and improved communicative and learning skills in

Table 9.1 Summary of studies examined by Schweizer, Knorth, and Spreen (2014)

Study	*Type of study*	*Gender*	*Age*	*Diagnosis*	*Duration of treatment*	*Art means and expression*	*Outcomes*
Bragge and Fenner, 2009	Theoretical study (art therapy theory and a model to evaluate practice). Examples from two cases	M[a]	7.5	HFA[a]	15 weeks, weekly sessions	Stereotyped images Representative images Broadening interests by exploring drawing and painting materials: Animals, landscape Sharing art experiences	Improved communication skills/social behaviour Improved self-image Transfer is not described
		F[a]	12.5	ASD[a] non-verbal	Unknown	Scribbling Kinaesthetic and sensory tactile play Sharing art experiences	Improved communication skills/social behaviour Explored art materials Transfer is not described
Elkis-Abuhoff, 2008	Case example with short theoretical founding	F	18	Before AT[a]: Social phobia After AT: Asperger	Seven months; once a week	Representative images Exploring a diversity of materials Tactile and playful experiences Themes from daily life, emotions Sharing art experiences Talking about the artwork is talking about her own functioning	Improved communication skills/social behaviour Improved self-image Improved learning skills
Emery, 2004	Case example in theoretical frame	M	6	ASD, normal intelligence	Seven months; frequency unknown	From kinaesthetic and pre-representative experiences, to representative drawing of people and daily life, including talking about it Sharing art experiences Also drawing at home and better eye contact	Improved communication skills/social behaviour Improved learning skills
Etherington, 2012	Chapter in a book about assessment in art therapy. Practice example	M	6	Asperger	Unknown	From pre representative and fragmented drawing and painting, to representative human figure Becoming more personal Shared experiences. Talking about the work	Improved communication skills/social behaviour

(*continued*)

Study	*Type of study*	*Gender*	*Age*	*Diagnosis*	*Duration of treatment*	*Art means and expression*	*Outcomes*
Evans, 1998	Practice-oriented and theoretical research with examples from practice	M	6	ASD, verbal and non-verbal	Treatment of two years; frequency unknown	From stereotype representative drawing to kinaesthetic and sensory experiences with materials Becoming more personal Sharing art experiences	Improved communication skills/social behaviour More flexible behaviour Development of learning skills
Evans and Dubovsky, 2001	Book about Art Therapy and children with diagnosis ASD; case examples in theoretical frame [i.e., early developmental psychology (Stern, 1985)]	F	8	ASD, non-verbal	55 sessions; frequency unknown	Drawing, painting, pre-representative scribbles Sharing art experiences	Improved communication skills/social behaviour No transfer of results mentioned
		M	9	ASD, verbal	Unknown	Representative drawing, painting animals, people Sharing art experiences Talking about the artwork	More attention, more playful, use more space in his paintings, more tolerance for new experiences Greater insight and understanding of his own autism Improved self-image Transfer of results is not mentioned
		M	7	ASD, non-verbal	Two years; frequency is not mentioned	Pre-representative scribbling Kinaesthetic and sensory play in the space and with crayon, paper and water Sharing art experiences	Hardly any development Developed new play with water Great need of governing the situation No transfer mentioned

Study	*Type of study*	*Gender*	*Age*	*Diagnosis*	*Duration of treatment*	*Art means and expression*	*Outcomes*
Evans and Rutten-Saris, 1998	Chapter in book about art therapy with children with developmental problems. Examples from three cases in theoretical frame [i.e., early developmental psychology (Stern, 1985)]	M	10	ASD	Unknown	Representative drawing with increased control and awareness Pencils, crayons, paint, paper, water Animals, human figures Sharing art experiences	Improved communication skills/social behaviour Improved self-image Better regulation of anxiety and anger
		M	8	ASD	Unknown	Pre-representative scribbles Stockmar wax crayons, paper Kinaesthetic and sensory experiences Sharing art experiences	Improved communication skills/social behaviour Improved self-image More quality of life
		M	6–8	ASD	Unknown	Pre-representative scribbles Stockmar wax crayons, paper Kinaesthetic and sensory experiences Sharing art experiences	Improved communication skills/social behaviour Improved self-image Improved learning skills
Gabriels, 2003	Chapter in Handbook Art Therapy; theoretical overview with general practice examples	-	-	All types	Unknown	A diversity of art media, tools and activities Sensory and kinaesthetic experiences Shared experiences	Improved communication skills/social behaviour Better regulation of anger and anxiety Improved learning skills
Goucher, 2012	Chapter in a book about play based interventions for children with ASD	M	13 up to 17 years	Asperger	Group: Two years	Representative drawing and writing Broadened interests from stereotyped interests Expressed and talked about his insecurities and fears which diminished Sharing art experiences	Improved communication skills/social behaviour Improved self-image Increased flexibility Awareness of pleasure Reduced anxiety
		M	13 up to 17 years	ASD	Several years	Representative shaping with a variety of art materials Increased differentiation of images and symbols. From rainbows to animals, to portraits Sharing art experiences	Improved communication skills/social behaviour Improved self-image More control over art materials and more self-control

Study	*Type of study*	*Gender*	*Age*	*Diagnosis*	*Duration of treatment*	*Art means and expression*	*Outcomes*
Henley, 1999	A qualitative group study of five years of Art Therapy Summer Camps with 25 children with ASD and ADHD	M	Group: 6–12 Case: 7	ASD/ADHD	Five weeks, daily program	Representative and expressive play. Animals Every facet of the daily camp experience is a potential creative therapeutic experience Sharing art experiences with other children	Improved communication skills/social behaviour Improved self-image Transfer: Many children behaved better at home
Isserow, 2008	Theoretical study (art therapy theory; joint attention theory; psycho-analytical points of view). Examples from two cases	F	17	ASD non-verbal	Seven months AT, weekly sessions	Pre-representative sensory and kinaesthetic experiences Own saliva, water and paint Slightly awareness of materials and the other	Slightly more aware of the (verbal) other and of the material
		M	12	ASD high intelligence	Unknown	Representative and expressive shaping Claying a portrait with scared eyes Talking about experiences in art and in daily life	Improved communication skills/social behaviour Improved self-image Reduced anxiety
Kornreich and Schimmel, 1991	Case study	M	11	DSM III: Early infantile Autism with schizophrenic features and functional mental retardation	Two years, once a week	Representative stereotype figures are becoming more personal with drawing and painting materials, water clay and tissue paper Themes from the world around him: Family members, animals, landscape seen from the window Talking about drawings and daily life	Improved communication skills/social behaviour, also at home and in school Better regulation of anger and anxiety Improved learning skills Improved self-image
Lu et al., 2010	Action research and theoretical frame of Jungian sandplay therapy. Case vignettes illustrating descriptions of development of play skills	Two girls, 23 boys	7–12	ASD at different levels of functioning	Ten weeks intervention, once a week 60 min, 5–10 min Opening and closing rituals Both individually and in small groups	Sensoric and symbolic experiences in sandtray with sand and colourful figurines and building materials, water Stimulating sensory play and symbolic expression Sharing art experiences	Improved communication skills/social behaviour Better regulation of anger and anxiety More flexible behaviour Improved learning skills

Study	*Type of study*	*Gender*	*Age*	*Diagnosis*	*Duration of treatment*	*Art means and expression*	*Outcomes*
Martin, 2009a	Qualitative study. Theory and practice based	Unknown	Unknown	ASD at different levels of functioning	Unknown	The whole range of expressive materials and possibilities to stimulate sensory and expressive experiences	Unknown
Martin, 2009b	Practice based and theory based.	Numerous examples from practice	experiences	≥2	ASD at different levels of functioning	?	Often pre-representative stadium and kinaesthetic stimulus Diversity of painting materials, drawing materials, clay, textile, found objects
Improved communication skills/social behaviour Improved learning skills More flexible behaviour Better self-image							
Schweizer, 1997[b]	Case examples in theoretical frame [i.e., early developmental psychology (Stern, 1985)]	M	8	PDD-NOS[a]	1.5 year 2× weekly treatment	Representative images: Drawing stereotyped figures from his own scary fantasy world to a more crafts-like shaping Experiences with different art materials to a safer symbolic work Talking about the techniques and safety here and now	Improved communication skills/social behaviour Improved self-image More flexible behaviour Better regulation of anger and anxiety
Schweizer, 2014[b]	Theory based on interviews with eight art therapists about their practice examples	M, F	6 up to 12 years	ASD	Unknown	Representative and pre-representative expressions Thematic/symbolic expressions Sensory experiences Broad diversity of materials, techniques and expressions Sharing art experiences	Improved communication skills/social behaviour Improved self-image Better regulation of anger and anxiety More flexible behaviour Showing the child's art to enjoy life Better planning skills

Study	*Type of study*	*Gender*	*Age*	*Diagnosis*	*Duration of treatment*	*Art means and expression*	*Outcomes*
Van Zweden-Van Buren, 2007[b]	MA thesis, based on literature comparing art therapy with art education as interventions for children with ASD. Recommendations for art therapy	Unknown	Unknown	ASD at different levels of functioning	Unknown	Expressive materials are used to develop varied and deeper experiences and understanding of body and inner world	Improved self-image More flexible behaviour Better regulation of anger and anxiety Improved communication skills/social behaviour

Key:
[a] Explanation of abbreviations: M = male; F = female; HFA = High Functioning Autism; ASD = Autism Spectrum Disorder; PDD-NOS = Pervasive Developmental Disorder – Not Otherwise Specified; AT = Art Therapy.
[b] Study not included in the reference list.
Source: Schweizer, Knorth, and Spreen, 2014, pp. 580–589.

> children with ASD. Art therapy might be able to contribute in mitigating two main problem areas: social communicative problems, and restricted and repetitive behaviour patterns. Typical art therapeutic elements such as sensory experiences with sight and touch may improve social behavior, flexibility and attention-abilities of autistic children. (Schweizer, Knorth, & Spreen, 2014, p. 577).

In Malchiodi's (2011) book, *Handbook of Art Therapy*, Gabriels presented an overview of the research about the application of art therapy for autistics, noting that artistic activities could help autistics improve their fine motor skills when they use paintbrushes or pencils to draw objects. It can also help them develop their cognitive skills in terms of coordinating colours and shapes to illustrate rudimentary objects. For example, by placing a triangle on top of a big square then placing a smaller square in the centre at the base of the bigger square, an individual can symbolise a house. Alternatively, placing a cloud-like green shape on top of a brown rectangle can symbolise a tree. Art therapy can also help autistic children develop their social skills, especially if they have to cooperate when sharing artistic equipment with others or are asked to explain their artistic creations to their peers or their art instructors. Similarly, such interactions can help non-autistic peers learn about the autism spectrum, especially through learning how to cooperate and socialise with those who are autistic.

9.3.2 Evaluation of art therapy

Rating: Silver – Usually promising

Based on the studies examined we have rated the efficacy of art therapy for autistics as 'Silver – Usually promising'. We gave art therapy this rating because while autistics can obtain many different benefits from this therapy, such as improvements in social and fine motor skills, it remains unknown if all autistics can obtain the same benefits. Additionally, due to a lack of research it is unknown if the skills autistics develop during art therapy are maintained long-term.

9.3.3 Directions for research in the future about art therapy

Despite current indications that art therapy has potential to help autistics, there remains areas where more research can be conducted. First, it is unclear what component or combination of components in the art therapy program produces the most beneficial outcomes for autistics. In other words, we do not know what factors in the art therapy program helps autistics improve their social skills. Is it the interaction between the autistic participant and their artistic instructor or peers in the art therapy program? Is it the act of the autistic participant describing their art projects to their peers or instructor? Or is it a combination of these factors or another factor altogether?

Second, not much research has examined if autistics retain the skills, they have developed during the art therapy program after the program itself ends. To address this lack of research, researchers should re-examine a participant's acquired skills during a follow-up period to assess if the benefits that they have obtained from art therapy programs are retained long-term. If such research shows that the skills and abilities developed and refined during art therapy programs decline over the long-term then this would justify the usage of other autism supports. However, if the opposite result is discovered then the usage of other supports would not be warranted, saving autistics time and financial resources in using other support strategies and programs.

Third, autistic children have been the focus of most of the research about the therapeutic value of art therapy for autistics. Consequently, there is a scarcity of research about this topic for autistic adults. However, they most likely would have a greater need to participate in artistic activities than autistic children since they routinely engage in more complex and diverse social situations. Furthermore, unlike autistic children, who routinely rely on their parents for support, artistic activities may help autistic adults develop their independence.

Fourth, in comparison to non-autistics, autistics have greater rates of comorbid psychological conditions, such as depression and anxiety (Buck et al., 2014; Croen et al., 2015; Lugnegård, Hallerbäck, & Gillberg, 2011). While research has shown that art therapy can help improve an autistic's social and motor skills, it is unknown if it can also help them manage their comorbid psychological conditions. If research shows that it can help them manage such conditions, then it could complement traditional treatment approaches, or it might even have the potential to be an alternative form of support altogether.

9.3.4 Autistic views about art therapy

Have you personally taken part in art/drawing therapy as an autism therapy?

Out of the 206 respondents who completed our online survey, 56 (27.18%) answered the question 'Have you personally taken part in art/drawing therapy as an autism therapy?' Of those who answered this question, 30 (53.57%) selected 'No', 16 (28.57%) selected 'Yes I have taken part but it was not an autism therapy', and 10 (17.86%) selected 'Yes'.

Respondents' ratings of the efficacy of art/drawing therapy

Of the 52 respondents who made a comment about the efficacy of art/drawing therapy, nine (17.31%) selected the option 'enjoyed but did not find useful', eight (15.38%) selected the option 'enjoyed, found useful and was able to be more confident or confident after participating', and six (11.54%) selected the option 'enjoyed and found useful'. Based on the distribution of responses, the efficacy of art therapy for autistics as perceived by autistics was calculated as 3.5 stars.

Respondents' comments about art/drawing therapy

When asked 'How was your experience of art/drawing therapy?' 15 respondents provided a comment. Our analysis of their responses showed that most recalled that art/drawing therapy provided them with positive benefits, while three expressed the opposite view. Three respondents highlighted that it relaxed them.

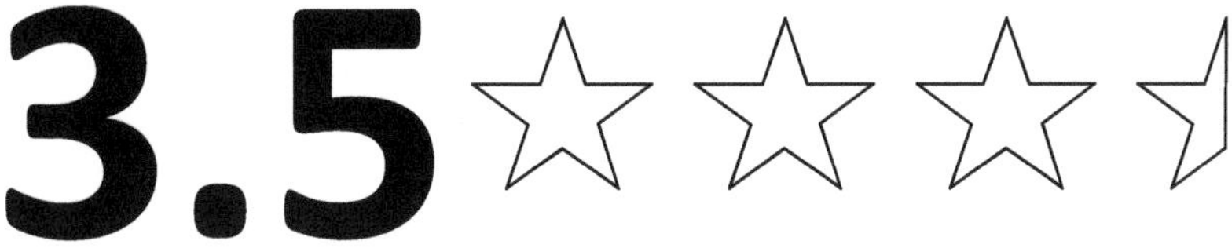

Figure 9.2 3.5 stars

> "I did art therapy when I was an inpatient in a psychiatric ward. I enjoyed it and found it was helpful for managing anxiety and improving my mood a little."
> "Able to use another part of my brain and feel more free."
> "Art relaxes me and when I am relaxed, I am more confident in interacting with the world."

While three respondents found art/drawing therapy relaxing, two found that it was a more effective form of communication than expressing comments using words.

> "Art is the most useful tool of all (next to my therapy dog). I can instantly shut out everything else, focusing only on my art. I can express myself in a way I can't with words (and I am fully verbal). I feel the colour and it reminds me of my value."
> "Best therapy for me. I'd communicate and share and it was not to intense. Even others sharing not too intense as I could doodle while I listened. Brilliant for me."
> In contrast, three respondents believed that art/drawing therapy was ineffective, they stated.
> "It was not clear to me how this would help. The creative therapist did not understand much about autism."
> "Therapist seemed to ascribe different meanings to things than I did."
> "The therapist used a shredder as part of the treatment. It was awful."

Our analysis of the respondents' comments showed that some found art/drawing therapy enjoyable and beneficial while others did not hold this view, although in all these cases it seemed to be the therapist rather than the art component that was problematic. Since art/drawing therapy appears not to be universally beneficial, autistics should be consulted about if they would like to participate in this therapy before they start art/drawing therapy.

9.4 Conclusion

This chapter examined the literature about the therapeutic benefits that music and art therapies might provide autistics. Based on the literature reviewed, art and music therapy were both rated as 'Silver – Usually promising' since there remain questions about its utility for autistic adults and whether or not the benefits obtained continue after the therapy program has ended. These limitations present potential opportunities for research in the future. Finally, the autistic perspectives presented in this chapter showed that artistic activities were generally experienced as a beneficial form of therapy as they enabled autistics the opportunity to express their sense of self and the wider world in unconventional and innovative ways that go beyond the more traditional allied health professional therapist-client interaction paradigm.

References

Boso, M., Emanuele, E., Minazzi, V., Abbamonte, M., & Politi, P. (2007). Effect of long-term interactive music therapy on behaviour profile and music skills in young adults with severe autism. *Journal of Alternative and Complementary Medicine*, 13(7), 709–712. doi:10.1089/acm.2006.6334.

Bragge, A., & Fenner, P. (2009). The emergence of the 'Interactive Square' as an approach to art therapy with children on the autistic spectrum. *International Journal of Art Therapy*, 14(1), 17–28. doi:10.1080/17454830903006323.

Buck, T. R., Viskochil, J., Farley, M., Coon, H., McMahon, W. M., Morgan, J., & Bilder, D. A. (2014). Psychiatric comorbidity and medication use in adults with autism spectrum disorder. *Journal of Autism and Developmental Disorders*, 44(12), 3063–3071. doi:10.1007/s10803-014-2170-2.

Campbell, M., Decker, K. P., Kruk, K., & Deaver, S. P. (2016). Art therapy and cognitive processing therapy for combat-related PTSD: A randomized controlled trial. *Art Therapy*, 33(4), 169–177. doi:10.1080/07421656.2016.1226643.

Croen, L. A., Zerbo, O., Qian, Y., Massolo, M. L., Rich, S., Sidney, S., & Kripke, C. (2015). The health status of adults on the autism spectrum. *Autism*, 19(7), 814–823. doi:10.1177/1362361315577517.

Elkis-Abuhoff, D. L. (2008). Art therapy applied to an adolescent with Asperger's syndrome. *The Arts in Psychotherapy*, 35(4), 262–270. doi:10.1016/j.aip.2008.06.007.

Emery, M. J. (2004). Art therapy as an intervention for autism. *Art Therapy*, 21(3), 143–147. doi:10.1080/07421656.2004.10129500.

Erkkilä, J., Punkanen, M., Fachner, J., Ala-Ruona, E., Pöntiö, I., Tervaniemi, M., … & Gold, C. (2011). Individual music therapy for depression: Randomised controlled trial. *The British Journal of Psychiatry*, 199(2), 132–139. doi:10.1192/bjp.bp.110.085431.

Etherington, A. (2012). Assessing a young autistic boy in art therapy private practice . In *Assessment in Art Therapy* (pp. 117–121). Oxford: Routledge.

Evans, K. (1998). Shaping experience and sharing meaning art therapy for children with autism. *International Journal of Art Therapy: Inscape*, 3(1), 17–25. doi:10.1080/17454839808413055.

Evans, K., & Dubowski, J. (2001). *Art therapy with children on the autistic spectrum: Beyond words*. London: Jessica Kingsley Publishers.

Evans, K., & Rutten-Saris, M. (1998). Shaping vitality affects, enriching communication: Art therapy for children with autism. In *Development and diversity: New applications in art therapy*, 57–77.

Gabriels, R. L. (2003). Art therapy with children who have autism and their families . In Malchiodi, C. A. (Ed.) *Handbook of art therapy* (pp. 193–206). New York, NY: The Guilford Press.

Geretsegger, M., Elefant, C., Mössler, K. A., & Gold, C. (2014). Music therapy for people with autism spectrum disorder. *Cochrane Database of Systematic Reviews*, 2014(6). doi:10.1002/14651858.CD004381.pub3.

Goucher, C. (2012). Art therapy: Connecting and communicating. In *Play-based interventions for children and adolescents with autism spectrum disorders* (pp. 295–315).

Haase, U. (2012). Thoughts on WFMT's definition of music therapy. *Nordic Journal of Music Therapy*, 21(2), 194–195.

Henley, D. (1999). Facilitating socialization within a therapeutic camp setting for children with attention deficits utilizing the expressive therapies. *American Journal of Art Therapy*, 38(2), 40.

Isserow, J. (2008). Looking together: Joint attention in art therapy. *International Journal of Art Therapy*, 13(1), 34–42. doi:10.1080/17454830802002894.

James, R., Sigafoos, J., Green, V. A., Lancioni, G. E., O'Reilly, M. F., Lang, R., … & Marschik, P. B. (2015). Music therapy for individuals with autism spectrum disorder: A systematic review. *Review Journal of Autism and Developmental Disorders*, 2(1), 39–54. doi:10.1007/s40489-014-0035-4.

Katagiri, J. (2009). The effect of background music and song texts on emotional understanding of children with autism. *Journal of Music Therapy*, 46(1), 15–31. doi:10.1093/jmt/46.1.15.

Kern, P., Wakeford, L., & Aldridge, D. (2007). Improving the performance of a young child with autism during self-care tasks using embedded song interventions: A case study. *Music Therapy Perspectives*, 25(1), 43–51. doi:10.1093/mtp/25.1.43.

Kopytin, A., & Lebedev, A. (2013). Humor, self-attitude, emotions, and cognitions in group art therapy with war veterans. *Art Therapy*, 30(1), 20–29. doi:10.1080/07421656.2013.757758.

Kornreich, T. Z., & Schimmel, B. F. (1991). The world is attacked by great big snowflakes-art-therapy with an autistic boy. *American Journal of Art Therapy*, 29(3), 77–84.

Lim, H. A., & Draper, E. (2011). The effects of music therapy incorporated with applied behavior analysis verbal behavior approach for children with autism spectrum disorders. *Journal of Music Therapy*, 48(4), 532–550. doi:10.1093/jmt/48.4.532.

Lu, L., Petersen, F., Lacroix, L., & Rousseau, C. (2010). Stimulating creative play in children with autism through sandplay. *The Arts in Psychotherapy*, 37(1), 56–64. doi:10.1016/j.aip.2009.09.003.

Lugnegård, T., Hallerbäck, M. U., & Gillberg, C. (2011). Psychiatric comorbidity in young adults with a clinical diagnosis of Asperger syndrome. *Research in Developmental Disabilities*, 32(5), 1910–1917. doi:10.1016/j.ridd.2011.03.025.

Malchiodi, C. A. (Ed.). (2011). *Handbook of art therapy*. New York, NY: Guilford Press.

Martin, N. (2009a). Art therapy and autism: Overview and recommendations. *Art Therapy*, 26 (4), 187–190. doi:10.1080/07421656.2009.10129616.

Martin, N. (2009b). *Art as an early intervention tool for children with autism*. London: Jessica Kingsley Publishers.

Pasiali, V. (2004). The use of prescriptive therapeutic songs in a homebased environment to promote social skills acquisition by children with autism: Three case studies. *Music Therapy Perspectives*, 22(1), 11–20. doi:10.1093/mtp/22.1.11.

Särkämö, T., Tervaniemi, M., Laitinen, S., Numminen, A., Kurki, M., Johnson, J. K., & Rantanen, P. (2014). Cognitive, emotional, and social benefits of regular musical activities in early dementia: Randomized controlled study. *The Gerontologist*, 54(4), 634–650. doi:10.1093/geront/gnt100.

Schouten, K. A., de Niet, G. J., Knipscheer, J. W., Kleber, R. J., & Hutschemaekers, G. J. (2015). The effectiveness of art therapy in the treatment of traumatized adults: A systematic review on art therapy and trauma. *Trauma, Violence and Abuse*, 16(2), 220–228. doi:10.1177/1524838014555032.

Schweizer, C., Knorth, E. J., & Spreen, M. (2014). Art therapy with children with Autism Spectrum Disorders: A review of clinical case descriptions on 'what works'. *The Arts in Psychotherapy*, 41(5), 577–593. doi:10.1016/j.aip.2014.10.009.

Shi, Z. M., Lin, G. H., & Xie, Q. (2016). Effects of music therapy on mood, language, behavior, and social skills in children with autism: A meta-analysis. *Chinese Nursing Research*, 3(3), 137–141. doi:10.1016/j.cnre.2016.06.018.

Skeffington, P. M., & Browne, M. (2014). Art therapy, trauma and substance misuse: Using imagery to explore a difficult past with a complex client. *International Journal of Art Therapy*, 19(3), 114–121. doi:10.1080/17454832.2014.910816.

van Wijck, F., Knox, D., Dodds, C., Cassidy, G., Alexander, G., & MacDonald, R. (2012). Making music after stroke: Using musical activities to enhance arm function. *Annals of the New York Academy of Sciences*, 1252(1), 305–311doi:10.1111/j.1749-6632.2011.06403.x.

Walker, M. S., Kaimal, G., Koffman, R., & DeGraba, T. J. (2016). Art therapy for PTSD and TBI: A senior active duty military service member's therapeutic journey. *The Arts in Psychotherapy*, 49, 10–18. doi:10.1016/j.aip.2016.05.015.

Chapter 10

Psychotropic medications

10.1 Introduction

This chapter begins with a brief overview of the most common psychotropic medications used to treat the depression, insomnia, irritability, and attention deficit hyperactivity disorder (ADHD) that some autistics experience. Where a medication has not been reviewed, it is because there was a dearth of research around the usage of the medication specifically with autistics. Each following section contains the same three sub-sections; (1) an introduction to the co-morbid mental condition in the autistic population, (2) a summary and evaluation of the literature about the common psychotropic medication or medications that are often used to treat that specific condition, and (3) recommendations for research in the future about the psychotropic medication for autistics. This chapter also reviews the literature about Chelation therapy, a dangerous and potentially life-threatening treatment. With the exception of Chelation therapy, the efficacy of the psychotropic medications reviewed are not rated because each autistic's interaction with the prescription medication is different and should be overseen by a medical doctor. Therefore, it is not possible to rate the probable efficacy of each of the medications, as what works for one person may have no effect or indeed a negative impact on another person. This chapter concludes with a series of views from a group of autistics about their usage of prescription and non-prescription medications.

10.2 Literature review into studies about psychotropic medications for autistics

Currently, there are publications that have examined studies on a range of different psychotropic medications used to treat co-morbid mental conditions commonly experienced by autistics (Benvenuto et al., 2013; Fitzpatrick et al., 2016; Fung et al., 2012; Mohiuddin & Ghaziuddin, 2013; Siegel & Beaulieu, 2012). An examination of these publications revealed that there were ten main psychotropic medications used to treat four main mental health conditions (See Table 10.1). The literature exploring the effects of autistics using these common medications to treat these conditions is presented.

Table 10.1 Common psychotropic medications used to treat co-morbid mental conditions found in autistics

Co-morbid mental condition	*Psychotropic medication used to treat the co-morbid mental condition*
Depression	Selective Serotonin Reuptake Inhibitors (SSRIs) (i.e., fluoxetine, fluvoxamine, fenfluramine, citalopram, sertraline, paroxetineor, esctalopram)
Insomnia	Melatonin
Irritability	Risperidone, Aripiprazole
Attention deficit hyperactivity disorder (ADHD)	Atomoxetine, Clonidine, Methylphenidate

10.3 Depression

10.3.1 Overview of depression in the autistic population

The World Health Organization (2019) has defined depression as:

> a common mental disorder, characterized by persistent sadness and a loss of interest in activities that you normally enjoy, accompanied by an inability to carry out daily activities, for at least two weeks.

At higher rates than the general population, autistics can experience depression and suicidal ideation (Bennett, 2016). Depending on the definition and the study's sampling and methodological processes, the prevalence of depression in the autistic population can vary between 18 to 22% (Stewart et al., 2006). Aside from statistics, Stewart et al. (2006) found that most studies on depression in autism presented quantitative data (e.g., age when diagnosed with depression, number of depressive episodes) instead of qualitative experiences (e.g., personal experiences and views about depression). In response to this statistical focus, Bennett (2016) has emphasised that researchers should pay more attention to exploring the depression and suicidal ideation experiences of autistic adults.

10.3.2 Selective Serotonin Reuptake Inhibitors (SSRIs)

One of the most commonly researched family of medications used to treat depression, regardless of whether or not the patient is autistic, are Selective Serotonin Reuptake Inhibitors (SSRIs) (e.g., sertraline, paroxetine, esctalopram, fluoxetine, fluvoxamine, fenfluramine, and citalopram).

In 2013, Williams et al. examined nine Randomized Controlled Trials (RCTs) on SSRI being used by autistics to treat their depression, aggression, and anxiety. Collectively, 320 participants and four different medications in the SSRI family of medications were examined (i.e., fluoxetine, fluvoxamine, fenfluramine, and citalopram). Five studies examined the effect of SSRIs on autistic children and four examined their effect on autistic adults. In terms of treating depression, two studies examined the therapeutic potential that fluoxetine had in helping autistic adults manage their depression (Buchsbaum et al., 2001; Hollander et al., 2012).Both Buchsbaum et al. (2001) and

Hollander et al. (2012) reported that fluoxetine did not help reduce depression among autistic adults, as indicated by there being no observed difference between the treatment and control groups in regard to depression scores (mean difference 3.83, SD 3.87, P = 0.06).

Previously, Kolevzon, Mathewson, and Hollander (2006) published a review of studies about the tolerability and efficacy of SSRIs for autistics. They examined three RCTs (Buchsbaum et al., 2001; Hollander et al., 2004; McDougle et al., 1996) and ten open-label trials or retrospective chart reviews (Cook et al., 1992; DeLong, Ritch, & Burch, 2002; DeLong, Teague, & Kamran, 1998; Fatemi et al., 1998; Hellings et al., 1996; Martin et al., 2003; McDougle et al., 1998; Namerow et al., 2003; Owley et al., 2005; Steingard et al., 1997). Five medications in the SSRI family were examined; fluoxetine (Buchsbaum et al., 2001; DeLong, Ritch, & Burch, 2002; DeLong, Teague, & Kamran, 1998; Fatemi et al., 1998; Hollander et al., 2004), sertraline (Cook et al., 1992; Hellings et al., 1996; McDougle et al., 1998; Steingard et al., 1997), fluvoxamine (Martin et al., 2003; McDougle et al., 1996), citalopram (Namerow et al., 2003), and escitalopram (Owley et al., 2005). Based on the volume of literature examined, they concluded that:

> Although SSRIs [Selective Serotonin Reuptake Inhibitors] may demonstrate therapeutic benefit in autism spectrum disorder, methodological weaknesses of many of the clinical trials suggest the need for additional randomized controlled trials. Furthermore, given the increased awareness of the dangers associated with SSRI-induced activation and agitation, the presence of these side effects in the autistic population warrants closer attention to dosage, titration, and subject selection issues. (Kolevzon, Mathewson, & Hollander, 2006, p. 407).

Despite SSRIs being relatively commonplace as a treatment of depression and anxiety in both autistic children and adults there is currently a dearth of evidence supporting their efficacy in treating mood disorders within this population with most of the validation being extrapolated from studies of non-autistic individuals (Howes et al., 2018). Also of note the literature tends to suggest that SSRIs are less well tolerated by autistics with many studies indicating a significantly higher incidence of adverse effects for autistics on SSRIs. Hence, it is recommended and clinically prudent to start at the lowest possible dose followed by a slow dose titration coupled with regular reviews and close monitoring particularly of adverse effects (Howes et al., 2018).

The choice of SSRI is very individual with regards to efficacy and side-effect profile and hence is often a case of 'trial and error' although the use of shorter half-life ($t^1/_2$) antidepressants such as paroxetine are less commonly used due to side-effect liability and high risk of discontinuation syndrome with missed doses and/or abrupt cessation.

Citalopram is racemic, i.e., a combination of 'S' & 'R' – enantiomers (enantiomers by definition are non-superimposable mirror-images of each other – the fact they are not superimposable means they bind differently to receptors). Consequently the 'S' enantiomer of citalopram is estimated to be approximately 150 times greater potency for the serotonin-transporter in comparison to the 'R' enantiomer. Hence, 'S' – citalopram accounts for most of 'citalopram's' pharmacotherapeutic activity and because it is highly selective as an inhibitor of serotonin activity it tends to have less 'off-target' binding which (in theory at least) reduces adverse effects. There is some evidence to suggest that the 'R' enantiomer of citalopram may actually counteract the efficacy of the 'S' enantiomer molecule (Schatzberg & Nemeroff, 2013).

It is possible that in the future genetic studies may help inform more targeted psychotropic use in autistics. Currently only the use of fluoxetine has been studied in adult autistics with depression, which showed no change in depressive symptoms following treatment. However, fluoxetine was demonstrated to possibly reduce some symptoms of obsessive-compulsive disorder in adult autistics (Buchsbaum et al., 2001). The literature shows that in certain situations, some individual autistics may benefit from the use of SSRIs. However, due to a lack of research it is not possible at this stage to definitively claim that SSRIs can help most autistics manage depression.

10.3.3 Recommendations for research in the future about Selective Serotonin Reuptake Inhibitors (SSRIs)

There is currently a small amount of literature that has examined the role which SSRIs play in helping autistics manage their depression. Areas where research in the future could be conducted relate to the efficacy, side effects and interactions with additional supports.

Howes et al. (2018), noted that our understanding of the efficacy of SSRIs for autistics is based on studies about their efficacy for non-autistics. Consequently, future research should examine at what dose, with which medication, therapeutic efficacy may present for individual autistics when treating the depression that individual autistics experience. This research is complicated by an autistic's biology including age, weight, other co-occurring health conditions and varying absorption and metabolic rates of different medications.

The side effects that autistics can develop after long-term exposure to SSRIs remains predominantly unknown. For instance, all nine RCTs that Williams et al. (2013) reviewed, examined the efficacy of SSRIs for autistics from the beginning of the study until trial completion, which was a maximum duration of 12 weeks. Due to a lack of longitudinal research, the side effects that autistics develop from prolonged SSRI usage remains unknown. In the interest of protecting the health of future generations of autistics, longitudinal research that uncovers the potential consequences for autistics of prolonged SSRI usage should be conducted. Furthermore, such longitudinal research can help explain if medications in the SSRI family become ineffective over time, or if side effects become more problematic over time and subsequently would need to be discontinued.

Additionally, the handful of studies which have examined the therapeutic benefits of SSRIs in treating depression in autistics have not stated if the participants were receiving supplementary supports whilst taking SSRIs. To examine whether the therapeutic benefits of SSRIs can be enhanced it would be wise to study if combining SSRIs with other approaches that have been proven to reduce depression, such as physical exercise, can help autistics overcome depression more readily than a single strategy or approach. In the interests of confirming current results, as well as developing a more sophisticated understanding about the efficacy of different SSRIs in helping autistics manage their depression, more research about the role SSRIs have in specifically helping autistics should be conducted.

10.3.4 A note of caution about Selective Serotonin Reuptake Inhibitors (SSRIs)

Currently, there are still many gaps in our knowledge about the efficacy of SSRIs for treating the depression that autistics experience. SSRI medications should only be used on the advice of a medical professional, following a consultation and prescription for the specific medication. Individuals and treating practitioners should also take into consideration any potential side effects associated with SSRI usage, the costs associated with SSRI treatment, and all relevant medical history (e.g., previous physiological and psychological responses to antidepressant medications), as well as possible executive functioning difficulties that may make it difficult for an individual to remember to take the medication appropriately.

10.4 Insomnia

10.4.1 Overview of insomnia in the autistic population

In a rudimentary sense, insomnia is the inability to fall asleep or maintain sleep (Roth, 2007). It is widely believed that 30% of the adult population has at some point experienced symptoms of insomnia, such as difficulties with initiating or maintaining sleep, waking up too early, or low-quality sleep (Ancoli-Israel & Roth, 1999). It has been known for many years that there are significant negative consequences associated with insomnia in adulthood, including a greater likelihood of having industrial accidents, along with decreased work productivity (e.g., greater rates of absenteeism, decreased periods of concentration, and difficulty completing work tasks by deadlines) (Kuppermann et al., 1995).

Studies have shown that many autistics experience insomnia (Deliens et al., 2015; Mannion & Leader, 2014), and that their insomnia can be triggered or exacerbated by electronic media usage before bedtime and sensory sensitivities during bedtime. In 2013, Engelhardt, Mazurek, and Sohl used questionnaires to obtain information from 49 autistic boys, 38 boys with ADHD, and 41 typically developing boys about daily hours of media use, bedroom access to media, and average sleep hours per night. Irrespective of the diagnostic group, they found that media usage in the bedroom contributed to less time spent sleeping per night. Additionally, the usage of a television or computer before bedtime was more strongly associated with reduced sleep among autistic boys than boys with ADHD or typically developing boys.

Another factor that can exacerbate the insomnia that autistics experience is hypersensitivities to touch. As reported by Tzischinsky et al. (2018), an autistic's hypersensitivity to touch can potentially interfere with their sleep onset and maintenance. The autistic psychologist and educational consultant interviewed, confirmed this research finding stating:

"I can't sleep if the room is too hot, or the covers too heavy" and "As a child, I couldn't sleep unless I was wedged between the mattress and the wall, squished tight."

Incidentally, the autistic psychologist commented on the high levels of insomnia in the autistic children and adults that they worked with, and the significant impact of this on educational and social outcomes for the individuals. They suggested that the tendency of autistics to perseverate and analyse "everything that has ever gone wrong", contributes significantly to not being able to fall asleep. They both felt that the use of electronic devices at bedtime could be useful, acting "as a distractor, to block out all those ruminating negative thoughts", enabling autistics to fall asleep sooner.

10.4.2 Melatonin

Melatonin is often used to help autistics manage their insomnia (Andersen et al., 2008; Galli-Carminati, Deriaz, & Bertschy, 2009; Wright et al., 2011). There is a growing body of evidence supporting the use of exogenous melatonin (i.e., tablets) to augment the effects of its endogenous (naturally occurring in the body) counterpart in manipulating the sleep/wake cycle (i.e., circadian rhythms) which, in turn, improves the sleep/wake cycle for autistic children (Rossignol & Frye, 2011). In particular, the use of melatonin tablets appears to help improve sleep initiation by reducing the latency, or delay, in the onset of sleep. The efficacy demonstrated by the use of melatonin tablets in treating insomnia in autistic children appears to suggest that insufficient melatonin production and/or secretion and/or receptor response underpins the development of insomnia. Thus, given this evidence it seems reasonable that implementing environmental strategies designed to stimulate the increased production and release of endogenous melatonin from the pineal gland, such as eliminating light and avoiding the use of lighting emitting electronic devices, such as tablet computers and cell phones, are also important in helping to treat insomnia.

There are personal accounts of autistics using melatonin. For example, in Hayashi's (2000) study, a 14-year-old autistic male documented in a diary the impact that consuming melatonin had on his sleep/wake cycle. Parents have also described the sleep/wake effects that melatonin has had on their autistic children (Andersen et al., 2008). In 2011, Guénolé and colleagues published a systematic review in which they examined studies about the efficacy and safety of melatonin in the treatment of sleep disturbances among autistics. They examined three retrospective studies (Andersen et al., 2008; Galli-Carminatti, Deriaz, & Bertschy, 2009; Gupta & Hutchins, 2005), two open-label clinical trials (Giannotti et al., 2006; Paavonen et al., 2003), and three placebo-controlled trials (Garstang & Wallis, 2006; Wirojanan et al., 2009; Wright et al., 2011). Based on the studies that they examined, they concluded:

> As a whole, we found that the literature supports the existence of a beneficial effect of melatonin on sleep in individuals with ASD, with only few and minor side effects. However, considering the small number of studies and their methodological limits, these conclusions cannot yet be regarded as evidence-based. Randomized controlled trials and long-term follow-up data are still lacking to better assess efficacy and safety of exogenous melatonin for disordered sleep in individuals with ASD. (Guénolé et al., 2011, p. 379).

In 2011, Rossignol and Frye published a systematic review and meta-analysis about studies that examined the benefits that autistics obtained from melatonin. Out of the 18 studies that they examined, they found that one sampled autistic adults (Galli-Carminati, Deriaz, & Bertschy, 2009), another reported the effects of melatonin usage for individuals between three and 28 years (Ishizaki, Sugama, & Takeuchi, 1999), and the remaining 16 only measured the effects of melatonin usage on autistic children. Furthermore, the dosage of melatonin in the studies that Rossignol and Frye examined ranged from 0.75 mg per day (Galli-Carminati, Deriaz, & Bertschy, 2009) to 25 mg per day (Jan & O'Donnell, 1996). The length of time of melatonin exposure was wide ranging from 14 days (Paavonen et al., 2003) to four years (Jan & O'Donnell, 1996). Out of the 18 studies examined, nine provided ambiguous conclusions and nine concluded that melatonin usage resulted in improvements in sleep quality (Andersen et al., 2008; Galli-Carminati, Deriaz, & Bertschy, 2009; Hayashi, 2000; Horrigan & Barnhill, 1997; Ishizaki, Sugama, & Takeuchi, 1999; Jan & O'Donnell, 1996; Jan et al., 2004; Kulman et al., 2000; Miyamoto et al., 1999). Rossignol and Frye (2011, p. 792) concluded:

> The meta-analysis found that the use of melatonin in ASD is associated with significantly improved sleep parameters (sleep duration and sleep onset latency). Furthermore, melatonin appears to improve daytime behavior in some individuals with ASD and has minimal to no side effects.

Based on the research examined, melatonin has been found to significantly improve the sleep quality of some autistic children. Most of the research collected has examined the relationships between melatonin usage and sleep quality and duration for autistic children. Consequently, the potential melatonin has in helping autistics manage other problems, such as their irritability, remains unknown. It is possible that melatonin itself does not reduce irritability directly. Instead irritability may simply decrease as a result of increased sleep quality and duration.

Melatonin has been found to be safe and effective for some autistic children in reducing their insomnia. However, the same outcomes cannot be known for autistic adults since there is insufficient literature on the use of melatonin by adult autistics. However, it is always advisable to consult with medical professionals and take into consideration any potential side effects and other factors, such as the costs associated with melatonin, medical history and personal context before starting or stopping any medications or non-prescription tablets/liquids to aid with sleep (i.e., previous physiological responses to melatonin and other medications).

10.4.3 Recommendations for research in the future about melatonin

There is a considerable amount of research about the role melatonin has had in helping autistic children manage their insomnia. Despite this vast amount of literature, there are still two areas where more research would be useful. First, as highlighted by Rossignol and Frye (2011), few studies have examined if melatonin can help autistic adults manage their insomnia. It is important that the potential therapeutic value that melatonin gives autistic adults be explored so that they have more options to help them develop healthy sleep/wake patterns. Second, Cortesi et al. (2012) reported that the combination of cognitive behavioural therapy (CBT) and melatonin can produce more optimal outcomes in reducing insomnia than either melatonin or CBT alone. In the future, there should be more high-quality research designed to compared the efficacy of melatonin alone, melatonin and CBT, and CBT alone +/- placebo in treating symptoms of insomnia specifically in the autistic population. In light of the comments by the interviewed autistic psychologist and educational consultant, it may be useful for research to be conducted on what autistics are doing and thinking when they are struggling to fall asleep. Other research could focus on minimizing ruminating thoughts at bedtime, and the effect on insomnia in both autistic children and adults.

10.4.4 A note of caution about melatonin

While most of the research shows that melatonin can help some autistics manage their insomnia, in particular autistic children, it is prudent to consult with medical professionals. Individuals should also be vigilant in noting and reporting any potential side effects of melatonin to their treating doctor. Other factors to consider are the costs associated with using melatonin, which in many countries is a prescription only medication.

10.5 Irritability

10.5.1 Irritability in the autistic population

Lecavalier (2006) has stated that three of the most commonly observed challenging behaviours exhibited by autistics are irritability, aggression, self-injury and 'severe tantrums'. According to Mayes et al. (2011), maladaptive/dysregulated behaviours considered to be irritability are more common in those who have untreated co-morbid mood disorders. Hence, identifying and treating co-existing psychopathologies, such as depression with or without anxiety, is essential to ensure both diagnostic clarity and to help inform the most appropriate treatment options. This approach is particularly important since autistics might experience a higher incidence of side effects with psychotropic medications (Deb et al., 2014; Douglas-Hall et al., 2011).

While there is no cure for irritability, there are many approaches that can be used to reduce it. The mainstay of managing symptoms suggestive of irritability in autistics are firstly to identify possible precipitants and implement behavioural strategies and/or modify the environment, with the aim to eliminate irritability or at least minimise the frequency of episodes and/or intensity of the episodes. O'Nions et al. (2018), for instance, identified nine approaches that parents can use to help their autistic children manage their irritability;

1 accommodate the child
2 modify the environment
3 provide structure, routines, and occupation
4 supervise and monitor
5 manage non-compliance within everyday tasks
6 respond to problem behaviour
7 manage distress
8 maintain safety
9 analysis and planning.

Once all of these non-psychopharmacological strategies have been exhausted, and other coexisting psychopathologies have been identified and treated, often the next step is to trial a medication designed to treat irritability (Douglas-Hall et al., 2011). Next, we examine the findings in literature reviews and meta-analysis studies about the benefits that aripiprazole and risperidone can give autistics in managing their irritability.

10.5.2 Aripiprazole

There are three literature reviews that contain studies about the efficacy of aripiprazole in helping autistics manage their irritability and other conditions (Deb et al., 2014; Douglas-Hall et al., 2011; Maneeton et al., 2018). Douglas-Hall et al. (2011) examined two randomised double-blind placebo-controlled trials (See Table 10.2), four non-randomised open trials using aripiprazole to alleviate the behavioural symptoms of autism in children and adolescents (See Table 10.3), and two case studies using aripiprazole to alleviate the behavioural symptoms associated with autism in children and adolescents (See Table 10.4). Based on the studies reviewed, they concluded that:

> It is suggested that aripiprazole should be reserved for treating irritability associated with autism in children and adolescents where behavioural and educational therapies alone have failed to have an impact and it is felt that the behaviour is severe enough to warrant the use of an antipsychotic. (Douglas-Hall et al., 2011, p. 151).

This is in contrast to a literature review in which studies about the effects of aripiprazole on the disruptive behaviours of autistic children and adolescents was published by Ghanizadeh, Tordjman, and Jaafari in 2015, who concluded:

> This systematic review of double-blind controlled RCTs [Randomized Controlled Trials] showed convincing evidence of effectiveness and, therefore, supported the recommendations for the use of aripiprazole for treating irritability associated with autism. Other reviews that include open label or retrospective trials also have shown similar results.

One of the most recent literature reviews in which studies about the efficacy, acceptability, and tolerability of aripiprazole in assisting autistic children and adolescents was published by Maneeton and colleagues (2018). Maneeton et al. concluded that aripiprazole was safe, acceptable, and tolerable for autistic children and adolescents, to help reduce irritability, hyperactivity, inappropriate speech, and stereotypic behaviours. However, it did not improve lethargy or social withdrawal.

There are also studies in which the effectiveness and safety of aripiprazole in helping autistics manage their irritability has been compared against risperidone (Cohen et al., 2013; Ghanizadeh, Sahraeizadeh, & Berk, 2014). In Ghanizadeh, Sahraeizadeh, and Berk's (2014) study, 59 autistic children were randomly assigned to one of two groups. Over the course of two months one group received aripiprazole and the other group received risperidone. All participants completed all five ABC subscales (i.e., irritability, hyperactivity, lethargy, stereotypy, and speech) before receiving treatment and at one and two months after receiving treatment. They found that aripiprazole and risperidone were both effective in reducing irritability, hyperactivity, lethargy, and stereotypy.

Studies have measured what dosage of aripiprazole can produce optimal benefits for autistics (Aman et al., 2010; Benton, 2011; Marcus et al., 2009). Aman et al.'s (2010) study was a *post hoc* analysis of data from two eight-week, randomised, double-blind, multi-centre trials that evaluated the efficacy of different aripiprazole doses; flexible dosage (2–15 mg/day, n=47), fixed doses (5 mg/day, n=52; 10 mg/day, n=59; and 15

Table 10.2 Randomised double-blind placebo-controlled trials using aripiprazole to alleviate the behavioural symptoms of ASD in children and adolescents examined by Douglas-Hall et al. (2011)

Study	*Study design*	*Study duration*	*Age years diagnosis*	*Number of patients recruited (completed)*	*Main efficacy measure*	*Outcome*
Marcus et al., 2009	R db pc fixed dose 5 mg, 10 mg, 15 mg	Eight weeks	Six to 17 autistic disorder	218 (178)	ABC-I CGI-I	Significantly greater reduction in ABC-I scores for all doses compared with placebo
Owen et al., 2009	r db pc flexible dosing	Eight weeks	Six to 17 autistic disorder	98 (75)	ABC-I CGI-I	Significantly greater reduction in ABC-I scores for the aripiprazole group compared with placebo

Source: Douglas-Hall et al., 2011, p. 146.

r db pc, randomised double-blind placebo-controlled trial; ABC-I, Aberrant Behaviour Checklist irritability subscale; CGI-I, Clinical Global Impression improvement score.

Table 10.3 Non-randomised open trials using aripiprazole to alleviate the behavioural symptoms of ASD in children and adolescents examined by Douglas-Hall et al. (2011)

Study	*Study design*	*Study duration*	*Age years diagnosis*	*Number of patients recruited (completed)*	*Main efficacy measure*	*Outcome*
Masi et al., 2009	Retrospective naturalistic follow up	All patients had aripiprazole for at least 12 weeks and were followed for four to 12 months	4 to 15 autistic disorder PDD NOS	34 (ten had autistic disorder)	CGI-I	Four of the autism group were deemed responders to treatment.
Valicenti-McDermott and Demb, 2006	Retrospective chart review	Range of aripiprazole usage was six to 15 months	5 to 19 any developmental disability	32 (16 had autism +/- other co-morbid conditions)	CGI-I	Aripiprazole found to be effective in five of the 16 children with autism.
Gibson et al., 2007	Naturalistic retrospective	Aripiprazole for at least two weeks	11 to 18 Any mental disorder	45 (three had autism or PDD)	CGI-I CGI-S (chart extracted)	No specific results given for autism.
Rugino and Janvier, 2005	Retrospective chart review and Pros OL	Range of 14 to 210 days	5 to 17 Any mental disorder	17 (six had autism)	CGI-I and ABI-I CGI-S	One autism patient reported as responding to treatment (reduction in aggression).

Key:
PROS OL, prospective open label study; CGI-I, Clinical Global Impression improvement score; CGI-S, Clinical Global Impression severity of illness score.

Source: Douglas-Hall et al., 2011, p. 147.

Table 10.4 Case studies using aripiprazole to alleviate the behavioural symptoms of ASD in children and adolescents examined by Douglas-Hall et al. (2011)

Study	*Number of patients*	*Age/Years/Diagnosis*	*Main efficacy measure*	*Dose per day*	*Outcome*
Huang, Tsai, and Yang, 2010	Three	1 = Male 9 years PDD-NOS	CBCL	5 mg	Improvements in behaviour
		2 = Male 7 years autistic disorder	CBCL	5 mg	Improvement in behaviour
		3 = Male 11 years PDD-NOS	CBCL	20 mg	Improvement in behaviour
Stigler, Posey, and McDougle, 2004	Five	1 = male 11 years autistic disorder	CGI-I	15 mg	Much improved
		2 = male 18 years, autistic disorder and mod MR	CGI-I	15 mg	Very much improved
		3 = male 16 years Asperger's	CGI-I	10 mg	Much improved
		4 = male 5 years autistic disorder	CGI-I	10 mg	Very much improved
		5 = male 11 years Autism	CGI-I	10 mg	Much improved

Key:
CBCL, child behaviour checklist; CGI-I, Clinical Global Impression improvement

Source: Douglas-Hall et al., 2011, p. 148.

mg/day, n=53), flexible placebo dose (n=49), and fixed placebo dose (n=49). They found that aripiprazole reduced irritability, as indicated by the ABC-Irritability total subscale score and on the following individual ABC-Irritability items: Mood changes quickly, inappropriate cries/screams, and stamps feet/bangs objects. Aman et al. concluded that:

> Aripiprazole is efficacious in the treatment of irritability in children and adolescents with autistic disorder, particularly with respect to symptoms associated with tantrum behaviour. (2010, p. 415).

In 2011, Benton measured the effectiveness of fixed doses of aripiprazole against placebo doses. In their study, 218 participants aged six to 17 years with a *Diagnostic and Statistical Manual of Mental Disorders – Fourth Edition, Text Revision* diagnosis of autistic disorder and demonstrated behaviours of concern (i.e., irritability, agitation, and self-injurious behaviours) were randomly assigned to one of four treatment groups (i.e., 5 mg/day; 10 mg/day; 15 mg/day; and placebo group). When compared to the placebo group, participants in all aripiprazole dosage groups exhibited significant reductions in irritability after eight weeks of aripiprazole usage. Benton also found that aripiprazole was well tolerated and safe. However, the most commonly reported adverse side effects were sedation, extrapyramidal symptoms, and weight gain. These adverse side effects, however, were not severe enough to warrant a discontinuation of treatment. Significantly greater weight gain occurred across all groups receiving aripiprazole treatment compared with the placebo group, with a mean weight gain in the aripiprazole group over the duration of the study ranging from 1.3 to 1.5 kilograms. Despite these findings Benton stressed that since their study only lasted eight weeks, it was not possible to formulate any conclusions about the safety and efficacy of long-term aripiprazole usage.

In 2009, Marcus and colleagues examined the impact that different doses of aripiprazole had on reducing the irritation that autistics exhibited. In their study, 218 participants aged six to 17 years with autistic disorder and with a history of tantrums, aggression, or self-injurious behaviours were randomly assigned to one of four treatment groups; 5 mg/day of aripiprazole, 10 mg/day of aripiprazole, 15 mg/day of aripiprazole, or placebo. During their eight-week, double-blind, randomised, placebo-controlled, parallel-group study the caregivers completed the ABC – Irritability subscale. Additionally, clinicians who monitored the participants completed the *Clinical Global Impressions – Improvement* (CGI-I) scale. Marcus et al. found that aripiprazole, regardless of the dosage, resulted in significantly greater improvement than placebo in the mean ABC – Irritability subscale scores (5 mg/day = -12.4; 10 mg/day = -13.2; 15 mg/day = -14.4; versus placebo = -8.4). Additionally, at week eight all doses of aripiprazole resulted in significantly greater improvements in mean CGI-I scores than placebo. The most common adverse side effect noted was sedation. However, presyncope and aggression were also observed. Finally, across all test groups participants had increased weight gain; placebo + 0.3 kilograms; 5 mg/day of aripiprazole + 1.3 kilograms; 10 mg/day of aripiprazole + 1.3 kilograms; and 15 mg/day of aripiprazole + 1.5 kilograms.

Most studies about the risks and benefits of aripiprazole usage for autistics have been conducted in English speaking countries. However, there are studies about the efficacy of this medication for autistics who live in non-English speaking countries. Ichikawa et al.'s (2017) study evaluated the efficacy and safety of aripiprazole to treat irritability in autistic children aged six to 17 years who lived in Japan. Their study was a randomised, double-blind, placebo-controlled trial which lasted eight weeks. In their study, 92 participants were randomly assigned to either a placebo (n=45) or aripiprazole (n=47) group. Participants received flexible doses of aripiprazole between 1 to 15 mg/day or a placebo dosage. According to the parent/caregiver-rated scores from the irritability subscales of the Japanese version of the *Aberrant Behavior Checklist*, those in the aripiprazole group displayed reduced irritability relative to those in the placebo group from week three through to week eight. No serious side effects were reported in the group receiving aripiprazole. Based on these results, Ichikawan et al. concluded:

> Aripiprazole was effective and generally safe and well-tolerated in the treatment of irritability associated with ASD in Japanese children and adolescents. (2017, p. 804).

The studies that Douglas-Hall et al. (2011) and Deb et al. (2014) examined, documented the side effects that autistics experienced whilst taking aripiprazole. In Douglas-Hall et al.'s paper they listed the top ten treatment-emergent adverse-events occurring in 5% or more of patients studied. As listed in Table 10.5, for autistics taking aripiprazole the top ten side effects in order of prevalence were: Sedation, fatigue, vomiting, increased appetite, somnolence, tremor, pyrexia, drooling, headache, and extrapyramidal disorder.

Unlike Douglas-Hall et al.'s study, Deb et al. (2014) reported side effects in the studies that they examined. For example, they reported the findings in Owen et al.'s (2009) study that found that 21% of autistics who took aripiprazole reported feeling fatigue compared to 4% of autistics in the placebo group (See Table 10.6).

In summary, most of the literature has shown that despite some significant but non-life-threatening side effects, aripiprazole is predominantly safe and can reduce some irritability exhibited by autistics (Aman et al., 2010; Benton, 2011; Ichikawa et al., 2017). The literature also shows that for autistics aripiprazole can also reduce their

Table 10.5 Pooled top 10 treatment-emergent adverse events occurring in 5% or more of participants in the studies examined by Douglas-Hall et al.'s (2011) study

Adverse event	*Placebo (n = 101) n (%)*	*Aripiprazole (n = 212) n (%)*
Sedation	4 (3.96)	44 (20.75)
Fatigue	2 (1.98)	35 (16.51)
Vomiting	6 (5.94)	29 (13.68)
Increased appetite	7 (6.93)	27 (12.74)
Somnolence	4 (3.96)	22 (10.38)
Tremor	0 (0)	21 (9.91)
Pyrexia	1 (0.99)	19 (8.96)
Drooling	0 (0)	19 (8.96)
Headache	10 (9.90)	16 (7.55)
Extrapyramidal disorder	0 (0)	13 (6.13)

Source: Douglas-Hall et al., 2011, p. 149.

Table 10.6 Adverse effects described in the studies examined by Deb et al. (2014)

Study	*Adverse effects*
Owen et al., 2009	Fatigue: Aripiprazole: 21%; Placebo: 4% Somnolence: Aripiprazole: 17%; Placebo: 4% Vomiting: Aripiprazole: 15%; Placebo: 4% Increased appetite: Aripiprazole: 15%; Placebo: 10% Sedation: Aripiprazole: 11%; Placebo: 2% Headache: Aripiprazole: 6%; Placebo: 16% (Differences between treatment and placebo were not statistically significant)
Marcus et al., 2009	Sedation: Aripiprazole: 23%; Placebo: 6% Fatigue: Aripiprazole: 14%; Placebo: 0% Vomiting: Aripiprazole: 13%; Placebo: 8% Increased appetite: Aripiprazole: 12%; Placebo: 4% Tremor: Aripiprazole: 10%; Placebo: 0% Drooling: Aripiprazole: 9%; Placebo: 0% Somnolence: Aripiprazole: 8%; Placebo: 4% Headache: Aripiprazole: 7%; Placebo: 4% (Differences between treatment and placebo were not statistically significant)
Marcus et al., 2011	Refers to adverse effects in Marcus et al. (2009)
Stigler et al., 2009	Tiredness: 60% Cough: 48% Increased appetite: 44% Nausea/vomiting: 40% Rhinitis: 40% Diarrhoea: 36%
Erickson et al., 2011	Tiredness: 44% Nausea/vomiting: 25% Drooling: 25% Insomnia: 19%
Masi et al., 2009	Agitation: 26% Sleep disorders: 15% Tremors: 3% Weight gain: 3%
Valicenti-McDermott and Demb, 2006	Drowsiness: 19% Weight gain: 12% Abdominal pain: 6% Aggression: 6%
Basgul and Uneri, 2011	No details of adverse effects
Hellings et al., 2011	Four individuals (19%) experienced significant increases in appetite and weight
Stigler, Posey, and McDougle, 2004	Case 1: Moderate daytime sedation for first 14 days Case 3: Mild dizziness
Kültür, Tiryaki, and Tasgin, 2009	Salivation Constipation Decreased sleep Weight gain

Study	*Adverse effects*
Stigler et al., 2011	BMI change: 17 ± 2.1 to 20.3 ± 2.6 (p = 0.0001) 10/12 Mild drooling 1/12 Mild muscle twitching 1/12 Mild tremor Fatigue Mild headache Increased appetite Cough Mild vomiting
Fung et al., 2012	11/13 Increased appetite 6/13 Sedation/tiredness 2/13 Drooling 1/13 Skin rash 1/13 Lower extremity tremor 1/13 Slurred speech 1/13 Olfactory abnormality Weight gain (0.9–12 kg) (5.2 ± 3.9 kg)
Ishitobi et al., 2012	One developed insomnia 2/2 Daytime sleepiness improved 7/11 Obesity improved 3/3 Hyperprolactinaemia improved 1/1 Amenorrhoea improved Improvements were recorded after switching to aripiprazole in a number of adverse effects that appeared in a number of patients after treatment with risperidone
Jordan et al., 2012	One patient developed akathisia who received 30 mg aripiprazole a day This patient's ASD symptoms also got worse with aripiprazole treatment
Huang, Tsai, and Yang, 2010	Case 1, 2, and 3: No adverse effects
Dratcu et al., 2007	No adverse effects
Shashtri, Alla, and Sabaratnam, 2006	Tremors in upper limbs after four months of treatment at 15 mg dosage
Staller, 2003	Minor fatigue
Pardini, Guida, and Gialloreti, 2010	No adverse effects

Source: Deb et al., 2014, p. 720.

sensory sensitivities (Fung et al., 2012) and challenging behaviours (Jordan et al., 2012). However, despite these benefits, aripiprazole usage can cause some significant negative side effects, including sedation, fatigue, vomiting, increased appetite, tremors, headaches, and weight gain (Deb et al., 2014; Douglas-Hall et al., 2011).

Although risperidone and aripiprazole are classified as second-generation (SGA) or atypical 'antipsychotics' and both dampen dopaminergic activity they do so via different mechanisms of action. The primary mechanism of action of risperidone appears to be via antagonism of both dopamine at dopamine-2 receptors (D2) and serotonin at serotonin-2A receptors (5-HT2A) with a higher affinity for 5-HT2A. While aripiprazole appears to reduce dopaminergic activity by acting as a partial agonist at both D2 and 5-HT1A receptors, in addition it also antagonises serotonin (5-HT) at 5-HT2A receptors. Although both drugs seem to be equally efficacious in reducing irritability the difference in receptor binding translates into significant differences in their side-effect profile and hence their tolerability especially in the early phase of treatment. The persistent side-effects seen with long-term risperidone therapy include weight gain, mild sedation, hypersalivation/drooling and hyperprolactinaemia. In turn, although the side-effect profile of aripiprazole long-term is similar to that of risperidone it demonstrates no discernible increase in plasma prolactin levels making it the preferred agent should hyperprolactinaemia be issue with risperidone. Elevated plasma prolactin levels is associated with sexual dysregulation, gynaecomastia, galactorrhea and longer-term bone demineralisation.

10.5.3 Risperidone

Studies about the effectiveness of risperidone in reducing the irritability exhibited by autistics have been published (Nagaraj, Singhi, & Malhi, 2006; Pandina et al., 2007). Nagaraj, Singhi, and Malhi (2006) examined if risperidone helped reduce the irritability, aggressiveness, and hyperactivity that children with autism experienced and if it also increased their emotional responsiveness and communication skills. In their study, 40 children with autism who were aged between two to nine years were randomly assigned to one of two groups; 20 were allocated to a group that orally received 1mg/day of risperidone and the other 20 were allocated to a group that received an oral placebo. To examine the behavioural effects that risperidone produced, before the initiation of risperidone therapy and every eight weeks thereafter until the end of the six-month study, each child completed the *Childhood Autism Rating Scale* (CARS) and the *Children's Global Assessment Scale* (CGAS). At the end of the study, 19 children remained in the risperidone group and 20 remained in the placebo group. Nagaraj, Singhi, and Malhi found that 12 out of 19 children in the group that received risperidone demonstrated improvements according to the CARS test and 17 of these children showed improvements according to the CGAS test. In contrast, none of the 20 children in the placebo group demonstrated improvements according to the CARS test and two of these children demonstrated improvements as measured by the CGAS test. Nagaraj, Singhi, and Malhi concluded that for children with autism, risperidone improved global functioning and social responsiveness while simultaneously reducing irritability, hyperactivity, and aggression.

There are studies about the tolerability, safety, and benefits of long-term exposure to risperidone in treating the irritability experienced by autistic children. Aman et al. (2015) reported that long-term exposure to risperidone helped reduce maladaptive behaviours including the core symptoms associated with autism, as indicated by the social skills subscale of the *Vineland Adaptive Behavior* scale. Additionally, prolonged exposure to risperidone also reduced the irritability, as indicated by the parent-rated *Aberrant Behavior Checklist* irritability subscale scores. They concluded that despite increased appetite, weight gain, and enuresis these risks were not significant to discontinue treatment. However individual autistics and/or their families may find some of these side effects unacceptable.

There are also studies about the therapeutic effectiveness that different doses of risperidone can give autistics in treating their irritability. Kent et al. (2013) compared the effectiveness and safety of a high-dose of risperidone (1.25 mg/day [20 to <45kg]; 1.75 mg/day [>45kg]), a low-dose of risperidone (0.125 mg/day [20 to <45kg]; 0.175 mg/day [>45kg]), and a placebo. They found that high doses of risperidone (i.e.,1.25 and 1.75 mg/day) were efficacious, whilst doses of <0.25 mg/day did not reduce the irritability and related behaviours exhibited by autistics. However, in the high-dose group, somnolence, sedation, and increased appetite occurred more frequently than in the low-dose group.

Multiple studies have shown that autistics usually gain weight as a consequence of taking risperidone (Martin et al., 2004; McCracken et al., 2002; Nagaraj, Singhi, & Malhi, 2006; Pandina et al., 2007; Scahill et al., 2016). McCracken et al. (2002) reported that during their study autistics taking risperidone had an average weight gain of 2.7 ± 2.9 kilograms compared to autistics in the placebo group, who had an average weight gain of 0.8 ± 2.2 kilograms. Scahill et al. (2016) reported that over their 24-week study there was a 5.4 ± 3.4 kilograms average weight gain in 97 autistic children who on average had 22.9 ± 2.8 weeks of risperidone exposure. Additionally, at the beginning of their study, 59 of the 97 autistic children (60.8%) were classified as having a normal body weight. However, by the end of their 24-week study, only 25 of the original 85 autistic participants remaining in the study (29.4%) had a normal body weight. Furthermore, over the course of their study, the waist circumference of these 97 autistic children increased on average from 60.7 ± 10.4 centimetres at the start of their study to 66.8 ± 11.3 centimetres at week 24. Currently, most of the literature concludes that autistics gain weight as a consequence of taking risperidone.

10.5.4 Recommendations for research in the future about risperidone and aripiprazole

While there is a large amount of research about the efficacy of risperidone and aripiprazole in helping autistics manage their irritability, there are two areas where more research can be conducted.

First, there are few studies that have examined if the effectiveness of risperidone and aripiprazole are enhanced if they are combined with other medications (Akhondzadeh et al., 2010; Ghaleiha et al., 2013; Ghanizadeh & Ayoobzadehshirazi, 2015). For example, Akhondzadeh et al. (2010) found that pentoxifylline added to risperidone helped reduce the aberrant behaviour exhibited by children with autism. Additionally, there is not much research about the efficacy of risperidone and aripiprazole if it is combined with non-pharmacological supports. Consequently, studies in the future can examine if risperidone or aripiprazole combined with mindfulness-based activities can reduce the irritability that some autistics exhibit. Such studies might be beneficial because if a combination of supports can be found to be effective, then it can enhance the desired treatment outcomes of using risperidone and aripiprazole.

Second, studies have shown that autistics often gain weight whilst taking risperidone (Martin et al., 2004; Scahill et al., 2016). Since weight gain can contribute to the development of poor health, it is important that researchers explore ways that autistics can minimise weight gain during risperidone usage. Diets and physical exercise are two potential approaches that might help autistics taking risperidone maintain a healthy weight. Hence, studies should examine the relationships between diets, physical exercise, and risperidone usage. This might be accomplished by conducting a study that compares weight fluctuations for four groups; (1) risperidone only, (2) risperidone and diet, (3) risperidone and physical exercise, and (4) risperidone, diet, and physical exercise. To examine long-term weight changes, weight measurements could be recorded once every week for twelve months. Furthermore, the dosage and frequency of risperidone administration should be standardised between groups so that its dosage and frequency does not distort the results. If results from this hypothetical study were to show that diets and/or exercise can offset the weight gains that risperidone causes, then this result can lead to better health outcomes for autistics.

10.5.5 A note of caution about risperidone and aripiprazole

Overall there is a considerable amount of research which concludes that risperidone and aripiprazole can help autistic children manage their irritability. However, as with any medication, risperidone and aripiprazole should be used judiciously with clear treatment targets which require regular evaluation of both therapeutic gains and side-effects. Despite these benefits, risperidone and aripiprazole usage can result in uncomfortable non-life-threatening side effects (See Table 10.7).

Deb et al. (2014) and Douglas-Hall et al. (2011) found that aripiprazole can cause sedation, fatigue, vomiting, increased appetite, tremors, headaches, and weight gain. McCracken et al. (2002), Nagaraj, Singhi, and Malhi (2006), and Scahill et al. (2016) reported that autistics gained weight while taking risperidone. Due to these side effects, before using risperidone or aripiprazole autistic adults, or the parents/caregivers of autistic children, should consult with medical professionals and ensure the potential side effects of these medications are monitored. Again, additional factors to consider are; the costs associated with using these medications, and the patient's medical history (i.e., previous physiological responses to risperidone and aripiprazole). Furthermore, according to the National Institute of Health and Care Excellence (NICE) the use of risperidone and other antipsychotic medications can be used to manage the challenging behaviours exhibited by autistic children and adults. However, NICE recommends that risperidone and other antipsychotics should only be used after other interventions have been found to be ineffective or if other interventions cannot be delivered due to the

Table 10.7 Relative adverse effects of antipsychotic drugs

Drug	*Sedation*	*Weight gain*	*Akathisia*	
Aripiprazole	-	-	+	
Risperidone	+	++	+	
Drug	**Parkinsonism**	**Anticholinergic**	**Hypertension**	**Prolactin elevation**
Aripiprazole	-	-	-	-
Risperidone	+	+	++	+++

Source: Taylor, Barnes, and Young, 2018, p. 39.

+++ high incidence / severity; ++ moderate; + low; - very low patient's circumstances and/or challenging behaviours. NICE also recommends that antipsychotics should only be used under very strict conditions and under the ongoing supervision and careful monitoring of a suitably qualified and experienced medical professional, such as a paediatrician or psychiatrist (Research Autism, 2019).

10.6 Attention Deficit Hyperactivity Disorder (ADHD)

10.6.1 ADHD in the autistic population

In the American Psychiatric Association's (APA) Diagnostic and Statistical Manual of Mental Disorders – Fifth Edition (DSM-5), ADHD is defined as 'a persistent (at least six month) pattern of inattention and/or hyperactivity-impulsivity that interferes with functioning or development'. In a rudimentary sense, ADHD can be defined by three characteristics; inattentiveness, hyperactivity, and impulsivity (Schrimsher et al., 2002). ADHD first appeared in the second edition of the APA's *Diagnostic and Statistical Manual of Mental Disorders* under the term 'Hyperkinetic Reaction of Childhood'. In 1980, the third edition of this manual was released, and this disorder was renamed 'Attention Deficit Disorder – (with and without Hyperactivity)'. This name was a result of a reconceptualisation of the condition with an emphasis on problems with attention, impulsivity, and hyperactivity. With the release of the revised edition of the third edition of this manual the term ADHD was used and the option of no hyperactivity was eliminated. In the fourth edition of this manual the term ADHD was retained, but it was split into three subtypes (i.e., Predominantly Inattentive, Predominantly Hyperactive-Impulsive, and Combined). Finally, in May 2013 the fifth edition of this manual was released and in this edition the APA published modifications to the diagnostic criteria but retained the name ADHD (Epstein & Loren, 2013).

Although the prevalence of ADHD in the autistic population has not been measured, there are studies that have shown that self-reported rates of ADHD among autistic adults is significantly higher than the general adult population (Johnston et al., 2013). Despite a lack of statistical information, the impacts of ADHD for non-autistics have been studied in detail. ADHD has been found to decrease concentration levels which can cause poor academic and work performance (Nydén, Myrén, & Gillberg, 2008). Atomoxetine and methylphenidate are psychotropic medications that are often prescribed to help autistics manage their ADHD. In the next section, we review studies about the safety and efficacy of these medications in helping autistics manage their ADHD.

10.6.2 Methylphenidate

Methylphenidate is one of the most commonly prescribed medications used to treat ADHD, with both slow release and fast release versions prescribed. In their literature review, Howes et al. (2018) reported evidence that the response rate to methylphenidate in individuals with autism and ADHD was lower than in individuals with ADHD without autism. The Research Units on Pediatric Psychopharmacology (RUPP) Autism Network (2005) reported a 50% response rate for children with ADHD and autism, compared to response rates of 70–80% in children with ADHD without ASD. Despite increased response rates, side effects may also be greater in autistic individuals with

ADHD in comparison to non-autistic individuals with ADHD, with discontinuation rates due to side effects much higher for autistics (18%) than non-autistics (1.4%) (RUPP Autism Network, 2005). The most commonly reported side effects of methylphenidate usage were; sleeping difficulties, abdominal discomfort, decreased appetite, social withdrawal, irritability, and emotional outbursts. Thus, the research suggests that "although effective, methylphenidate may not be as effective" in autistics with ADHD and that these individuals are more likely to experience more significant side effects (Howes et al., 2018).

10.6.3 Atomoxetine

Atomoxetine is an alternative non-stimulant medication for ADHD. Researchers have measured atomoxetine's effectiveness in reducing ADHD symptoms exhibited by autistic children (Arnold et al., 2006; Charnsil, 2011; Harfterkamp et al., 2012; Niederhofer et al., 2006). Ghanizadeh (2012) examined six studies about the use of atomoxetine for treating ADHD among autistic children and adolescents. They concluded that:

> There are not enough controlled clinical trials for showing the efficacy of atomoxetine for treatment of ADHD symptoms in autism. Although evidence suggests potential efficacy of atomoxetine, the current evidences are not conclusive. (Ghanizadeh, 2012, p. 635).

Researchers have examined if long-term usage of atomoxetine results in a reduction in ADHD symptoms exhibited by autistics (Harfterkamp et al., 2013). In Harfterkamp et al.'s (2013) longitudinal study, 88 autistic participants who were aged between six to 17 years received 1.2 mg/kg/day of atomoxetine for 20 weeks. The *ADHD Rating Scale* was used to measure if atomoxetine reduced ADHD symptoms. Based on the results, Harfterkamp et al. (2013, p. 194) concluded:

> the results of the present analysis suggest that continued treatment with atomoxetine up to 28 weeks further improve ADHD symptoms in children and adolescents with ASD, while adverse events tend to subside.

The role that parent training programs can play in improving the therapeutic benefits that atomoxetine gives autistics in reducing their ADHD symptoms has been researched (Handen et al., 2015; Smith et al., 2016). In Handen et al.'s (2015) study, 128 autistic children aged between five to 14 years with ADHD were randomly assigned to one of four treatment groups; atomoxetine treatment-only group (ATX), atomoxetine treatment and parent training (ATX + PT), placebo and parent training, or placebo only. The dosage of atomoxetine was gradually adjusted so that it was tailored to each participant, but was capped at 1.8 mg/kg/day for a period of six weeks and then maintained for an additional four weeks. Whilst the autistic children were taking atomoxetine or a placebo their parents attended nine parent-training sessions. The *Swanson, Nolan and Pelham* (SNAP) and the *Home Situations Questionnaire* (HSQ) were both used to gauge the effectiveness of these four combinations of interventions (i.e., ATX, ATX + PT, placebo and parent training, and placebo only). Results from the

SNAP and HSQ showed that a combination of ATX and parent training resulted in the most significant reduction in ADHD symptoms.

10.6.4 Recommendations for research in the future about methylphenidate and atomoxetine

An examination of the research shows that there are two areas where additional research can be conducted on the role that methylphenidate and atomoxetine plays in helping autistics manage their ADHD. First, Handen et al. (2015) reported that combining atomoxetine with parent training was a more effective approach in helping young autistics manage their ADHD than just prescribing atomoxetine by itself. In the future, studies should examine if the therapeutic benefits that methylphenidate and atomoxetine give autistics can be enhanced if they are combined with other support programs. For example, parent behaviour training or mindfulness training could be a viable complimentary support that increases the ability methylphenidate and/or atomoxetine has in helping autistics manage their ADHD. Second, most of the research about the therapeutic benefits of methylphenidate and/or atomoxetine for autistics have based their results on samples of autistic children. In the future, researchers should measure the efficacy of these medications on autistic adults to see if they too can also benefit from using these medications. By conducting research into this topic it could provide autistic adults with additional support options.

10.6.5 A note of caution about methylphenidate and atomoxetine

While most of the research shows that methylphenidate and atomoxetine can help autistics manage their ADHD, it is important to consult with medical professionals as these medications are prescription only and may have unexpected side-effects. You should also be vigilant against any potential side effects of methylphenidate and atomoxetine usage and be aware of the financial costs associated with taking methylphenidate and atomoxetine. Finally, before using methylphenidate and atomoxetine or non-prescription tablets/liquids to aid with ADHD the prescribing doctor will take into consideration medical history (i.e., physiological responses to methylphenidate, atomoxetine, and other medications).

10.7 Summary regarding psychotropic medications

In this chapter, we have not used our Gold, Silver, Bronze, or Tin rating system to rate the efficacy of psychotropic medications for autistics. This is because it would have been irresponsible to rate their efficacy since every autistic is different in terms of their physiology and life circumstances. In addition, it is important to note that no medication has demonstrated conclusive effectiveness for helping every autistic overcome their psychotropic challenges (Siegel & Beaulieu, 2012). In the United States only risperidone and aripiprazole have been approved by the Food and Drug Administration (FDA) for use to treat irritability and agitation in autism. Despite psychotropic medications often being prescribed off label, with particularly high rates of antipsychotics, antidepressants, and stimulants (Langworthy-Lam, Aman, & Van Bourgondien, 2002), autistics using psychotropic medications have remained controversial, especially for children, due to the lack of research on the safety and efficacy for this population (Barnard-Brak et al., 2016).

However, autistics may be more sensitive to experiencing negative side effects of psychotropic medications and may have a higher or lower sensitivity to the medication itself. Decisions to trial a psychotropic medication should be based on a risk/benefit analysis following an open and honest discussion of the pros and cons of possible medications. Side effects should be clearly communicated to the patient and/or family and monitored. Dosages may need to be significantly lower or higher than for non-autistics.

While the FDA has approved risperidone and aripiprazole for treating irritability and agitation exhibited by autistics, we have taken a more cautious approach, in line with the NICE guidelines. We have stressed at every opportunity that autistics and their families should consult with medical professionals both prior to using a psychotropic medication and regularly whilst using the medication to monitor for any side effects and evaluate efficacy. During an initial consultation the patient's medical history, the benefits associated with the possible treatment plan, and the potential side effects should be discussed. Since some of the side effects associated with using the medications examined can be severe, medical practitioners should clearly communicate to the patient and/or their family all possible side effects so that they know what to be aware of. Finally, since autistics may have a higher or lower sensitivity to the medication itself, dosages may need to be adjusted significantly.

10.8 Chelation: A dangerous and ineffective medications/treatment

10.8.1 Chelation therapy

Multiple studies have shown that exposure to mercury, from vaccines containing thimerosal, does not contribute to the development of autism (Andrews et al., 2004; Bennett et al., 2018; Hviid et al., 2003; Madsen et al., 2003; Parker et al., 2004; Price et al., 2010; Stehr-Green et al., 2003; Uno et al., 2015). However, despite this incontrovertible evidence, there are still some who recommend that chelation therapy should be used to remove mercury and other heavy metals from autistics. It is believed that removing these heavy metals will cause a reduction in autistic symptomology that will improve the overall functioning and quality of life of autistics. According to Brent (2013), in the United States of America over half a million autistics are treated with chelation therapy annually.

Chelation therapy involves a patient consuming medication that causes heavy metals to be excreted via urine (Risher & Amler, 2005). The chemicals used in chelation therapy can result in serious health difficulties, including fever, vomiting, diarrhoea, loss of appetite, hypertension, haemorrhoid symptoms, hypotension, cardiac arrhythmias, hypocalcaemia. These side effects can also contribute to a person's death. For example, in 2005 a five-year-old autistic boy died from cardiac arrest caused by hypocalcaemia while receiving chelation intravenously (Beauchamp et al., 2006). Additionally, the safety risks associated with chelation therapy have resulted in the suspension of a chelation therapy trial for autistics (Mitka, 2008).

Despite the risks associated with chelation therapy, Green et al. (2006) found that 7.4% of parents reported that their child had received this therapy. In another study,

Harrington et al. (2006) found that out of their sample of 64 parents raising autistic children, eight (13%) claimed that they have used chelation treatment to treat their child's autism. From the perspective of medical professionals, Golnik and Ireland (2009) reported that no physician recommended the use of chelation therapy for treating the symptoms associated with the autism spectrum. However, 26% reported that they did not have enough knowledge about chelation therapy to discuss its effectiveness or safety, or lack of.

To the best of Davis et al.'s (2013) knowledge, a literature review about the effects of chelation treatment on the symptoms associated with the autism spectrum has never been published. To fill this gap in the literature, they published a literature review in which they described the characteristics and results of five studies about the impact of chelation treatment on autistics (Adams et al., 2009; Eppright, Sanfacon, & Horwitz, 1996; Geier & Geier, 2006; Patel & Curtis, 2007; Senel, 2010). Of the collected studies, one was a case-study (Eppright, Sanfacon, & Horwitz, 1996), and four examined groups of autistic children (Adams et al., 2009; Geier & Geier, 2006; Patel & Curtis, 2007; Senel, 2010). With the exception of Senel's (2010) study, the type of chelation treatment used was described. The duration of the chelation program ranged from 1.5 to seven months and the frequency of administration ranged from one to 12 times per week. In four studies, chelation treatment was one part of the treatment program (Adams et al., 2009; Eppright, Sanfacon, & Horwitz, 1996; Geier & Geier, 2006; Patel & Curtis, 2007). For example, other treatment components included an organic diet and nutritional supplements (i.e., vitamins, minerals, amino acids, and peptides) (Patel & Curtis, 2007), or intramuscular injections of LUPRON DEPOT® (Geier & Geier, 2006). Based on these collected studies, Davis et al. (2013, p. 54) recommended that:

> Based on the results of this review, evidence to support the use of chelation as a treatment for children with ASD is extremely weak. The weakness of the evidence base, the lack of a sound rationale for use of chelation as an ASD treatment, and the potential negative side effects strongly argue against the use of chelation treatment for ASD.

10.8.2 Evaluation of Chelation therapy

Rating: Tin – Dangerous and potentially life threatening

The use of chelating agents is problematic due to the serious side effects, mainly attributable to disturbing metal ion homeostasis and dislocation of complexed metal ions to dangerous body sites. For this reason, chelation therapy should only be limited to specific critical heavy metal toxicity situations and needs to be closely monitored within a medical/clinical context (Crisponi et al., 2015). The literature has shown that chelation therapy is ineffective for autistics (Adams et al., 2009; Davis et al., 2013; Geier & Geier, 2006; Patel & Curtis, 2007; Senel, 2010). Additionally, this treatment can produce significantly detrimental side effects (Beauchamp et al., 2006; Doja & Roberts, 2006), and has caused death (Beauchamp et al., 2006). Due to these severe side effects we have rated the efficacy of chelation therapy for autistics as 'Tin – Dangerous and potentially life threatening'. Additionally, since Chelation therapy is extremely dangerous no more research should be conducted on its use for autistics.

10.9 Autistic views about medications

10.9.1 Autistic views about using prescription medications

Out of the 201 respondents who completed our survey, 35 provided a comment about their usage of prescription medications. Most comments were very brief, however, four were longer with two describing instances in which prescription medication did not help because the respondents were misdiagnosed and two described the side effects associated with using prescription medication.

Two respondents explained that the prescription medication that they were taking was ineffective and caused potential side effects because they were misdiagnosed.

> "I was misdiagnosed with ADHD when I was seven and put on Ritalin and that had horrible side effects that lasted for many years after I stopped taking it. I'm very against medication for this reason."
>
> "At age 30 I first tried medication to help with what was then thought to be 'depression' – Zoloft. It 'sort of' helped at the time, but not that much really. I wasn't really depressed. It was 'Autistic burnout' really and not knowing that I was Autistic. I also had recurring nightmares from my time at high school being bullied from Year 7 – also PTSD. The only medication that managed to get me functioning again was Seroquel. With the support of a fantastic Psychiatrist we went through every psychotropic medication until we found one that worked. I then slowly started to overcome my Autistic burnout. I am no longer taking Seroquel or any other medications and have recovered from trauma of school bullying and supporting an unwell partner through an alcohol addiction."

Another theme that we discovered as we were examining the comments collected was that sometimes prescription medication usage produced unforeseen side effects. Two participants revealed such experiences.

> "Many different anti-psychotic, risperidone Seroquel etc. – did not like taking them gave me bad side effects felt sluggish and not myself and massive weight gain doubled my body weight."
>
> "I took Effexor for a short time and absolutely hated it. I will go so far as to say I feel like it nearly ruined my life. It took a long time to get off it and an even longer time to feel ok again. Never again."

However, one of the autistic professionals interviewed talked about how much medication had helped them return to calm.

> "I couldn't believe how this little tablet could take away all my distress in 20 minutes, when normally, if I was at that level of distress it would last for four to 12 hours"

The themes presented in this chapter emphasise the need to ensure that autistics are accurately diagnosed in terms of any co-occurring mental health conditions and that they and their families make sure to monitor side effects and seek medical support as necessary. Failure to accurately diagnose mental health conditions in autistics or to be aware of the potential side effects associated with prescription medication usage can result in autistics being injured, complicating their health and quality of life.

10.9.2 Autistic views about using non-prescription medications

Respondents who completed our survey were asked, "Have you ever used and type of non-prescribed or recreational drugs or alcohol to self-medicate or self-manage any aspect of your autism?" The purpose of this question was to provide the respondent with the opportunity to explain their experiences of using non-prescription medications. Out of 206 respondents who completed our survey, 22 provided a comment to this question. Our examination of their comments revealed that most respondents consumed either alcohol or marijuana to help them cope with situations in life.

Our analysis of the comments collected revealed that nine contained a sufficient amount of detail about the benefits or drawbacks of alcohol consumption. Of these, six respondents expressed unease about their consumption of alcohol.

> "I have used alcohol to dumb my senses when they are really hyper and I can't even access my own house anymore. I wouldn't recommend this because drinking alcohol is a short term solution which does more damage than good."
>
> "I drank as a teenager to cope with peer social pressure. Once I reached adulthood I stopped. Hate alcohol and will not succumb to peer pressure of that kind even if it makes me extremely unpopular."
>
> "Alcohol helps to relax in social situations but I get really sick the next day. So I stopped using it."
>
> "I used to drink a lot to feel better and more relaxed but it became a problem and I quit in 2012 and haven't had a drink since."
>
> "In social situations, I find that a limited amount of alcohol does make me less socially anxious. I dislike being drunk, so I moderate my intake very carefully."
>
> "... my brain gets too overloaded which all of my combined therapies cannot alleviate so I've found if I get drunk it 'resets' my brain and the overload. I have no understanding why but it has always been this way. It's not something I prefer to do though as it can make me anxious so I only do it in dire overload."

In contrast, three respondents explained the benefits that alcohol provided.

> "Never get drunk but the occasional glass of wine or rum and coke relieves anxiety better than anything else. I use in moderation and only three to four times a week."
>
> "I also find alcohol can be helpful to manage social anxiety and allow me to relax in social situations."
>
> "I enjoy drinking alcohol socially, but not for autism. In some situations, it can reduce the anxiety and overwhelm but not often."

The eclectic collection of comments presented here shows that the choice to consume alcohol is an individual one. It is advised that autistics familiarise themselves with typical alcoholic beverages and the effects of mixing different types of alcohol, so that they can minimise the likelihood of widely known consequences, such as feeling nauseous, or getting a hangover.

The other non-prescribed substance that respondents reported using was marijuana. Two respondents explained their experiences with this drug.

> "Medical marijuana. Finding high quality, high Marijuana edibles helped calm neuro system from inside out. Amazing to experience that. Using a 50/50 inhaler, when I go nonverbal, it helps me be able to speak again in about ten minutes. Calms neuro tics or repetitive motions. I like how other senses slowly increase in being noticed, and over used senses get to calm. Now I mostly use at times for numerous reasons and aids."
>
> "Marijuana was my drug of choice for a long time. It is the only thing that ever made my brain feel calm. Eventually (after decades of heavy use) I started to notice feelings of paranoia and had to concede that it was no longer my friend. I decided one day to stop and I have not touched it since, however I miss having something that could switch off my brain and help me sleep. I used to worry about smoking though so I feel better now I'm not worried about smoking. I was never a big drinker but I don't mind the odd drink. It doesn't feel therapeutic to me though. I never have more than three or four drinks because I don't enjoy the sensory feeling associated with a hangover and I also have a strong aversion / fear of vomiting."

Finally, two respondents explained that in the past they have used a combination of non-prescribed substances.

> "I used alcohol and illicit substances (ranging from cannabis to opioids) for many years to self-medicate. It ended with me as a psychiatric inpatient twice. I am now 3.5 years sober. At the time I felt it helped with anxiety and social interaction, but it actually made me worse."
>
> "Speed helped me slow my brain down OR feel that my fast overthinking was ok as other speed users matched me. I no longer use this. Alcohol dulls my overthinking and makes me feel slowed down. It makes me feel more relaxed."

The insights provided by the respondents illustrate the need to provide education about the short- and long-term benefits and issues of consuming alcohol and marijuana. In particular, the range of different effects of drinking alcohol or consuming marijuana both immediately and in the short- and long-term.

10.10 Conclusion

This chapter examined the literature about medications that are often used to treat common co-morbid conditions that autistics experience. The medications examined were Selective Serotonin Reuptake Inhibitors (SSRIs) (used to treat depression), melatonin (used to treat insomnia), aripiprazole and risperidone (used to treat irritability), and atomoxetine and methylphenidate (used to treat ADHD). The literature about chelation therapy was explored and it was rated as 'Tin – Dangerous and potentially life threatening'. This chapter concluded with a collection of quotes from autistics about their insights and experiences of prescription and non-prescription medications.

References

Adams, J. B., Baral, M., Geis, E., Mitchell, J., Ingram, J., Hensley, A., ... & Mitchell, K. (2009). Safety and efficacy of oral DMSA therapy for children with autism spectrum disorders: Part A-Medical results. *BMC Clinical Pharmacology*, 9(1), 16. doi:10.1186/1472-6904-9-16.

Akhondzadeh, S., Fallah, J., Mohammadi, M. R., Imani, R., Mohammadi, M., Salehi, B., ... & Forghani, S. (2010). Double-blind placebo-controlled trial of pentoxifylline added to risperidone: Effects on aberrant behavior in children with autism. *Progress in Neuro-Psychopharmacology and Biological Psychiatry*, 34(1), 32–36. doi:10.1016/j.pnpbp.2009.09.012.

Aman, M. G., Kasper, W., Manos, G., Mathew, S., Marcus, R., Owen, R., & Mankoski, R. (2010). Line-item analysis of the aberrant behavior checklist: Results from two studies of aripiprazole in the treatment of irritability associated with autistic disorder. *Journal of Child and Adolescent Psychopharmacology*, 20(5), 415–422. doi:10.1089/cap.2009.0120.

Aman, M., Rettiganti, M., Nagaraja, H. N., Hollway, J. A., McCracken, J., McDougle, C. J., ... & Posey, D. J. (2015). Tolerability, safety, and benefits of risperidone in children and adolescents with autism: 21-month follow-up after 8-week placebo-controlled trial. *Journal of Child and Adolescent Psychopharmacology*, 25(6), 482–493. doi:10.1089/cap.2015.0005.

Ancoli-Israel, S., & Roth, T. (1999). Characteristics of insomnia in the United States: Results of the 1991 National Sleep Foundation Survey. I. *Sleep*, 22, S347–353.

Andersen, I. M., Kaczmarska, J., McGrew, S. G., & Malow, B. A. (2008). Melatonin for insomnia in children with autism spectrum disorders. *Journal of Child Neurology*, 23(5), 482–485. doi:10.1177/0883073807309783.

Andrews, N., Miller, E., Grant, A., Stowe, J., Osborne, V., & Taylor, B. (2004). Thimerosal exposure in infants and developmental disorders: A retrospective cohort study in the United Kingdom does not support a causal association. *Pediatrics*, 114(3), 584–591. doi:10.1542/peds.2003-1177-L.

Arnold, L. E., Aman, M. G., Cook, A. M., Witwer, A. N., Hall, K. L., Thompson, S., & Ramadan, Y. (2006). Atomoxetine for hyperactivity in autism spectrum disorders: Placebo-controlled crossover pilot trial. *Journal of the American Academy of Child & Adolescent Psychiatry*, 45(10), 1196–1205. doi:10.1097/01.chi.0000231976.28719.2a.

Barnard-Brak, L., Davis, T. N., Schmidt, M., & Richman, D. M. (2016). Effects associated with on-and off-label stimulant treatment of core autism and ADHD symptoms exhibited by children with autism spectrum disorder. *Developmental Neurorehabilitation*, 19(1), 46–53. doi:10.3109/17518423.2014.904949.

Basgul, S. S., & Uneri, O. (2011). Use of aripiprazole in children and adolescents: Case reports. *Child and Adolescent Psychiatry*, 20(S1), S7–S223.

Beauchamp, R. A., Willis, T. M., Betz, T. G., Villanacci, J., Leiker, R. D., Rozin, L., ... & Morta, T. (2006). Deaths associated with hypocalcemia from chelation therapy – Texas, Pennsylvania, and Oregon, 2003–2005. *Journal of the American Medical Association*, 295(18), 2131–2133.

Bennett, M. (2016). The importance of interviewing adults on the autism spectrum about their depression and suicidal ideation experiences. *Journal of Autism and Developmental Disorders*, 46(4), 1492–1493. doi:10.1007/s10803-015-2674-4.

Bennett, M., Webster, A. A., Goodall, E., & Rowland, S. (2018). Challenging the Public's Perception of Life on Autism Spectrum: The Impact of the Vaccination Myth. In *Life on the Autism Spectrum* (pp. 37–60). Springer, Singapore. doi:10.1007/978-981-13-3359-0_3.

Benton, T. D. (2011). Aripiprazole to treat irritability associated with autism: A placebo-controlled, fixed-dose trial. *Current Psychiatry Reports*, 13(2), 77–79. doi:10.1007/s11920-010-0172-0.

Benvenuto, A., Battan, B., Porfirio, M. C., & Curatolo, P. (2013). Pharmacotherapy of autism spectrum disorders. *Brain and Development*, 35(2), 119–127. doi:10.1016/j.braindev.2012.03.015.

Brent, J. (2013). Commentary on the abuse of metal chelation therapy in patients with autism spectrum disorders. *Journal of Medical Toxicology* 9(4), 370–372. doi:10.1007/s13181-013-0345-4.

Buchsbaum, M. S., Hollander, E., Mehmet Haznedar, M., Tang, C., Spiegel-Cohen, J., Wei, T. C., … & Cartwright, C. (2001). Effect of fluoxetine on regional cerebral metabolism in autistic spectrum disorders: A pilot study. *International Journal of Neuropsychopharmacology*, 4(2), 119–125. doi:10.1017/S1461145701002280.

Charnsil, C. (2011). Efficacy of atomoxetine in children with severe autistic disorders and symptoms of ADHD: An open-label study. *Journal of Attention Disorders*, 15(8), 684–689. doi:10.1177/1087054710376907.

Cohen, D., Raffin, M., Canitano, R., Bodeau, N., Bonnot, O., Périsse, D., … & Laurent, C. (2013). Risperidone or aripiprazole in children and adolescents with autism and/or intellectual disability: A Bayesian meta-analysis of efficacy and secondary effects. *Research in Autism Spectrum Disorders*, 7(1), 167–175. doi:10.1016/j.rasd.2012.08.001.

Cook Jr, E. H., Rowlett, R., Jaselskis, C., & Leventhal, B. L. (1992). Fluoxetine treatment of children and adults with autistic disorder and mental retardation. *Journal of the American Academy of Child & Adolescent Psychiatry*, 31(4), 739–745. doi:10.1097/00004583-199207000-00024.

Cortesi, F., Giannotti, F., Sebastiani, T., Panunzi, S., & Valente, D. (2012). Controlled-release melatonin, singly and combined with cognitive behavioural therapy, for persistent insomnia in children with autism spectrum disorders: A randomized placebo-controlled trial. *Journal of Sleep Research*, 21(6), 700–709. doi:10.1111/j.1365-2869.2012.01021.x.

Crisponi, G., Nurchi, V. M., Lachowicz, J. I., Crespo-Alonso, M., Zoroddu, M. A., & Peana, M. (2015). Kill or cure: Misuse of chelation therapy for human diseases. *Coordination Chemistry Reviews*, 284, 278–285. doi:10.1016/j.ccr.2014.04.023.

Davis, T. N., O'Reilly, M., Kang, S., Lang, R., Rispoli, M., Sigafoos, J., … & Mulloy, A. (2013). Chelation treatment for autism spectrum disorders: A systematic review. *Research in Autism Spectrum Disorders*, 7(1), 49–55. doi:10.1016/j.rasd.2012.06.005.

Deb, S., Farmah, B. K., Arshad, E., Deb, T., Roy, M., & Unwin, G. L. (2014). The effectiveness of aripiprazole in the management of problem behaviour in people with intellectual disabilities, developmental disabilities and/or autistic spectrum disorder–A systematic review. *Research in Developmental Disabilities*, 35(3), 711–725. doi:10.1016/j.ridd.2013.12.004.

Deliens, G., Leproult, R., Schmitz, R., Destrebecqz, A., & Peigneux, P. (2015). Sleep disturbances in autism spectrum disorders. *Review Journal of Autism and Developmental Disorders*, 2(4), 343–356. doi:10.1007/s40489-015-0057-6.

DeLong, G. R., Ritch, C. R., & Burch, S. (2002). Fluoxetine response in children with autistic spectrum disorders: Correlation with familial major affective disorder and intellectual achievement. *Developmental Medicine and Child Neurology*, 44(10), 652–659. doi:10.1017/S0012162201002717.

DeLong, G. R., Teague, L. A., & Kamran, M. M. (1998). Effects of fluoxetine treatment in young children with idiopathic autism. *Developmental Medicine & Child Neurology*, 40(8), 551–562. doi:10.1111/j.1469-8749.1998.tb15414.x.

Doja, A., & Roberts, W. (2006). Immunizations and autism: A review of the literature. *Canadian Journal of Neurological Sciences*, 33(4), 341–346. doi:10.1017/S031716710000528X.

Douglas-Hall, P., Curran, S., Bird, V., & Taylor, D. (2011). Aripiprazole: A review of its use in the treatment of irritability associated with autistic disorder patients aged 6–17. *Journal of Central Nervous System Disease*, 3, JCNSD-S4140. doi:10.4137/JCNSD.S4140.

Dratcu, L., McKay, G., Singaravelu, V., & Krishnamurthy, V. (2007). Aripiprazole treatment of Asperger's syndrome in the acute psychiatric setting: Case report. *Neuropsychiatric Disease and Treatment*, 3(1), 173. doi:10.2147/nedt.2007.3.1.173.

Engelhardt, C. R., Mazurek, M. O., & Sohl, K. (2013). Media use and sleep among boys with autism spectrum disorder, ADHD, or typical development. *Pediatrics*, 132(6), 1081–1089. doi:10.1542/peds.2013-2066.

Eppright, T. D., Sanfacon, J. A., & Horwitz, E. A. (1996). Attention deficit hyperactivity disorder, infantile autism, and elevated blood-lead: A possible relationship. *Missouri Medicine*, 93 (3), 136–138.

Epstein, J. N., & Loren, R. E. (2013). Changes in the definition of ADHD in DSM-5: Subtle but important. *Neuropsychiatry*, 3(5), 455–458. doi:10.2217/npy.13.59.

Erickson, C. A., Stigler, K. A., Wink, L. K., Mullett, J. E., Kohn, A., Posey, D. J., & McDougle, C. J. (2011). A prospective open-label study of aripiprazole in fragile X syndrome. *Psychopharmacology*, 216(1), 85–90. doi:10.1007/s00213-011-2194-7.

Fatemi, S. H., Realmuto, G. M., Khan, L., & Thuras, P. (1998). Fluoxetine in treatment of adolescent patients with autism: A longitudinal open trial. *Journal of Autism and Developmental Disorders*, 28(4), 303–307. doi:10.1023/A:1026008602540.

Fitzpatrick, S. E., Srivorakiat, L., Wink, L. K., Pedapati, E. V., & Erickson, C. A. (2016). Aggression in autism spectrum disorder: Presentation and treatment options. *Neuropsychiatric Disease and Treatment*, 12, 1525–1538. doi:10.2147/NDT.S84585.

Fung, L. K., Chahal, L., Libove, R. A., Bivas, R., & Hardan, A. Y. (2012). A retrospective review of the effectiveness of aripiprazole in the treatment of sensory abnormalities in autism. *Journal of Child and Adolescent Psychopharmacology*, 22(3), 245–248. doi:10.1089/cap.2010.0103.

Galli-Carminati, G. M., Deriaz, N., & Bertschy, G. (2009). Melatonin in treatment of chronic sleep disorders in adults with autism: A retrospective study. *Swiss Medical Weekly*, 139(19–20),293–296. doi:10.4414/smw.2009.12342.

Garstang, J., & Wallis, M. (2006). Randomized controlled trial of melatonin for children with autistic spectrum disorders and sleep problems. *Child: Care, Health and Development*, 32(5), 585–589. doi:10.1111/j.1365-2214.2006.00616.x.

Geier, D. A., & Geier, M. R. (2006). A clinical trial of combined anti-androgen and anti-heavy metal therapy in autistic disorders. *Neuroendocrinology Letters*, 27(6), 833–838.

Ghaleiha, A., Mohammadi, E., Mohammadi, M. R., Farokhnia, M., Modabbernia, A., Yekehtaz, H., … & Akhondzadeh, S. (2013). Riluzole as an adjunctive therapy to risperidone for the treatment of irritability in children with autistic disorder: A double-blind, placebo-controlled, randomized trial. *Pediatric Drugs*, 15(6), 505–514. doi:10.1007/s40272-013-0036-2.

Ghanizadeh, A. (2012). Atomoxetine for treating ADHD symptoms in autism: A systematic review. *Journal of Attention Disorders*, 17(8), 635–640. doi:10.1177/1087054712443154.

Ghanizadeh, A., & Ayoobzadehshirazi, A. (2015). A randomized double-blind placebo-controlled clinical trial of adjuvant buspirone for irritability in autism. *Pediatric Neurology*, 52(1), 77–81. doi:10.1016/j.pediatrneurol.2014.09.017.

Ghanizadeh, A., Sahraeizadeh, A., & Berk, M. (2014). A head-to-head comparison of aripiprazole and risperidone for safety and treating autistic disorders, a randomized double blind clinical trial. *Child Psychiatry & Human Development*, 45(2), 185–192. doi:10.1007/s10578-013-0390-x.

Ghanizadeh, A., Tordjman, S., & Jaafari, N. (2015). Aripiprazole for treating irritability in children & adolescents with autism: A systematic review. *The Indian Journal of Medical Research*, 142(3), 269. doi:10.4103/0971-5916.166584.

Giannotti, F., Cortesi, F., Cerquiglini, A., & Bernabei, P. (2006). An open-label study of controlled-release melatonin in treatment of sleep disorders in children with autism. *Journal of Autism and Developmental Disorders*, 36(6), 741–752. doi:10.1007/s10803-006-0116-z.

Gibson, A. P., Crismon, M. L., Mican, L. M., & Fischer, C. (2007). Effectiveness and tolerability of aripiprazole in child and adolescent inpatients: A retrospective evaluation. *International Clinical Psychopharmacology*, 22(2), 101–105. doi:10.1097/YIC.0b013e3280119e0c.

Golnik, A. E., & Ireland, M. (2009). Complementary alternative medicine for children with autism: A physician survey. *Journal of Autism and Developmental Disorders*, 39(7), 996–1005. doi:10.1007/s10803-009-0714-7.

Green, V. A., Pituch, K. A., Itchon, J., Choi, A., O'Reilly, M., & Sigafoos, J. (2006). Internet survey of treatments used by parents of children with autism. *Research in Developmental Disabilities*, 27(1), 70–84. doi:10.1016/j.ridd.2004.12.002.

Guénolé, F., Godbout, R., Nicolas, A., Franco, P., Claustrat, B., & Baleyte, J. M. (2011). Melatonin for disordered sleep in individuals with autism spectrum disorders: Systematic review and discussion. *Sleep Medicine Reviews*, 15(6), 379–387. doi:10.1016/j.smrv.2011.02.001.

Gupta, R., & Hutchins, J. (2005). Melatonin: A panacea for desperate parents? (Hype or truth). *Archives of Disease in Childhood*, 90(9), 986–987. doi:10.1136/adc.2005.075218.

Handen, B. L., Aman, M. G., Arnold, L. E., Hyman, S. L., Tumuluru, R. V., Lecavalier, L., ... & Silverman, L. B. (2015). Atomoxetine, parent training, and their combination in children with autism spectrum disorder and attention-deficit/hyperactivity disorder. *Journal of the American Academy of Child & Adolescent Psychiatry*, 54(11), 905–915. doi:10.1016/j.jaac.2015.08.013.

Harfterkamp, M., Buitelaar, J. K., Minderaa, R. B., van de Loo-Neus, G., van der Gaag, R. J., & Hoekstra, P. J. (2013). Long-term treatment with atomoxetine for attention-deficit/hyperactivity disorder symptoms in children and adolescents with autism spectrum disorder: An open-label extension study. *Journal of Child and Adolescent Psychopharmacology*, 23(3), 194–199. doi:10.1089/cap.2012.0012.

Harfterkamp, M., van de Loo-Neus, G., Minderaa, R. B., van der Gaag, R. J., Escobar, R., Schacht, A., ... & Hoekstra, P. J. (2012). A randomized double-blind study of atomoxetine versus placebo for attention-deficit/hyperactivity disorder symptoms in children with autism spectrum disorder. *Journal of the American Academy of Child and Adolescent Psychiatry*, 51(7), 733–741. doi:10.1016/j.jaac.2012.04.011.

Harrington, J. W., Patrick, P. A., Edwards, K. S., & Brand, D. A. (2006). Parental beliefs about autism: Implications for the treating physician. *Autism*, 10(5), 452–462. doi:10.1177/1362361306066609.

Hayashi, E. (2000). Effect of melatonin on sleep–wake rhythm: The sleep diary of an autistic male. *Psychiatry and Clinical Neurosciences*, 54(3), 383–384. doi:10.1046/j.1440-1819.2000.00725.x.

Hellings, J. A., Boehm, D., Yeh, H. W., Butler, M. G., & Schroeder, S. R. (2011). Long-term aripiprazole in youth with developmental disabilities including autism. *Journal of Mental Health Research in Intellectual Disabilities*, 4(1), 40–52. doi:10.1080/19315864.2010.542274.

Hellings, J. A., Kelley, L. A., Gabrielli, W. F., Kilgore, E., & Shah, P. (1996). Sertraline response in adults with mental retardation and autistic disorder. *The Journal of Clinical Psychiatry*, 57 (8), 333–336.

Hollander, E., Phillips, A., King, B. H., Guthrie, D., Aman, M. G., Law, P., ... & Robinson, R. (2004). Impact of recent findings on study design of future autism clinical trials. *CNS Spectrums*, 9(1), 49–56. doi:10.1017/S109285290000835X.

Hollander, E., Soorya, L., Chaplin, W., Anagnostou, E., Taylor, B. P., Ferretti, C. J., ... & Settipani, C. (2012). A double-blind placebo-controlled trial of fluoxetine for repetitive behaviors and global severity in adult autism spectrum disorders. *American Journal of Psychiatry*, 169 (3), 292–299. doi:10.1176/appi.ajp.2011.10050764.

Horrigan, J. P., & Barnhill, L. J. (1997). More on melatonin. *Journal of the American Academy of Child & Adolescent Psychiatry*, 36(8), 1014. doi:10.1097/00004583-199708000-00002.

Howes, O. D., Rogdaki, M., Findon, J. L., Wichers, R. H., Charman, T., King, B. H., ... & Povey, C. (2018). Autism spectrum disorder: Consensus guidelines on assessment, treatment and research from the British Association for Psychopharmacology. *Journal of Psychopharmacology*, 32(1), 3–29. doi:10.1177/0269881117741766.

Huang, S. C., Tsai, S. J., & Yang, H. J. (2010). Aripiprazole improves social interaction in Taiwanese children with pervasive developmental disorder. *Chang Gung Med J*, 33(2), 211.

Hviid, A., Stellfeld, M., Wohlfahrt, J., & Melbye, M. (2003). Association between thimerosal-containing vaccine and autism. *Journal of American Medical Association*, 290(13), 1763–1766. doi:10.1001/jama.290.13.1763.

Ichikawa, H., Mikami, K., Okada, T., Yamashita, Y., Ishizaki, Y., Tomoda, A., ... & Tadori, Y. (2017). Aripiprazole in the treatment of irritability in children and adolescents with autism spectrum disorder in Japan: A randomized, double-blind, placebo-controlled study. *Child Psychiatry & Human Development*, 48(5), 796–806. doi:10.1007/s10578-016-0704-x.

Ishitobi, M., Hiratani, M., Kosaka, H., Takahashi, T., Mizuno, T., Asano, M., ... & Wada, Y. (2012). Switching to aripiprazole in subjects with Pervasive Developmental Disorders showing tolerability issues with risperidone. *Progress in Neuro-Psychopharmacology and Biological Psychiatry*, 37(1), 128–131. doi:10.1016/j.pnpbp.2011.12.015.

Ishizaki, A., Sugama, M., & Takeuchi, N. (1999). Usefulness of melatonin for developmental sleep and emotional/behavior disorders–studies of melatonin trial on 50 patients with developmental disorders. *Brain and Development*, 31(5), 428–437.

Jan, J. E., & O'Donnell, M. E. (1996). Use of melatonin in the treatment of paediatric sleep disorders: Mini Review. *Journal of Pineal Research*, 21(4), 193–199. doi:10.1111/j.1600-079X.1996.tb00286.x.

Jan, J. E., Freeman, R. D., Wasdell, M. B., & Bomben, M. M. (2004). A child with severe night terrors and sleep-walking responds to melatonin therapy. *Developmental Medicine and Child Neurology*, 46(11), 789–789. doi:10.1017/S0012162204231358.

Johnston, K., Dittner, A., Bramham, J., Murphy, C., Knight, A., & Russell, A. (2013). Attention deficit hyperactivity disorder symptoms in adults with autism spectrum disorders. *Autism Research*, 6(4), 225–236. doi:10.1002/aur.1283.

Jordan, I., Robertson, D., Catani, M., Craig, M., & Murphy, D. (2012). Aripiprazole in the treatment of challenging behaviour in adults with autism spectrum disorder. *Psychopharmacology*, 223(3), 357–360. doi:10.1007/s00213-012-2723-z.

Kent, J. M., Kushner, S., Ning, X., Karcher, K., Ness, S., Aman, M., ... & Hough, D. (2013). Risperidone dosing in children and adolescents with autistic disorder: A double-blind, placebo-controlled study. *Journal of Autism and Developmental Disorders*, 43(8), 1773–1783. doi:10.1007/s10803-012-1723-5.

Kolevzon, A., Mathewson, K. A., & Hollander, E. (2006). Selective serotonin reuptake inhibitors in autism: A review of efficacy and tolerability. *The Journal of Clinical Psychiatry*, 67(3), 407–414. doi:10.4088/jcp.v67n0311.

Kulman, G., Lissoni, P., Rovelli, F., Roselli, M. G., Brivio, F., & Sequeri, P. (2000). Evidence of pineal endocrine hypofunction in autistic children. *Neuro Endocrinology Letters*, 21(1), 31–34.

Kültür, S. E. C., Tiryaki, A., & Tasgin, E. (2009). Aripiprazole for maladaptive behavior in mental retardation: Case reports. *Bulletin in Clinical Psychopharmacology*, 19(3), 294–297.

Kuppermann, M., Lubeck, D. P., Mazonson, P. D., Patrick, D. L., Stewart, A. L., Buesching, D. P., & Filer, S. K. (1995). Sleep problems and their correlates in a working population. *Journal of General Internal Medicine*, 10(1), 25–32. doi:10.1007/BF02599573.

Langworthy-Lam, K. S., Aman, M. G., & Van Bourgondien, M. E. (2002). Prevalence and patterns of use of psychoactive medicines in individuals with autism in the Autism Society of North Carolina. *Journal of Child and Adolescent Psychopharmacology*, 12(4), 311–321. doi:10.1089/104454602762599853.

Lecavalier, L. (2006). Behavioral and emotional problems in young people with pervasive developmental disorders: Relative prevalence, effects of subject characteristics, and empirical classification. *Journal of Autism and Developmental Disorders*, 36(8), 1101–1114. doi:10.1007/s10803-006-0147-5.

Madsen, K. M., Lauritsen, M. B., Pedersen, C. B., Thorsen, P., Plesner, A. M., Andersen, P. H., & Mortensen, P. B. (2003). Thimerosal and the occurrence of autism: Negative ecological evidence from Danish population-based data. *Pediatrics*, 112(3), 604–606. doi:10.1542/peds.112.3.604.

Maneeton, N., Maneeton, B., Putthisri, S., Suttajit, S., Likhitsathian, S., & Srisurapanont, M. (2018). Aripiprazole in acute treatment of children and adolescents with autism spectrum disorder: A systematic review and meta-analysis. *Neuropsychiatric Disease and Treatment*, 14, 3063–3072. doi:10.2147/NDT.S174622.

Mannion, A., & Leader, G. (2014). Sleep problems in autism spectrum disorder: A literature review. *Review Journal of Autism and Developmental Disorders*, 1(2), 101–109. doi:10.1007/s40489-013-0009-y.

Marcus, R. N., Owen, R., Kamen, L., Manos, G., McQuade, R. D., Carson, W. H., & Aman, M. G. (2009). A placebo-controlled, fixed-dose study of aripiprazole in children and adolescents with irritability associated with autistic disorder. *Journal of the American Academy of Child & Adolescent Psychiatry*, 48(11), 1110–1119. doi:10.1097/CHI.0b013e3181b76658.

Marcus, R. N., Owen, R., Manos, G., Mankoski, R., Kamen, L., McQuade, R. D., ... & Aman, M. G. (2011). Aripiprazole in the treatment of irritability in pediatric patients (aged 6–17 years) with autistic disorder: Results from a 52-week, open-label study. *Journal of Child and Adolescent Psychopharmacology*, 21(3), 229–236. doi:10.1089/cap.2009.0121.

Martin, A., Koenig, K., Anderson, G. M., & Scahill, L. (2003). Low-dose fluvoxamine treatment of children and adolescents with pervasive developmental disorders: A prospective, open-label study. *Journal of Autism and Developmental Disorders*, 33(1), 77–85. doi:10.1023/A:1022234605695.

Martin, A., Scahill, L., Anderson, G. M., Aman, M., Arnold, L. E., McCracken, J., ... & Research Units on Pediatric PsychopharmacologyAutism Network. (2004). Weight and leptin changes among risperidone-treated youths with autism: 6-month prospective data. *American Journal of Psychiatry*, 161(6), 1125–1127. doi:10.1176/appi.ajp.161.6.1125.

Masi, G., Cosenza, A., Millepiedi, S., Muratori, F., Pari, C., & Salvadori, F. (2009). Aripiprazole monotherapy in children and young adolescents with pervasive developmental disorders. *CNS Drugs*, 23(6), 511–521. doi:10.2165/00023210-200923060-00005.

Mayes, S. D., Calhoun, S. L., Murray, M. J., Ahuja, M., & Smith, L. A. (2011). Anxiety, depression, and irritability in children with autism relative to other neuropsychiatric disorders and typical development. *Research in Autism Spectrum Disorders*, 5(1), 474–485. doi:10.1016/j.rasd.2010.06.012.

McCracken, J. T., McGough, J., Shah, B., Cronin, P., Hong, D., Aman, M. G., ... & McDougle, C. J. (2002). Risperidone in children with autism and serious behavioral problems. *New England Journal of Medicine*, 347(5), 314–321. doi:10.1056/NEJMoa013171.

McDougle, C. J., Brodkin, E. S., Naylor, S. T., Carlson, D. C., Cohen, D. J., & Price, L. H. (1998). Sertraline in adults with pervasive developmental disorders: A prospective open-label investigation. *Journal of Clinical Psychopharmacology*, 18(1), 62–66.

McDougle, C. J., Naylor, S. T., Cohen, D. J., Volkmar, F. R., Heninger, G. R., & Price, L. H. (1996). A double-blind, placebo-controlled study of fluvoxamine in adults with autistic disorder. *Archives of General Psychiatry*, 53(11), 1001–1008. doi:10.1001/archpsyc.1996.01830110037005.

Mitka, M. (2008). Chelation therapy trials halted. *Journal of the American Medical Association*, 300, 2236. doi:10.1001/jama.2008.607.

Miyamoto, A., Oki, J., Takahashi, S., & Okuno, A. (1999). Serum melatonin kinetics and long-term melatonin treatment for sleep disorders in Rett syndrome. *Brain and Development*, 21(1), 59–62. doi:10.1016/S0387-7604(98)00072-2.

Mohiuddin, S., & Ghaziuddin, M. (2013). Psychopharmacology of autism spectrum disorders: A selective review. *Autism*, 17(6), 645–654. doi:10.1177/1362361312453776.

Nagaraj, R., Singhi, P., & Malhi, P. (2006). Risperidone in children with autism: Randomized, placebo-controlled, double-blind study. *Journal of Child Neurology*, 21(6), 450–455. doi:10.1177/08830738060210060801.

Namerow, L. B., Thomas, P., Bostic, J. Q., Prince, J., & Monuteaux, M. C. (2003). Use of citalopram in pervasive developmental disorders. *Journal of Developmental & Behavioral Pediatrics*, 24(2), 104–108.

Niederhofer, H., Damodharan, S. K., Joji, R., & Corfield, A. (2006). Atomoxetine treating patients with Autistic disorder. *Autism*, 10(6), 647–648. doi:10.1177/1362361306073001.

Nydén, A., Myrén, K. J., & Gillberg, C. (2008). Long-term psychosocial and health economy consequences of ADHD, autism, and reading-writing disorder: A prospective service evaluation project. *Journal of Attention Disorders*, 12(2), 141–148. doi:10.1177/1087054707306116.

O'Nions, E., Happé, F., Evers, K., Boonen, H., & Noens, I. (2018). How do parents manage irritability, challenging behaviour, non-compliance and anxiety in children with autism spectrum disorders? A meta-synthesis. *Journal of Autism and Developmental Disorders*, 48(4), 1272–1286. doi:10.1007/s10803-017-3361-4.

Owen, R., Sikich, L., Marcus, R. N., Corey-Lisle, P., Manos, G., McQuade, R. D., ... & Findling, R. L. (2009). Aripiprazole in the treatment of irritability in children and adolescents with autistic disorder. *Pediatrics*, 124(6), 1533–1540. doi:10.1542/peds.2008-3782.

Owley, T., Walton, L., Salt, J., Guter Jr, S. J., Winnega, M., Leventhal, B. L., & Cook Jr, E. H. (2005). An open-label trial of escitalopram in pervasive developmental disorders. *Journal of the American Academy of Child & Adolescent Psychiatry*, 44(4), 343–348. doi:10.1097/01.chi.0000153229.80215.a0.

Paavonen, E. J., Nieminen-von Wendt, T., Vanhala, R., Aronen, E. T., & von Wendt, L. (2003). Effectiveness of melatonin in the treatment of sleep disturbances in children with Asperger disorder. *Journal of Child and Adolescent Psychopharmacology*, 13(1), 83–95. doi:10.1089/104454603321666225.

Pandina, G. J., Bossie, C. A., Youssef, E., Zhu, Y., & Dunbar, F. (2007). Risperidone improves behavioral symptoms in children with autism in a randomized, double-blind, placebo-controlled trial. *Journal of Autism and Developmental Disorders*, 37(2), 367–373. doi:10.1007/s10803-006-0234-7.

Pardini, M., Guida, S., & Gialloreti, L. E. (2010). Aripiprazole treatment for coprophagia in autistic disorder. *The Journal of Neuropsychiatry and Clinical Neurosciences*, 22(4), 451–e33. doi:10.1176/jnp.2010.22.4.451.e33.

Parker, S. K., Schwartz, B., Todd, J., & Pickering, L. K. (2004). Thimerosal-containing vaccines and autistic spectrum disorder: A critical review of published original data. *Pediatrics*, 114(3), 793–804. doi:10.1542/peds.2004-0434.

Patel, K., & Curtis, L. T. (2007). A comprehensive approach to treating autism and attention-deficit hyperactivity disorder: A prepilot study. *The Journal of Alternative and Complementary Medicine*, 13(10), 1091–1098. doi:10.1089/acm.2007.0611.

Price, C. S., Thompson, W. W., Goodson, B., Weintraub, E. S., Croen, L. A., Hinrichsen, V. L., ... & Bernal, P. (2010). Prenatal and infant exposure to thimerosal from vaccines and immunoglobulins and risk of autism. *Pediatrics*, 126(4), 656–664. doi:10.1542/peds.2010-0309.

Research Autism. (2019, December 5). *Risperidone and Autism*. Retrieved from http://www.researchautism.net/interventions/43/risperidone-and-autism.

Research Units on Pediatric Psychopharmacology (RUPP) Autism Network (2005). Randomized, controlled, crossover trial of methylphenidate in pervasive developmental disorders with hyperactivity. *Archives Of General Psychiatry*, 62(11), 1266–1274. doi:10.1001/archpsyc.62.11.1266.

Risher, J. F., & Amler, S. N. (2005). Mercury exposure: Evaluation and intervention: The inappropriate use of chelating agents in the diagnosis and treatment of putative mercury poisoning. *Neurotoxicology*, 269(4), 691–699. doi:10.1016/j.neuro.2005.05.004.

Rossignol, D. A., & Frye, R. E. (2011). Melatonin in autism spectrum disorders: A systematic review and meta-analysis. *Developmental Medicine & Child Neurology*, 53(9), 783–792. doi:10.1111/j.1469-8749.2011.03980.x.

Roth, T. (2007). Insomnia: Definition, prevalence, etiology, and consequences. *Journal of Clinical Sleep Medicine*, 3(5 Suppl), S7.

Rugino, T. A., & Janvier, Y. M. (2005). Aripiprazole in children and adolescents: Clinical experience. *Journal of Child Neurology*, 20(7), 603–610. doi:10.1177/08830738050200071301.

Scahill, L., Jeon, S., Boorin, S. J., McDougle, C. J., Aman, M. G., Dziura, J., … & Deng, Y. (2016). Weight gain and metabolic consequences of risperidone in young children with autism spectrum disorder. *Journal of the American Academy of Child and Adolescent Psychiatry*, 55 (5), 415–423. doi:10.1016/j.jaac.2016.02.016.

Schatzberg, A. F., & Nemeroff, C. B. (Eds.). (2013). *Essentials of clinical psychopharmacology*. Arlington, VA: American Psychiatric Pub.

Schrimsher, G. W., Billingsley, R. L., Jackson, E. F., & Moore, B. D. (2002). Caudate nucleus volume asymmetry predicts attention-deficit hyperactivity disorder (ADHD) symptomatology in children. *Journal of Child Neurology*, 17(12), 877–884. doi:10.1177/08830738020170122001.

Şenel, H. G. (2010). Parents' views and experiences about complementary and alternative medicine treatments for their children with autistic spectrum disorder. *Journal of Autism and Developmental Disorders*, 40(4), 494–503. doi:10.1007/s10803-009-0891-4.

Shastri, M., Alla, L., & Sabaratnam, M. (2006). Aripiprazole use in individuals with intellectual disability and psychotic or behavioural disorders: A case series. *Journal of Psychopharmacology*, 20(6), 863–867. doi:10.1177/0269881106067765.

Siegel, M., & Beaulieu, A. A. (2012). Psychotropic medications in children with autism spectrum disorders: A systematic review and synthesis for evidence-based practice. *Journal of Autism and Developmental Disorders*, 42(8), 1592–1605. doi:10.1007/s10803-011-1399-2.

Smith, T., Aman, M. G., Arnold, L. E., Silverman, L. B., Lecavalier, L., Hollway, J., … & Rice Jr, R. R. (2016). Atomoxetine and parent training for children with autism and attention-deficit/hyperactivity disorder: A 24-week extension study. *Journal of the American Academy of Child & Adolescent Psychiatry*, 55(10), 868–876. doi:10.1016/j.jaac.2016.06.015.

Staller, J. A. (2003). Aripiprazole in an adult with Asperger disorder. *Annals of Pharmacotherapy*, 37(11), 1628–1631. doi:10.1345/aph.1D147.

Stehr-Green, P., Tull, P., Stellfeld, M., Mortenson, P. B., & Simpson, D. (2003). Autism and thimerosal-containing vaccines. *American Journal of Preventive Medicine*, 25(2), 101–106. doi:10.1016/s0749-3797(03)00113-2.

Steingard, R. J., Zimnitzky, B., DeMASO, D. R., Bauman, M. L., & Bucci, J. P. (1997). Sertraline treatment of transition-associated anxiety and agitation in children with autistic disorder. *Journal of Child and Adolescent Psychopharmacology*, 7(1), 9–15. doi:10.1089/cap.1997.7.9.

Stewart, M. E., Barnard, L., Pearson, J., Hasan, R., & O'Brien, G. (2006). Presentation of depression in autism and Asperger syndrome: A review. *Autism*, 10(1), 103–116. doi:10.1177/1362361306062013.

Stigler, K. A., Diener, J. T., Kohn, A. E., Li, L., Erickson, C. A., Posey, D. J., & McDougle, C. J. (2009). Aripiprazole in pervasive developmental disorder not otherwise specified and Asperger's disorder: A 14-week, prospective, open-label study. *Journal of Child and Adolescent Psychopharmacology*, 19(3), 265–274. doi:10.1089/cap.2008.093.

Stigler, K. A., Mcdougle, C. J., Scahill, L., Aman, M. G., Eugene, A. L., Johnson, C., et al. (2011). Medication and parent training in children with pervasive developmental disorders and serious behavior problems: Effectiveness and tolerability of aripiprazole in risperidone nonresponders. *Neuropsychopharmacology*, 36, S228.

Stigler, K. A., Posey, D. J., & McDougle, C. J. (2004). Aripiprazole for maladaptive behavior in pervasive developmental disorders. *Journal of Child & Adolescent Psychopharmacology*, 14(3), 455–463. doi:10.1089/cap.2004.14.455.

Taylor, D. M., Barnes, T. R., & Young, A. H. (2018). *The Maudsley prescribing guidelines in psychiatry.* John Wiley & Sons.

Tzischinsky, O., Meiri, G., Manelis, L., Bar-Sinai, A., Flusser, H., Michaelovski, A. … & Dinstein, I. (2018). Sleep disturbances are associated with specific sensory sensitivities in children with autism. *Molecular Autism*, 9(1), 22. doi:10.1186/s13229-018-0206-8.

Uno, Y., Uchiyama, T., Kurosawa, M., Aleksic, B., & Ozaki, N. (2015). Early exposure to the combined measles-mumps-rubella vaccine and thimerosal-containing vaccines and risk of autism spectrum disorder. *Vaccine*, 33(21), 2511–2516. doi:10.1016/j.vaccine.2014.12.036.

Valicenti-McDermott, M. R., & Demb, H. (2006). Clinical effects and adverse reactions of off-label use of aripiprazole in children and adolescents with developmental disabilities. *Journal of Child & Adolescent Psychopharmacology*, 16(5), 549–560. doi:10.1089/cap.2006.16.549.

Williams, K., Brignell, A., Randall, M., Silove, N., & Hazell, P. (2013). Selective serotonin reuptake inhibitors (SSRIs) for autism spectrum disorders (ASD). *Cochrane Database of Systematic Reviews*, 2013(8). doi:10.1002/14651858.CD004677.pub3.

Wirojanan, J., Jacquemont, S., Diaz, R., Bacalman, S., Anders, T. F., Hagerman, R. J., & Goodlin-Jones, B. L. (2009). The efficacy of melatonin for sleep problems in children with autism, fragile X syndrome, or autism and fragile X syndrome. *Journal of Clinical Sleep Medicine*, 5(2), 145–150.

World Health Organization. (2019, December 5). *Depression: Let's talk*. Retrieved from https://www.who.int/mental_health/management/depression/en/.

Wright, B., Sims, D., Smart, S., Alwazeer, A., Alderson-Day, B., Allgar, V. … & McCaffrey, N. (2011). Melatonin versus placebo in children with autism spectrum conditions and severe sleep problems not amenable to behaviour management strategies: A randomised controlled cross-over trial. *Journal of Autism and Developmental Disorders*, 41(2), 175–184. doi:10.1007/s10803-010-1036-5.

Chapter 11

Cognitive-based strategies

11.1 Introduction

This chapter reviews the research about the therapeutic benefits that autistics can obtain from mindfulness programs and cognitive behaviour therapy (CBT). It begins with a brief overview of mindfulness, including interoception, and then examines the contents of several studies about the efficacy of mindfulness and interoception for autistics. The support's efficacy for autistics is then rated followed by several recommendations for research in the future. The contents in studies about the efficacy of CBT for autistics is then examined, followed by a rating of the efficacy of CBT for autistics and several recommendations for where research can be conducted in the future. After presenting these recommendations this chapter presents some views and experiences about mindfulness programs and CBT from a group of autistics.

11.2 Mindfulness activities/interoception

11.2.1 Mindfulness activities

Mindfulness activities are broadly defined as activities in which one focuses all of their attention on the present moment, either on internal or external stimuli. Such activities have a diverse range of applications. They can help reduce the burnout rates of healthcare professionals (Goodman & Schorling, 2012), help support people with intellectual disabilities (Harper, Webb, & Rayner, 2013; Singh et al., 2013), and maintain or improve the physical and mental health of caregivers raising autistic children (Jones et al., 2018; Rayan & Ahman, 2016, 2017, 2018). In over 200 South Australian schools, mindful body awareness activities are taught two to three times a day and referred to as 'interoception activities', which have been found to help autistics develop self-regulation skills (Davies et al., 2017; Goodall, 2018). During our review of the general literature about supports for autistics, we identified four studies about the value of mindfulness activities for autistics and one literature review on interoception and autism.

In their study, which combined a systematic literature review and narrative analysis, Cachia, Anderson, and Moore (2016a) examined studies about the efficacy of mindfulness activities in helping autistics decrease their stress, anxiety, depression, rumination and aggression, and increase their psychological well-being. They used the *Evaluative Method for Determining Evidence-Based Practices in Autism* (Reichow,

Volkmar, & Cicchetti, 2008) to assess the quality of the six studies they collected. They rated three studies as 'weak', because they did not use a control group, one was rated as 'adequate', and two were rated as 'strong'. Based on this finding, they concluded that:

> This review assessing the effects of mindfulness-based interventions with persons with ASD analysed a range of participants, methodologies and measures adopted across studies corroborating the robustness of mindfulness interventions resulting in positive psychological changes in individuals with ASD. The body of literature discussed highlights the potential application of mindfulness with individuals with ASD; however, mindfulness research in this population is weak relative to other clinical and non-clinical group designs. (Cachia, Anderson, & Moore, 2016a, pp. 176–177).

Collectively, the studies examined by Cachia, Anderson, and Moore indicated that mindfulness programs can help autistics of all ages. For autistic children, such programs can help reduce instances of challenging behaviours and anxiety (Hwang et al., 2015). For autistic adolescents, they can help them reduce their aggression and increase their social responsiveness and psychological well-being (Singh et al., 2011a, 2011b). Finally, for autistic adults, they can reduce their anxiety, depression, and rumination (Kiep, Spek, & Hoeben, 2015; Spek, van Ham, & Nyklíček, 2013).

Most studies about the efficacy of mindfulness programs for autistics have not examined if the benefits of such programs are sustainable. Kiep, Spek, and Hoeben (2015) addressed this gap in the literature. In their study, 50 autistic adults participated in a nine-week mindfulness therapy program. Self-reported behaviours were evaluated at three intervals; (1) before the first session (i.e., pre-intervention,) (2) after the last session (i.e., post-intervention), and (3) nine weeks after the last session (i.e., follow-up). They found that during the mindfulness program participants exhibited a decline in anxiety, depression, agoraphobia, somatisation, distrust of others, interpersonal sensitivity, sleeping problems, and rumination. Additionally, there was a significant increase in affect (i.e., that is the ability to express one's emotions via their face). However, feelings of hostility did not significantly decline. They also found that from post-intervention to follow-up all measured symptoms remained stable and that rumination was an important mediating factor. They concluded that the mindfulness program that they examined can help autistics reduce psychological difficulties and that these benefits were retained nine weeks after the program ended.

While these findings appear promising, Kiep, Spek, and Hoeben have stressed that their results should be interpreted with caution because their study contained several limitations. First, since there was no control group it is unknown if the mindfulness program itself or some unknown factor not related to the mindfulness program produced positive benefits. Second, they only examined the therapeutic benefits that the mindfulness program gave autistic adults with average to above-average intelligence. Due to this sample composition, it is not possible to conclude if autistics who do not fit the profile of the people sampled and examined, such as those with below-average intelligence, would achieve the same outcomes.

Most studies which have measured the therapeutic benefits of mindfulness programs in relation to autism have either examined the utility of such programs with autistics

(Singh et al., 2011a) or their parents/caregivers (Cachia, Anderson, & Moore, 2016b; Conner & White, 2014; Jones et al., 2018; Rayan & Ahmad, 2016, 2017, 2018). However, there are some studies that have examined the efficacy of a mindfulness program for both autistic adolescents and their parents. In de Bruin et al.'s (2015) study, 23 autistic adolescents received nine weekly sessions of mindfulness called *MYmind*. At the same time their parents (18 mothers, 11 fathers) participated in a mindfulness program, called *Mindful Parenting*. To measure the effects of these programs, de Bruin et al. collected data about the participant's quality of life at pre-test, post-test, and at nine-weeks after the program ended. In terms of the effectiveness of *MYmind*, they found that adolescents reported that they experienced an increase in their quality of life and a decrease in rumination. However, they did not find any changes to their level of worry, core autistic symptoms, or mindful awareness. From the perspective of their parents, they thought that their adolescent children exhibited improvements with social responsiveness, social communication, social cognition, preoccupations, and social motivation. In terms of the effectiveness of *Mindful Parenting*, the parents reported that their parenting skills improved and that the quality of their life increased.

While the findings from de Bruin et al.'s study are promising, their study contained several limitations that could compromise the results reached. First, their findings are based on a small sample of autistic adolescents (n = 23) and a small sample of parents (18 mothers, 11 fathers). Due to these small sample sizes, it was not possible to generalise the results collected to autistic adolescents of their parents in general. Second, they did not use a control group which meant that it was not possible to determine the efficacy of their program against other factors, such as school lessons on coping skills that autistic adolescents could use to improve their lives. Third, data about the efficacy of *MYmind* and *Mindful Parenting* came from the participants completing questionnaires. Such data collection is extremely subjective and biased since respondents might be influenced by the placebo effect; believing the mindfulness program is working when it actually is not. Triangulating the data collected from parents and autistic adolescents with data collected from more objective sources, such as a clinician's observations, might help validate the conclusions drawn. Collectively, these limitations make it difficult to accurately determine the efficacy of their mindfulness program for autistic adolescents and their parents.

One way to examine the benefits of mindfulness activities is to compare the effectiveness of such activities to other strategies and approaches. Sizoo and Kuiper (2017) examined if mindfulness-based stress reduction (MBSR) and CBT were both equally effective in reducing the anxiety and depression exhibited by autistic adults. In their study, 59 autistic adults who had anxiety and depression scores above seven on the *Hospital Anxiety and Depression Scale* participated; with 27 being allocated to a CBT program and 32 being allocated to a MBSR program. Measurements about the participant's anxiety and depression, autism symptoms, rumination, and global mood were collected at the start of the study, at the end of the 13-week study, and three months after the study concluded (i.e., follow-up period). The data collected indicated that MBSR and CBT both helped autistic adults reduce their anxiety and depression and that these benefits were maintained, as indicated by scores collected during the follow-up period. Based on these outcomes, Sizoo and Kuiper (2017, p. 47) concluded:

> Mindfulness and cognitive behavioral therapies are both promising treatment methods for reducing comorbid anxiety and depression in adults with ASD.

While Sizoo and Kuiper claimed that CBT and mindfulness activities can both equally provide autistics with benefits, their results need to be treated with caution. First, their study contained a small number of participants in the CBT (n = 22) and mindfulness (n = 32) groups. With such small sample sizes, it is not possible to generalise the results collected to the entire autistic population. Second, they did not use a control group in their study, which made it difficult to compare the efficacy of the CBT and mindfulness programs against a group which did not receive these supports.

Aside from comparing the efficacy of mindfulness activities to other approaches there are studies that have examined if combining mindfulness activities with other approaches can produce benefits for autistics. Semple (2018) reviewed eight peer-reviewed studies that examined the combined effects of mindfulness activities and yoga. They found that such a combined approach improved a participant's self-control, quality of life, social responsiveness, social communication, social cognition, social motivation, and imitative behaviours (See Table 11.1). Additionally, such a combined approach also helped increase the participant's tolerance of adults entering their personal space and helped reduced their aggressive behaviours, irritability, lethargy, social withdrawal, and noncompliance. Despite these positive findings, Semple (2018, p. 1) concluded that:

> the empirical evidence to support the efficacy of yoga and mindfulness-based interventions for children and adolescents with ASD is inconclusive. The current body of research has significant limitations, including small sample sizes, no fidelity measures, and no control groups. Each of the eight studies, however, reported some positive effects on social, emotional, or behavioral metrics. These early results are promising and sufficient to warrant support for further research.

Recently, Hartley, Dorstyn, and Due (2019) examined studies about the benefits autistics obtained from mindfulness activities. They located ten studies that collectively involved a pool of 223 autistic participants and 241 caregivers. They used Reichow, Volkmar, and Cicchetti's (2008) *Evaluative Method for Determining Evidence-Based Practices in Autism* to determine the quality of the research collected. They found that mindfulness activities appear to mitigate many interpersonal and mental health issues that autistics experience. However, to confirm these promising results, they recommended that more quantitative research should be conducted. Such research can help improve the generalisability of the findings to the broader autistic population, as well as improve our understanding of intervention effects and the potential gender differences in treatment response.

11.2.2 Interoception

Interoception is colloquially known as the eighth sense, being the conscious perception of internal body states, or mindful body awareness. Neuroimaging studies focused on functional relationships between the insula and other primary sensory areas within the brain thought to be involved in interoception, have consistently demonstrated group differences in autistics (Barttfeld et al., 2012; Bernhardt et al., 2014; Di Martino et al., 2014; Ebisch et al., 2011; Uddin, Supekar, & Lynch, 2013). One study found reduced response or complete disconnection between the bilateral posterior insula to the anterior insula, and between corresponding somatosensory and limbic regions in adults with ASD (Ebisch et al., 2011). The posterior insula is considered the primary interoceptive cortex (Craig, 2004). DuBois et al.'s (2016, p. 104) literature review of interoception and autism found that interoception

> is atypical in ASD, but the degree and directionality of this abnormality is not yet clear due to the heterogeneity of the condition. Between-group interoceptive differences in individuals with and without ASD have been repeatedly demonstrated, with a slight tendency towards hyporeactivity in interoceptive awareness in individuals with ASD.

Goodall (2018) notes that good interoception is a prerequisite for developing the ability to manage emotions, which is an area of difficulty for many autistics of all ages and that engaging in interoception activities activates the parasympathetic nervous system, which acts to neurobiologically calm the individual (Craig, 2003).

There is little research on the benefits of interoception activities for autistics, other than Mahler's (2016) book on the link between improved interoception in autistics and improves self-awareness and social understanding of autistics. In addition, the research in South Australian Schools indicates that the benefits for children range from decreased dysregulation, through increased pro-social interactions and engagement in learning for both autistics and non-autistics (Department for Education, 2019). Interoception therapies are known to be effective in the treatment of trauma and Post Traumatic Stress Disorder (Payne, Levine, & Crane-Godreau, 2015) as well as more widely for improving emotion regulation (Price & Hooven, 2018).

11.2.3 Evaluation of mindfulness/interoception

Rating: Silver – Usually promising

Most of the research that we have examined has shown that mindfulness/interoception can give some autistics many benefits, including increased social communication and a reduction in anxiety and depression. Despite these findings the studies reviewed contained serious methodological flaws, such as small sample sizes and no control groups. These flaws have the potential to undermine the results collected. Due to these and other flaws, we cannot conclusively claim that mindfulness/interoception can help autistics. Therefore, we have rated such programs as 'Silver – Usually promising'.

11.2.4 Directions for research in the future about mindfulness/interoception

Most of the literature that we reviewed has concluded that mindfulness/interoception can provide some autistics with benefits, including a reduction in anxiety and depression, and increase in social communication. Despite these potential benefits, there remains three areas where more research can be conducted.

First, most studies reviewed did not contain a control group, which made it impossible to accurately measure the efficacy of the mindfulness activity against a non-treatment group. Similarly, with the exception of Sizoo and Kuiper's (2017) study, the benefits that mindfulness activities can give autistics have not been compared to the benefits that other supports can offer autistics (i.e., CBT). To determine the efficacy of mindfulness activities, in the future researchers should compare the benefits that a group of autistics participating in mindfulness obtain against a group of autistics who either do not receive any supports (i.e., control group) or who receive other types of supports.

Second, most of the studies examined the benefits that autistic children obtained from mindfulness activities. Consequently, there is a lack of knowledge about how such activities can help autistic adults. In the future studies should address this gap in our knowledge so that autistic adults, as well as those who support them, can have a better understanding about the potential benefits that they can deliver.

Third, with the exception of Semple's (2018) study, there is a lack of research that has explored if the benefits that mindfulness activities can produce can be enhanced if it is combined with other supports. In the future, it would be prudent to conduct more research into the benefits that autistics can obtain from participant in mindfulness activities that are combined with other supports. If such research shows promising benefits, then this will increase the number of support options available to autistics.

11.2.5 Autistic views about mindfulness activities

Respondents' ratings of the efficacy of mindfulness to manage any aspects of their autism

Most respondents (n = 10, 21.28%) rated mindfulness as either 'enjoyed, found useful and found that my well-being and mood were improved' or 'did not enjoy or find useful'. This was followed by 7 (14.89%) who selected the option 'did not enjoy but found useful', 6 (12.77%) who selected the option 'enjoyed and found useful', and 4 (8.51%) who selected the option 'enjoyed but did not find useful'. Based on the distribution of responses, the efficacy of mindfulness activities for autistics as perceived by autistics was calculated as 3.1 stars.

3.1 ☆☆☆

Figure 11.1 3.1 stars

Table 11.1 Summary of studies examined by Semple (2018)

Study	*Sample size, gender and age range*	*Indicator of level of functioning*	*Intervention*	*Research design*	*Main outcomes*
Radhakrishna, 2010	$N = 6$ with parents five males one female ages 8–14	DSM-IV diagnosis of ASD; IQ = 70 and above	Modified Integrated Approach to Yoga Therapy (IAYT) program. Five sessions per week for 10 months.	Uncontrolled open trial	Improvements in • Communication • Imitative behaviours • Motor control
Radhakrishna, Nagarathna, and Nagendra, 2010	$N = 6$ with parents five males one female ages 8–14	DSM-IV diagnosis of ASD; Mean IQ = 76.5	ABA plus modified IAYT program; 15 hours of ABA plus five hours of IAYT per week for two ten-month academic years.	Uncontrolled open trial [a]	Increased tolerance of • Sitting • Adult proximity • Subsequent socialisation Observation and anecdotal feedback suggested improvements in • Imitation skills • Verbal receptive skills • Expressions • Comprehension of spatial commands
Singh et al., 2011b	$N = 3$ all male ages 13–18	DSM-IV diagnosis of Asperger Syndrome with history of physical aggression	Meditation on the Soles of the Feet; five days of training followed by twice daily practice for 17–24 weeks.	Multiple baseline across subjects	• Reductions in aggressive behaviours • Improvements maintained over a four-year follow-up
Singh et al., 2011a	$N = 3$ all male ages 14–17	Diagnosis of ASD with history of physical aggression	Meditation on the Soles of the Feet; five days of training followed by twice daily practice for 23–30 weeks.	Multiple baseline across subjects	• Reductions in aggressive behaviours • Improvements maintained over a three-year follow-up

Study	*Sample size, gender and age range*	*Indicator of level of functioning*	*Intervention*	*Research design*	*Main outcomes*
Rosenblatt et al., 2011	$N = 24$ 22 males two females ages 3–16	Diagnosis of ASD	Eight-week multi-modal yoga, dance, and music therapy.	Uncontrolled open trial	Improvements on parent-reported BASC-2 • Behavioural Symptom Index (BSI) clinical scale • Atypicality subscale of the BSI
Koenig, Buckley-Reen, and Garg, 2012	$N = 46$ 37 males nine females ages 5–12	Diagnosis of ASD	Get Ready to Learn (GRTL) program; 16 weeks; daily sessions.	Nonrandomised trial with an "education-as-usual" comparison group	Reductions in • Irritability • Lethargy • Hyperactivity • Social withdrawal
Chan et al., 2013	$N = 46$ 36 males[b] four females ages 6–17	Diagnosis of ASD = 37 Diagnosis of PDD = 3 12 children (30%) had limited intelligence with IQ score below 70	Nei Yang Gong (NYG); four weeks; two training sessions per week; daily practice.	Age- and IQ-matched randomised trial with an active comparison group (Progressive Muscle Relaxation)	• Improvements in self-control • Less impulsivity in problem-solving
de Bruin et al., 2015	$N = 23$ 17 males six girls with 29 parents	ASD = 4 Asperger Syndrome = 8 Pervasive Developmental Disorder = 11 Educational level: Primary school = 1 Lower vocational secondary education = 10 High general secondary education = 4 Preuniversity = 5 College = 3	MYmind; nine weeks, 90 min sessions per week with concurrent Mindful Parenting Training.	Uncontrolled open trial	Adolescents reported • Improvements in quality of life • Decreases in rumination Parents reported improvements in • Social responsiveness • Social communication • Social cognition • Social motivation • Flexible thinking • Eye contact • Better peer contacts Parents reported decreases in • Preoccupations • Obsessive thinking

Key:
[a] Although Radhakrishna et al. (2010) indicated that six matched "ABA only" controls were also selected, no demographic or outcome data were provided for this group. Therefore, this study is described here as an uncontrolled open trial (n = 6).
[b] Demographic information was provided only for the completion sample (n = 40).
Source: Semple, 2018, pp. 3–4.

Respondents' comments about using mindfulness to manage any aspects of your autism

When asked 'How did you find using mindfulness to manage any aspects of your autism?' 18 respondents provided a comment. Our examination of the comments found a range of diverse experiences of mindfulness programs. Two respondents provided a very detailed explanation as to how mindfulness helped them develop a greater self-awareness.

> "Mindfulness has helped me to feel my body. Previously, I was always thinking and I could not stop my thoughts. I also found that it helped me connect my feelings to my body, something that I had never learned to do and due to school bullying I had only survived my high school years by suppressing all of my feelings so that I could face my bullies each day without crying. Mindfulness helped connect my thoughts, feelings, physiological responses to my body, and helped me to gain control over the overwhelming feelings that I'd had."
>
> "I have found it life changing to be able to know that what is happening now will come to an end. Before I would frequently get caught up in a 'now is forever' thinking loop which would increase distress."

Two respondents suggested that mindfulness did not help them because they did not receive proper training about mindfulness.

> "Yet to find a resource or teacher that can EXPLAIN mindfulness in any meaningful way. Personally, I find vague, analogy-based instructions that can't be explained in clear, simple language usually mean the instructor doesn't really know what they're doing, which gives me little faith in meditation or mindfulness."
>
> "Well I think mindfulness is being bandied around by a heap of people who have no real experience of how to practice it or guide others through it. I have practiced meditation and guided meditation since I was very young (6 or 7) and have only ever been frustrated when forced to be subjected to the droning voice of someone trying to sound like they know what they are doing when they clearly don't. I think you need a good 20 years of practice under your belt in order to guide people. It's not enough to simply have watched a Youtube video and read a book. As such it's become a bit of a fad and I have no respect for it."

Aside from a lack of training, one participant explained that other activities were more beneficial for them than mindfulness.

> "I worked with a psychologist on mindfulness to help manage anxiety. I didn't find the formal mindfulness stuff particularly useful – I think for me it's more useful to do something like dancing which is mindful anyway."

Interviewing an autistic psychologist, they talked about how difficult formal mindfulness is for some autistics, but focus on interest is very easy, which is similar to mindfulness.

> "I have seen mindfulness be a very powerful support for some autistics, who have learnt to notice their thoughts rather than get caught up in them. It can help to

> reframe life events whilst distancing from the emotive aspects. It can really help to challenge the 'now is forever' thinking so prevalent in autistics."

Since some respondents found mindfulness beneficial and others did not it is important that therapists take into consideration the needs of their individual autistic clients. It is possible that taking these views into consideration could show that some might find this type of support not beneficial.

11.3 Cognitive behavioural therapy (CBT)

11.3.1 Cognitive behavioural therapy (CBT)

One of the main aims of CBT is to deter the occurrence of maladaptive thinking that can cause disruptive behaviours (Marks et al., 2003). Patients who receive CBT learn strategies that they can use to recognise and mitigate any maladaptive or unhelpful thinking so that they prevent unhelpful behaviours. CBT can be used with patients individually or in a group, it can also be delivered via computer programs (Marks et al., 2003). CBT has been found to help people manage insomnia (Cheng & Dizon, 2012) and/or depression (Cuijpers et al., 2013). During our exploration of the literature about supports for autistics, we discovered several meta-analyses and literature reviews in which studies about the efficacy of CBT for autistics were examined.

Binnie and Blainey (2013) examined seven studies that examined the efficacy of CBT in helping autistic adults increase their social and communication skills. They found that the results in the studies they examined were mixed and that there was no definitive evidence that supported the hypothesis that CBT was effective for autistic adults. Furthermore, information about previous or concurrent supports or treatments that could have helped the participants was not explained in the analysed studies. With this information being omitted it was difficult to attribute any benefits obtained purely to CBT.

Sukhodolsky and colleagues (2013) published a meta-analysis in which they examined eight studies about the efficacy of CBT in helping children with high-functioning autism manage their anxiety. They found that CBT can be an effective strategy that can help reduce the anxiety that these autistic children exhibit. However, they noted that they examined a small number of studies and that they did not include case studies, single-case designs, and qualitative case reports. Examining such publications could have altered their findings.

Spain and colleagues (2015) published a review of the literature about the efficacy of CBT in helping autistic adults manage the symptoms of psychiatric co-morbid conditions. The six studies that they retrieved were conducted in different countries, used different CBT interventions, and examined the effectiveness of CBT on different co-morbid psychiatric diagnoses. They found that despite CBT programs having different durations (i.e., 6–26 weeks) and number of sessions (i.e., 6–16 sessions), they can be beneficial for members of the autistic population (See Table 11.2).

Spain et al. (2017) examined four case studies about the benefits that CBT can give autistics. They found that modifications to the structure and content of CBT programs can accommodate the specific needs of autistic patients. Examples of these modifications included detailed information about abstract concepts (e.g., anxiety), use of visual

Table 11.2 Summary of studies examined by Spain et al. (2015)

Study	*Method*	*Sample n, core and co-morbid diagnoses*	*Intervention*	*Outcome measures*	*Results*
Cardaciotto and Herbert, 2004	Case study	One male 26 years old Asperger syndrome Social phobia, depressive symptoms	*Number of sessions*: 14 *Session duration*: Not specified *Techniques*: Social skills training, skills rehearsal (role plays), cognitive restructuring	SPAI LSAS BDI-II CGI Behavioural assessment	Improvement in social anxiety and low mood symptoms
Hare, 1997	Case study	One male 23 years old Asperger syndrome Low mood, self-harm, excessive alcohol use	*Number of sessions*: 17 *Session duration*: 30–60 min *Techniques*: Emotional literacy, graded exposure, cognitive restructuring, relaxation and distraction	BDI Idiosyncratic record of self-harm incidents	Improvement in low mood symptoms Reduced frequency of self-harm
Russell et al., 2008	Quasi-experimental, non-randomised trial, CBT for OCD (n = 12) vs TAU (n = 12)	21 males, three females Mean age 23.8 (CBT) Mean age 32.1 (TAU) ASD diagnosis OCD Symptoms of anxiety or low mood	*Number of sessions*: Ten to 50 session (mean 27.5) *Session duration*: Not specified *Techniques*: Exposure-based tasks, cognitive restructuring	YBOCS BDI BAI	58% (n = 7) improved with CBT compared with 16% (n = 2) TAU group OCD symptom reduction more likely for CBT group No statistically significant changes or differences in BDI and BAI scores, between groups
Russell et al., 2013	RCT CBT for OCD (n = 20) vs anxiety management (AM) (n = 17) Manualised approach	35 adults Mean age 28.6 (CBT) Mean age 25.2 (AM) ASD diagnosis OCD diagnosis Symptoms of anxiety, or low mood	*Number of sessions*: Mean CBT: 17.4 Mean AM: 14.4 *Session duration*: 1 hour *Techniques*: Emotional literacy, exposure-based tasks, cognitive restructuring	YBOCS BDI BAI CGI WSAS	Improvements in OCD symptoms reported for CBT and AM conditions, 45% treatment responders (CBT) and 20% treatment responders (AM) No significant differences between groups pre- and post-treatment on other measures

Study	*Method*	*Sample n, core and co-morbid diagnoses*	*Intervention*	*Outcome measures*	*Results*
Spek, van Ham, and Nyklíček, 2013	RCT Mindfulness-based group (MBSR) (n = 20) vs wait list (WL) (21) Manualised approach	27 males, 14 females Mean age 44.4 (MBSR) Mean age: 40.1 (WL) ASD diagnosis Symptoms of anxiety, depression or rumination	*Number of sessions*: nine *Session duration*: 2.5 hour *Techniques*: Mindfulness-based techniques including meditation	SCL-90-R RRQ DGMS, positive affect sub-scale	Improvements in mood, rumination and anxiety symptoms following MBSR compared to wait list control, increase in positive affect Differences between groups, Cohen's d 0.76 (anxiety) and 1.25 (rumination)
Weiss and Lunsky, 2010	Group-based case series Manualised approach	Two males, one female Asperger syndrome Depression, PTSD, agoraphobia	*Number of sessions*: 12 *Session duration*: 60 min *Techniques*: Emotional literacy, cognitive restructuring, behavioural experiments, behavioural experiments	BDI-II BAI	Downward trend in anxiety symptoms, no significant change in self-report of mood pre- and post-treatment

Key:
TAU – treatment as usual, BDI – Beck Depression Inventory, BAI – Beck Anxiety Inventory, SPAI – Social Phobia and Anxiety Inventory, LSAS – Liebowitz Social Anxiety Scale, CGI – Clinical Global Impression, YBOCS – Yale-Brown Obsessive Compulsive Scale, SCL-90-R – Symptom checklist revised, RRQ – Rumination Reflection Questionnaire, DGMS – Global Mood Scale (Dutch version), WSAS – Work and Social Adjustment Scale.
Source: Spain et al., 2015, pp. 156–157.

aids (e.g., cue cards), and inclusion of social skills sessions. Each case study concluded that CBT can help reduce the participant's social anxiety and concerns about performance in social interactions. In terms of general mental health and emotional well-being, scores from the *Clinical Global Impression Scale* (Cardaciotto & Herbert, 2004) and the *Clinical Outcomes in Routine Evaluation Measure* (Turner & Hammond, 2016) changed from a rating of severe collected before the start of the CBT program to mid-range or milder after the CBT program. Based on these results, Spain et al. (2017, p. 44) concluded that:

> To date, the four case studies published (in English) indicate that cognitive and behavioural interventions are clinically useful for individuals with ASD and SA [Social Anxiety]. Future studies should seek to develop the intervention evidence base further.

Ung et al.'s (2015) study was both a systematic literature review and a meta-analysis. They examined 14 studies about the efficacy of CBT for treating anxiety for young autistics; 12 randomised controlled trials and two open trial studies. Based on the articles collected, they concluded that CBT was a useful therapeutic approach that can help reduce anxiety among high-functioning autistic children. However, Ung et al.'s findings need to be interpreted with caution since the studies they analysed did not have a consistent reporting of participant characteristics that may have influenced the effectiveness of the CBT program (e.g., anxiety diagnosis, medication usage).

11.4.2 Evaluation of cognitive behavioural therapy (CBT)

Rating: Silver – Usually promising

In our opinion, most of the studies examined contained minor methodological limitations. The overall conclusions drawn by most studies is mixed with conflicting suggestions as to whether CBT can provide autistics with many benefits, and it is uncertain if it can be effectively used with autistics who have different abilities and circumstances. Since there are questions about the efficacy of CBT for autistics we have rated it as 'Silver – Usually promising'.

11.3.3 Directions for research in the future about cognitive behavioural therapy (CBT)

As the literature about the benefits that CBT can give autistics is extensive with mixed findings there is a need for more research. In addition, the literature has only examined the benefits which autistic males have obtained from CBT. As a consequence, possible benefits that CBT for female or non-binary autistics remains an area that is under-researched. It might be that female or non-binary autistics would require more intense CBT than their male counterparts, especially considering that they may experience different demands and expectations in society than males. Second, a review of the literature showed that CBT is often conducted in isolation, and that few studies have examined if complementary supports, such as writing therapy or animal programs, can improve the efficacy of CBT for autistics. It could be that some specific supports in conjunction with CBT could produce more beneficial outcomes for autistics. For example, for autistics with depression a combination of CBT and animal programs could be an effective and valuable option. CBT can help them identify and manage depressive thoughts and an animal program could help them avoid the depression caused by social isolation by putting them into a position of interacting with others. Together they may help them build important social networks that can also help them manage their depression.

11.3.4 Autistic views about cognitive behavioural therapy (CBT)

Have you personally used cognitive behaviour therapy (CBT) to manage anything related to your autism?

Out of 206 respondents who completed our online survey, 51 (24.75%) answered the question 'Have you personally used cognitive behaviour therapy (CBT) to manage anything related to your autism?' Of the 51 who answered this question, 36 (70.59%) selected the option 'Yes' and 15 (29.41%) selected the option 'No'.

Respondents' ratings of the efficacy of using cognitive behaviour therapy (CBT) to manage anything related to your autism

Most respondents (n = 12, 26.09%) selected the option 'did not enjoy or find useful' when rating the efficacy of CBT, followed by nine (19.57%) who selected the option 'did not enjoy but found useful', and seven (15.22%) who selected the option 'enjoyed and found useful'. Finally, three (6.52%) selected either the option 'enjoyed but did not find useful' or 'enjoyed, found useful and found that my well-being and mood were improved'. Based on the distribution of responses, the efficacy of CBT for autistics as perceived by autistics was calculated as 2.6 stars.

Respondents' comments about using cognitive behaviour therapy (CBT) to manage anything related to your autism

When asked 'How did you find using cognitive behaviour therapy (CBT) to manage anything related to your autism?' 27 respondents provided a comment. Three participants described why they felt CBT was beneficial for them.

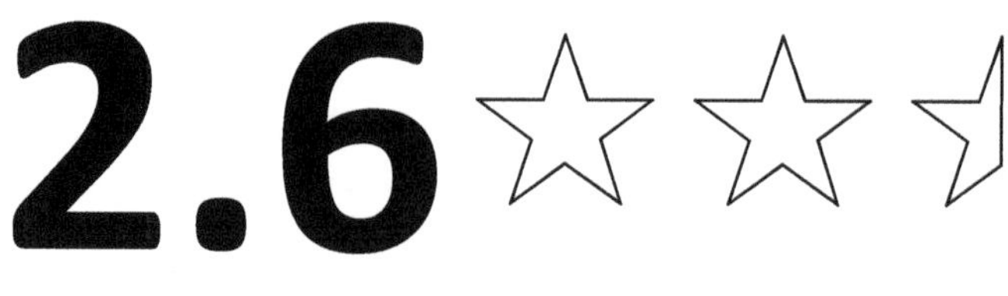

Figure 11.2 2.6 stars

> "I have done CBT for depression and anxiety, not targeted directly at treating autism but it's probably helped to address some of my unhelpful autism-related thinking styles (e.g. black-and-White thinking). It is helpful in some situations but not in others."
>
> "it was concrete, it provided skills that helped me function and manage my emotions better. It was practical and I definitely benefited from it."
>
> "As this was black and white I felt it gave me emotional rules/guidelines to live by in the neurotypicals world at work."

One respondent who believed CBT was not effective, felt that other forms of therapy were more beneficial for them.

> "CBT as a therapy may be useful for some people. For me though, it's underlying assumption that "I have dysfunctional thoughts" and 'cognitive errors' did not apply. What benefited me most was trauma-related therapies i.e. movement – walking, swimming, animal-assisted therapies – our pets, my music – listening to music and playing the piano, art – creating things; in addition to peer support from other Autistic adults."

Additionally, three respondents believed CBT either masked their anxiety or did not give them the tools to manage their challenges.

> "CBT taught me how to mask my anxiety so that it does not control my life. However, I still experience the anxiety. I just don't behave as though I do."
>
> "Had huge benefits initially as I developed insight but limited because it lacked practical application. I need strategies to manage on a daily basis even though I have heaps of insight."
>
> "Mostly for managing anxiety. I didn't find it useful as I could understand logically that it didn't make sense to worry about something, but the emotional part of my brain didn't understand that!"

An autistic psychologist reported that they had not found CBT to be particularly helpful for their autistic clients.

> "CBT can often leave autistics feeling judged or bad for who they are, which isn't helpful. I find Acceptance, Commitment Therapy much more useful, as it doesn't have the same feel."

Since some respondents found CBT beneficial while others did not experience benefits. Due to the dichotomy of views collected, it is important that clinicians take into consideration the views of their autistic clients. Such consultations might reveal that some would find this form of support not beneficial after one to two trial sessions.

11.4 Conclusion

This chapter reviewed the literature about the efficacy of mindfulness activities and CBT for autistics. Mindfulness activities and CBT were rated as 'Silver – Usually promising'. Despite some studies containing methodological weaknesses, for example, de Bruin et al.'s (2015) study about mindfulness did not use a control group, objective measurements or evaluations, most studies have shown that mindfulness and CBT can be effective supports for autistics. Despite their effectiveness, there still remain several areas in which research can be conducted in the future. For example, most research about mindfulness has based their results on samples of autistic children. As a consequence, not much is known about the effectiveness of this support for autistic adults. This chapter concluded with a series of views and experiences of autistics about CBT and mindfulness programs.

References

Barttfeld, P., Wicker, B., Cukier, S., Navarta, S., Lew, S., Leiguarda, R., & Sigman, M. (2012). State-dependent changes of connectivity patterns and functional brain network topology in autism spectrum disorder. *Neuropsychologia*, 50(14), 3653–3662. doi:10.1016/j.neuropsychologia.2012.09.047.

Bernhardt, B. C., Valk, S. L., Silani, G., Bird, G., Frith, U., & Singer, T. (2014). Selective disruption of sociocognitive structural brain networks in autism and alexithymia. *Cerebral Cortex*, 24(12), 3258–3267. doi:10.1093/cercor/bht182.

Binnie, J., & Blainey, S. (2013). The use of cognitive behavioural therapy for adults with autism spectrum disorders: A review of the evidence. *Mental Health Review Journal*, 18(2), 93–104. doi:10.1108/MHRJ-05-2013-0017.

Cachia, R. L., Anderson, A., & Moore, D. W. (2016a). Mindfulness in individuals with autism spectrum disorder: A systematic review and narrative analysis. *Review Journal of Autism and Developmental Disorders*, 3(2), 165–178. doi:10.1007/s40489-016-0074-0.

Cachia, R. L., Anderson, A., & Moore, D. W. (2016b). Mindfulness, stress and well-being in parents of children with autism spectrum disorder: A systematic review. *Journal of Child and Family Studies*, 25(1), 1–14. doi:10.1007/s10826-015-0193-8.

Cardaciotto, L., & Herbert, J. D. (2004). Cognitive behavior therapy for social anxiety disorder in the context of Asperger's syndrome: A single-subject report. *Cognitive and Behavioral Practice*, 11(1), 75–81. doi:10.1016/S1077-7229(04)80009-9.

Chan, A. S., Sze, S. L., Siu, N. Y., Lau, E. M., & Cheung, M. C. (2013). A Chinese mind-body exercise improves self-control of children with autism: A randomized controlled trial. *PLoS One*, 8(7), e68184. doi:10.1371/journal.pone.0068184.

Cheng, S. K., & Dizon, J. (2012). Computerised cognitive behavioural therapy for insomnia: A systematic review and meta-analysis. *Psychotherapy and Psychosomatics*, 81(4), 206–216. doi:10.1159/000335379.

Conner, C. M., & White, S. W. (2014). Stress in mothers of children with autism: Trait mindfulness as a protective factor. *Research in Autism Spectrum Disorders*, 8(6), 617–624. doi:10.1016/j.rasd.2014.02.001.

Craig, A. D. (2003). Interoception: The sense of the physiological condition of the body. *Current Opinion in Neurobiology*, 13(4), 500–505.

Craig, A. D. (Bud). (2004). Human feelings: Why are some more aware than others? *Trends in Cognitive Sciences*, 8(6), 239–241. doi:10.1016/j.tics.2004.04.004.

Cuijpers, P., Berking, M., Andersson, G., Quigley, L., Kleiboer, A., & Dobson, K. S. (2013). A meta-analysis of cognitive-behavioural therapy for adult depression, alone and in comparison with other treatments. *The Canadian Journal of Psychiatry*, 58(7), 376–385. doi:10.1177/070674371305800702.

Davies, C., Rodd, D., Parsons, K., & Goodall, E. (2017) The 8th sense: Interoception. *Department for Education and Child Development, Adelaide.*

de Bruin, E. I., Blom, R., Smit, F. M., van Steensel, F. J., & Bögels, S. M. (2015). MYmind: Mindfulness training for youngsters with autism spectrum disorders and their parents. *Autism*, 19(8), 906–914. doi:10.1177/1362361314553279.

Department for Education (2019). *Ready to Learn – Interoception kit*. Adelaide: Department for Education South Australia.

Di Martino, A., Yan, C. G., Li, Q., Denio, E., Castellanos, F. X., Alaerts, K., ... & Deen, B. (2014). The autism brain imaging data exchange: Towards a large-scale evaluation of the intrinsic brain architecture in autism. *Molecular Psychiatry*, 19(6), 659–667. doi:10.1038/mp.2013.78.

DuBois, D., Ameis, S. H., Lai, M. -C., Casanova, M. F., & Desarkar, P. (2016). Interoception in autism spectrum disorder: A review. *International Journal of Developmental Neuroscience*, 52, 104–111. doi:10.1016/j.ijdevneu.2016.05.001.

Ebisch, S. J. H., Gallese, V., Willems, R. M., Mantini, D., Groen, W. B., Romani, G. L., ... & Bekkering, H. (2011). Altered intrinsic functional connectivity of anterior and posterior insula regions in high-functioning participants with autism spectrum disorder. *Human Brain Mapping*, 32(7), 1013–1028. doi:10.1002/hbm.21085.

Goodall, E. (2018). *Understanding and facilitating the achievement of autistic potential*. Adelaide: Healthy Possibilities.

Goodman, M. J., & Schorling, J. B. (2012). A mindfulness course decreases burnout and improves well-being among healthcare providers. *The International Journal of Psychiatry in Medicine*, 43(2), 119–128. doi:10.2190/PM.43.2.b.

Hare, D. J. (1997). The use of cognitive-behavioural therapy with people with Asperger syndrome: A case study. *Autism*, 1(2), 215–225. doi:10.1177/1362361397012007.

Harper, S. K., Webb, T. L., & Rayner, K. (2013). The effectiveness of mindfulness-based interventions for supporting people with intellectual disabilities: A narrative review. *Behavior Modification*, 37(3), 431–453. doi:10.1177/0145445513476085.

Hartley, M., Dorstyn, D., & Due, C. (2019). Mindfulness for children and adults with autism spectrum disorder and their caregivers: A Meta-analysis. *Journal of Autism and Developmental Disorders*, 49(10), 4306–4319. doi:10.1007/s10803-019-04145-3.

Hwang, Y. S., Kearney, P., Klieve, H., Lang, W., & Roberts, J. (2015). Cultivating mind: Mindfulness interventions for children with autism spectrum disorder and problem behaviours, and their mothers. *Journal of Child and Family Studies*, 24(10), 3093–3106. doi:10.1007/s10826-015-0114-x.

Jones, L., Gold, E., Totsika, V., Hastings, R. P., Jones, M., Griffiths, A., & Silverton, S. (2018). A mindfulness parent well-being course: Evaluation of outcomes for parents of children with autism and related disabilities recruited through special schools. *European Journal of Special Needs Education*, 33(1), 16–30. doi:10.1080/08856257.2017.1297571.

Kiep, M., Spek, A. A., & Hoeben, L. (2015). Mindfulness-based therapy in adults with an autism spectrum disorder: Do treatment effects last? *Mindfulness*, 6(3), 637–644. doi:10.1007/s12671-014-0299-x.

Koenig, K. P., Buckley-Reen, A., & Garg, S. (2012). Efficacy of the get ready to learn yoga program among children with autism spectrum disorders: A pretest–posttest control group design. *American Journal of Occupational Therapy*, 66(5), 538–546. doi:10.5014/ajot.2012.004390.

Mahler, K. J. (2016). *Interoception: The eighth sensory system: Practical solutions for improving self-regulation, self-awareness and social understanding of individuals with autism spectrum and related disorders*. Kansas: AAPC Publishing.

Marks, I. M., Mataix-Cols, D., Kenwright, M., Cameron, R., Hirsch, S., & Gega, L. (2003). Pragmatic evaluation of computer-aided self-help for anxiety and depression. *The British Journal of Psychiatry*, 183(1), 57–65. doi:10.1192/bjp.183.1.57.

Payne, P., Levine, P. A., & Crane-Godreau, M. A. (2015). Somatic experiencing: Using interoception and proprioception as core elements of trauma therapy. *Frontiers in Psychology*, 6, 1–18. doi:10.3389/fpsyg.2015.00093.

Price, C. J., & Hooven, C. (2018). Interoceptive awareness skills for emotion regulation: Theory and approach of mindful awareness in body-oriented therapy (MABT). *Frontiers in Psychology*, 9. doi:10.3389/fpsyg.2018.00798.

Radhakrishna, S. (2010). Application of integrated yoga therapy to increase imitation skills in children with autism spectrum disorder. *International Journal of Yoga*, 3(1), 26–30. doi:10.4103/0973–6131.66775.

Radhakrishna, S., Nagarathna, R., & Nagendra, H. R. (2010). Integrated approach to yoga therapy and autism spectrum disorders. *Journal of Ayurveda and Integrative Medicine*, 1(2), 120–124. doi:10.4103/0975–9476.65089.

Rayan, A., & Ahmad, M. (2016). Effectiveness of mindfulness-based interventions on quality of life and positive reappraisal coping among parents of children with autism spectrum disorder. *Research in Developmental Disabilities*, 55, 185–196. doi:10.1016/j.ridd.2016.04.002.

Rayan, A., & Ahmad, M. (2017). Effectiveness of mindfulness-based intervention on perceived stress, anxiety, and depression among parents of children with autism spectrum disorder. *Mindfulness*, 8(3), 677–690. doi:10.1007/s12671-016-0595-8.

Rayan, A., & Ahmad, M. (2018). Psychological distress in Jordanian parents of children with autism spectrum disorder: The role of trait mindfulness. *Perspectives in Psychiatric Care*, 54 (1), 11–18. doi:10.1111/ppc.12187.

Reichow, B., Volkmar, F. R., & Cicchetti, D. V. (2008). Development of the evaluative method for evaluating and determining evidence-based practices in autism. *Journal of Autism and Developmental Disorders*, 38(7), 1311–1319. doi:10.1007/s10803-007-0517-7.

Rosenblatt, L. E., Gorantla, S., Torres, J. A., Yarmush, R. S., Rao, S., Park, E. R., … & Levine, J. B. (2011). Relaxation response–based yoga improves functioning in young children with autism: A pilot study. *The Journal of Alternative and Complementary Medicine*, 17(11), 1029–1035. doi:10.1089/acm.2010.0834.

Russell, A. J., Jassi, A., Fullana, M. A., Mack, H., Johnston, K., Heyman, I., … & Mataix-Cols, D. (2013). Cognitive behavior therapy for comorbid obsessive-compulsive disorder in high-functioning autism spectrum disorders: A randomized controlled trial. *Depression and Anxiety*, 30(8), 697–708. doi:10.1002/da.22053.

Russell, A. J., Mataix-Cols, D., Anson, M. A. W., & Murphy, D. G. M. (2008). Psychological treatment for obsessive-compulsive disorder in people with autism spectrum disorders-a pilot study. *Psychotherapy and Psychosomatics*, 78(1), 59.

Semple, R. J. (2018). Yoga and mindfulness for youth with autism spectrum disorder: Review of the current evidence. *Child and Adolescent Mental Health*, 24(1), 12–18. doi:10.1111/camh.12295.

Singh, N. N., Lancioni, G. E., Karazsia, B. T., Winton, A. S., Myers, R. E., Singh, A. N., … & Singh, J. (2013). Mindfulness-based treatment of aggression in individuals with mild intellectual disabilities: A waiting list control study. *Mindfulness*, 4(2), 158–167. doi:10.1007/s12671-012-0180-8.

Singh, N. N., Lancioni, G. E., Manikam, R., Winton, A. S., Singh, A. N., Singh, J., & Singh, A. D. (2011a). A mindfulness-based strategy for self-management of aggressive behavior in adolescents with autism. *Research in Autism Spectrum Disorders*, 5(3), 1153–1158. doi:10.1016/j.rasd.2010.12.012.

Singh, N. N., Lancioni, G. E., Singh, A. D., Winton, A. S., Singh, A. N., & Singh, J. (2011b). Adolescents with Asperger syndrome can use a mindfulness-based strategy to control their aggressive behavior. *Research in Autism Spectrum Disorders*, 5(3), 1103–1109. doi:10.1016/j.rasd.2010.12.006.

Sizoo, B. B., & Kuiper, E. (2017). Cognitive behavioural therapy and mindfulness based stress reduction may be equally effective in reducing anxiety and depression in adults with autism spectrum disorders. *Research in Developmental Disabilities*, 64, 47–55. doi:10.1016/j.ridd.2017.03.004.

Spain, D., Sin, J., Chalder, T., Murphy, D., & Happe, F. (2015). Cognitive behaviour therapy for adults with autism spectrum disorders and psychiatric co-morbidity: A review. *Research in Autism Spectrum Disorders*, 9, 151–162. doi:10.1016/j.rasd.2014.10.019.

Spain, D., Sin, J., Harwood, L., Mendez, M. A., & Happé, F. (2017). Cognitive behaviour therapy for social anxiety in autism spectrum disorder: A systematic review. *Advances in Autism*, 3 (1), 34–46. doi:10.1108/AIA-07-2016-0020.

Spek, A. A., van Ham, N. C., & Nyklíček, I. (2013). Mindfulness-based therapy in adults with an autism spectrum disorder: A randomized controlled trial. *Research in Developmental Disabilities*, 34(1), 246–253. doi:10.1016/j.ridd.2012.08.009.

Sukhodolsky, D. G., Bloch, M. H., Panza, K. E., & Reichow, B. (2013). Cognitive-behavioral therapy for anxiety in children with high-functioning autism: A meta-analysis. *Pediatrics*, 132 (5), e134–e1350. doi:10.1542/peds.2013-1193.

Turner, M. A., & Hammond, N. (2016). Cognitive behavioural therapy in the treatment of social skills deficits and social phobia in a man with an autism spectrum disorder: A single-case study. *The Cognitive Behaviour Therapist*, 9. doi:10.1017/S1754470X15000768.

Uddin, L., Supekar, K., & Lynch, C. (2013). Salience network–based classification and prediction of symptom severity in children with autism. *JAMA Psychiatry*, 70(8), 869–879. doi:10.1001/jamapsychiatry.2013.104.

Ung, D., Selles, R., Small, B. J., & Storch, E. A. (2015). A systematic review and meta-analysis of cognitive-behavioral therapy for anxiety in youth with high-functioning autism spectrum disorders. *Child Psychiatry and Human Development*, 46(4), 533–547. doi:10.1007/s10578-014-0494-y.

Weiss, J. A., & Lunsky, Y. (2010). Group cognitive behaviour therapy for adults with Asperger syndrome and anxiety or mood disorder: A case series. *Clinical Psychology & Psychotherapy*, 17(5), 438–446. doi:10.1002/cpp.694.

Chapter 12

Conclusion and final comments

In this book more than 30 different types of support programs for autistics were reviewed. For each support program, literature reviews, meta-analysis studies, and single academic studies were reviewed and summarised, with a rating of the support program's efficacy for autistics provided. Recommendations for where more research could be conducted in the future was then presented. Potential peer-reviewed studies of interest that were published in English were sourced from Google Scholar, Springer, Taylor & Francis, SAGE, and PubMed, with no restriction on date range. To ensure that only publications of the highest methodological quality were examined, the *Checklist for Systematic Reviews and Research Synthesis* (See Appendix 1) and the *Critical Review Form – Quantitative Studies* checklist (See Appendix 2) were used. Despite yielding a large number of creditable studies, our research processes did have some limitations. For example, studies published in languages other than English might have resulted in the supports being rated differently.

Unlike other books in this field, this one has the distinction of presenting the views and experiences from a group of autistics and people who self-identify as autistic about the efficacy of support programs. Their contributions have provided an added level of insight that other books or studies on this topic have not reached. Furthermore, the autistic contributors' recollections and views also revealed some unexplored perspectives about the potential unintended consequences or issues as well as not well-known benefits that support programs might provide.

While incorporating an 'autistic voice' into this work is a feature that distinguishes this book from others, there are some limitations that should be acknowledged. First, 194 people who were either autistic or who self-identified as autistic completed our online survey. Whilst their contributions were valuable, the small number of responses collected meant that the results drawn were not representative of the entire autistic population. Second, the data provided by the respondents were not corroborated by other people familiar with the participant's circumstances. Thus, it was not possible to confirm if the respondent's insights and experiences were authentic. In the future, this limitation might be mitigated if other people who are familiar with the respondent's experiences of autism supports, such as therapists, family members, or friends could provide input on their recollections of how the supports impacted the individual. Third, we decided to use an online survey because this method of information collection was accessible and did not require high levels of social interaction. Additionally, online surveys can provide autistics with an opportunity to reflect on their answers before they convey them. In contrast, face-to-face communication, such as a focus group or an in-depth interview, requires much quicker responses and a higher level of social communication skills. Despite the benefits of the online surveys, we were not in a position to ask the respondents for clarification. In the future this limitation can be mitigated if respondents provide their contact details, such as their email address. With these details, respondents can be contacted and asked for more details or a clarification of their answers.

Although this book is an important contribution to the field of autism supports each year there are new studies being published on existing or new supports and strategies. Since this book examines academic research up until 2019 it is important that readers have the tools to examine either new research or studies that were not included in this book. Using the checklists used to examine the research presented in this book may be helpful in evaluating the quality and applicability of new research (See Appendices 2 and 3).

While more than thirty different autism supports were reviewed, there were many that were not reviewed. Additionally, with each passing year new support programs for autistics are developed and advertised. With new autism support programs or existing programs that were not examined, it would be wise to study relevant research from many different perspectives. The list of questions from the National Autistic Society's *Researching Autism Program* checklist may be helpful for this (See Appendix 1).

On a final note, one rationale for including the views and experiences of autistics about support programs was because they are the ones who ultimately either reap the benefits or pay a price for participating in such strategies, supports or programs. Due to this, a range of autistics should be consulted during the development of autism supports as well as individual autistics being checked in with regularly when engaged in any therapy or support strategy.

Appendix 1

Researching autism program checklist from the National Autistic Society

Background questions

1 What is the full name of the support program? Does it have any other names?
2 How was the intervention developed? (For example, is it based on clinical or personal experience, religious or philosophical belief? Does it come from another field of medicine or disability?)
3 Were people on the autism spectrum actively involved in, or consulted on, its development?

Philosophy and aims

1 What is the aim of the intervention or programme?
2 What is the underlying idea or philosophy behind the intervention or programme?
3 What is the underlying mechanism, that is, how is it supposed to work?
4 Does it focus on one specific skill or problem or is it a general approach?
5 Are you happy with the philosophy and aims of the intervention or programme?

Key features of the support program

1 What type of intervention is it? (Is it a training programme, a special diet, a medication or a service?)
2 What are the major features of the intervention or programme? For example:

   a Who delivers the intervention?
   b Where is it delivered?
   c How is the intervention delivered?

3 Is the intervention or programme adapted to the needs of people on the autism spectrum? If so, how?
4 Is the intervention or programme personalised to the needs of the individual? If so, how?
5 How is it different to any similar interventions or programmes?
6 Will I have to undertake or stop other treatments or activities if I start this?

Evidence

1 What evidence is there for this intervention? (Research studies, personal accounts from other people?)
2 Are you happy with the level of evidence?

Participants

1 Which group of people is this intervention or programme supposed to help? (Anyone, people on the autism spectrum, children?)
2 Are there any people who should not undertake this intervention or programme - such as people with epilepsy or other medical conditions?

Supply and availability

1 Is this intervention available throughout the UK, only in certain places in the UK, or only overseas?
2 Which organisations and individuals provide this intervention or programme? If there is more than one supplier, what is the difference between the suppliers?
3 Is there a waiting list? If so, how long is it and do I have to make a payment to be put on it?

Training

1 Do I need any training in order to undertake this intervention or programme?
2 Who provides this training, what does it involve, how long does it take, and how much does it cost?

Equipment and materials

1 Do I need to buy or rent any special equipment or materials?
2 Do I need to make any special adaptations or modification to my home?

Time

1 How long does the intervention or programme last - days, weeks, months, years? (Maximum? Minimum?) How often does it take place (hourly, daily, weekly, monthly)?
2 How much time is involved over the course of a month (or year, including travel, training and any follow up activities) - for the participant, parents, carers, and professionals?

Costs

1 Do I have to pay for this intervention or programme? Can I get help to pay for this intervention from anywhere? If so, where?

2 How much in total does the intervention cost (including enrolment fee, training, materials or equipment (including renewals), fees, administration charges, travel costs, follow up or recurring costs such as re-registration, other additional costs)?
3 Can I get my money back if the intervention or programme is not effective?

Risks and safety

1 Does the intervention or programme use techniques that are:

   a painful or hazardous
   b distressing for the participants
   c socially unacceptable (such as sanction-based or restricting liberty)
   d illegal (such as physical assault, confinement or use of illegal substances)?

2 Does this intervention or programme have any side effects for the participants or effects for other members of the family (such as increased anxiety or stress)?

Staffing

1 What is the background of the programme director and staff?
2 Which staff will be working with me or my child and can I meet them before making my decision?
3 What experience do these staff have of working with people like me or my child?
4 Do programme staff co-ordinate their work for me or my child with other professionals?
5 Do all staff working with autistics:

   a work in partnership with autistic adults and/or children and, where appropriate, with their families, partners and carers?
   b offer support and care respectfully?
   c take time to build a trusting, supportive, empathic and non-judgemental relationship as an essential part of care?

6 Do all staff working with autistics understand the:

   a nature, development and course of autism?
   b impact on personal, social, educational and occupational functioning?
   c impact of the social and physical environment?

7 Do all health and social care professionals providing care and support for autistics:

   a aim to foster the person's autonomy, promote active participation in decisions about care and support self-management?
   b maintain continuity of individual relationships wherever possible?
   c ensure that comprehensive information about the nature of, and interventions and services for, their difficulties is available in an appropriate language or format including various visual, verbal and aural, easy-read, and different colour and font formats?
   d consider whether the person may benefit from access to a trained advocate?

8 Do all health and social care professionals providing care and support for autistics and their families, partners and carers:

   a ensure that they are easily identifiable (for example, by producing or wearing appropriate identification) and approachable?
   b clearly communicate their role and function?
   c address the person using the name and title they prefer?
   d clearly explain any clinical language and check that the person with autism understands what is being said?

9 Do all health and social care professionals providing care and support for autistics and their families, partners and carers ensure that they are:

   a familiar with recognised local and national sources (organisations and websites) of information and/or support for people with autism?
   b able to discuss and advise on how to access and engage with these resources?

10 Are all health and social care professionals providing care and support for autistics:

   a aware of under-reporting and under-recognition of physical disorders in people with autism?
   b vigilant for unusual likes and dislikes about food and/or lack of physical activity?
   c offering advice about the beneficial effects of a healthy diet and exercise, taking into account any hyper- and/or hypo-sensory sensitivities; if necessary, support referral to a GP or dietician?

Regulation and complaints

1 Is this intervention or programme regulated by an external organisation, such as a professional association or university? If so, when was the date of the last audit and what did it say?
2 Is there a complaints process? Have there been any complaints or legal disputes about the intervention or programme? What were the outcomes of those complaints or disputes?

Evaluation

1 What do people say about the intervention (including the providers, people on the spectrum, parents, independent professionals, research evidence)?
2 Are programme staff open to suggestions about improvements from people on the autism spectrum, families and other professionals?
3 Can I talk to other people (such as individuals on the autism spectrum, parents) who have been involved with the intervention?

Red flags

Red flags are signs that an intervention or programme may not be what it seems, examples of red flags include:

1. Celebrity endorsement (why should celebrities know more than you?)
2. Glitzy presentations (for example videos and PowerPoint presentations) which include bogus scientific data.
3. Commercialisation of the intervention or programme (expensive fees or opportunities for you to make money by becoming a reseller of the intervention).
4. 'Research' findings that have not been published in reputable peer-reviewed journals.
5. Use of outdated or incomplete research studies and reviews which don't show the full picture.
6. Hard-sell techniques (including emotional blackmail or special offers).
7. Use of words like 'miracle', 'faith', 'trust', 'cure', 'recovery'.
8. Claims of high success rates and rapid results.
9. Claims that the intervention is effective for many conditions, disorders, and diseases.
10. Claims that the intervention is easy to use, requiring little training or expertise.
11. Claims that other proven interventions are unnecessary, inferior, or harmful.
12. Promotional literature or websites which have incomplete contact details – such as a full postal address, landline phone number, etc.
13. Warnings and reprimands from appropriate organisations, such as the National Institute for Health and Care Excellence or the Advertising Standards Authority.

Remember: If an intervention looks too good to be true then it probably is.

Appendix 2

JBI critical appraisal checklist for systematic reviews and research syntheses

Reviewer: ______________________ Date of the review: ______________

Author of the publication: _________ Publication year: ______________

Record number: _________________________

Question	*Item*			
	Yes	*No*	*Unclear*	*Not applicable*
Is the review question clearly and explicitly stated?				
Were the inclusion criteria appropriate for the review question?				
Was the search strategy appropriate?				
Were the sources and resources used to search for studies adequate?				
Were the criteria for appraising studies appropriate?				
Was critical appraisal conducted by two or more reviewers independently?				
Were there methods to minimize errors in data extraction?				
Were the methods used to combine studies appropriate?				
Was the likelihood of publication bias assessed?				
Were recommendations for policy and/or practice supported by the reported data?				
Were the specific directives for new research appropriate?				

Overall appraisal: Include: ☐ Exclude: ☐ Seek further information: ☐

Comments (Including reason for exclusion)

Appendix 3

McMaster critical review form – Quantitative Studies

Study Purpose *Was the purpose stated clearly?* *Yes* □ *No* □	*Outline the purpose of the study. How does the study apply to occupational therapy and/or your research question?*
Literature *Was relevant background literature reviewed?* Yes □ No □	Describe the justification of the need for this study.
Design Randomized controlled trial □ Cohort □ Single case design □ Before and after □ Case-control □ Cross-sectional □ Case study □	Describe the study design. Was the design appropriate for the study question? (e.g., for knowledge level about this issue, outcomes, ethical issues, etc.) Specify any biases that may have been operating and the direction of their influence on the results.
Sample N = *Was the sample described in detail?* Yes □ No □ *Was sample size justified?* Yes □ No □ N/A □	Sampling (who; characteristics; how many; how was sampling done?) If more than one group, was there similarity between the groups? Describe ethics procedures. Was informed consent obtained?
Outcomes *Were the outcome measures reliable?* Yes □ No □ Not addressed □ *Were the outcome measures valid?* Yes □ No □ Not addressed □	Specify the frequency of outcome measurement (i.e., pre, post, follow-up) Outcome areas (e.g., self-care, productivity, leisure).

Intervention *Intervention was described in detail?* *Yes* ☐ *No* ☐ *Not addressed* ☐ *Contamination was avoided?* *Yes* ☐ *No* ☐ *Not addressed* ☐ *N/A* ☐ *Co-intervention was avoided?* *Yes* ☐ *No* ☐ *Not addressed* ☐ *N/A* ☐	*Provide a short description of the intervention (focus, who delivered it, how often, setting). Could the intervention be replicated in occupational therapy practice?*
Results *Results were reported in terms of statistical significance?* Yes ☐ No ☐ N/A ☐ Not addressed ☐ *Were the analysis method(s) appropriate?* Yes ☐ No ☐ Not addressed ☐ *Clinical importance was reported?* Yes ☐ No ☐ Not addressed ☐	What were the results? Were they statistically significant (i.e., $p < 0.05$)? If not statistically significant, was the study big enough to show an important difference if it should occur? If there were multiple outcomes, was that taken into account for the statistical analysis? What was the clinical importance of the results? Were differences between groups clinically meaningful? (If applicable)
Drop-outs were reported? Yes ☐ No ☐	Did any participants drop out from the study? Why? (Were reasons given and were drop-outs handled appropriately?)
Conclusions and clinical implications *Conclusions were appropriate given study methods and results* Yes ☐ No ☐	What did the study conclude? What are the implications of these results for occupational therapy practice? What were the main limitations or biases in the study?

Appendix 4

Survey questions

Question 1: Do you have a formal autism diagnosis?

- Yes
- No
- No, but I self-identify as autistic

Question 2: How old are you?

- Under 18
- 18–25
- 26–35
- 36–45
- 46–55
- 56–65
- 66–100

Question 3: Have you ever received any therapies or supports because of your autism?

- Yes
- No

Question 4: Where do you live?

Question 5: Have you personally been part of a social skills group for autistics?

- Yes, as an adult (over 18 years old)
- Yes, as a child (under 18 years old)
- No

Question 6: How was your experience of social skills groups?

- Did not enjoy or find useful
- Enjoyed but did not find useful
- Did not enjoy but found useful

- Enjoyed and found useful
- Enjoyed, found useful and was able to apply skills learnt to other situations
- N/A

Question 7: Have you personally had peer mentoring for autistics or taken part in any peer mediated activities?

- Yes, as an adult (over 18 years old)
- Yes, as a child (under 18 years old)
- No

Question 8: How was your experience of peer mentoring and/or peer mediated activities?

- Did not enjoy or find useful
- Enjoyed but did not find useful
- Did not enjoy but found useful
- Enjoyed and found useful
- Enjoyed, found useful and was able to apply skills learnt to other situations
- N/A

Question 9: Have you personally experienced pivotal response training (PRT) as a group on 1:1 with a therapist?

- Yes in a group, as an adult (over 18 years old)
- Yes, 1:1 with a therapist, as an adult (over 18 years old)
- Yes, in a group, as a child (under 18 years old)
- Yes, 1:1 with a therapist, as a child (under 18 years old)
- No

Question 10: How was your experience of pivotal response training?

- Did not enjoy or find useful
- Enjoyed but did not find useful
- Did not enjoy but found useful
- Enjoyed and found useful
- Enjoyed, found useful and was able to apply skills learnt to other situations
- N/A

Question 11: Have you personally experienced early intensive behavioural intervention (EIBI)?

- Yes, in a group, as an adult (over 18 years old)
- Yes, 1:1 with a therapist, as an adult (over 18 years old)
- Yes, in a group, as a child (under 18 years old)
- Yes, 1:1 with a therapist, as a child (under 18 years old)
- No

Question 12: How was your experience of early intensive behavioural intervention (EIBI)?

- Did not enjoy or find useful
- Enjoyed but did not find useful
- Did not enjoy but found useful
- Enjoyed and found useful
- Enjoyed, found useful, and was able to apply skills learnt to other situations
- N/A

Question 13: Have you personally taken part in the Denver Early Start Model?

- Yes, in a group, as an adult (over 18 years old)
- Yes, 1:1 with a therapist, as an adult (over 18 years old)
- Yes, in a group, as a child (under 18 years old)
- Yes, 1:1 with a therapist, as a child (under 18 years old)
- No

Question 14: How was your experience of the Denver Early Start Model?

- Did not enjoy or find useful
- Enjoyed but did not find useful
- Did not enjoy but found useful
- Enjoyed and found useful
- Enjoyed, found useful and was able to apply skills learnt to other situations
- N/A

Question 15: Have you personally used the Picture Exchange Communication System (PECS)?

- Yes, as a way for me to communicate
- Yes, in order to communicate with someone else who communicates using PECS
- No

Question 16: How did you, or do you, find using PECS?

- Difficult and not useful
- Easy but not useful
- Difficult but useful
- Easy and useful
- Easy and useful and helped me to communicate in a wide range of settings
- N/A

Question 17: Have people used social stories with you to help you understand or learn new things?

- Yes
- No

Question 18: What is your experience with social stories?

- Not helpful
- A bit helpful
- Helpful sometimes but not other times
- All the social stories were helpful
- Social stories were very helpful and I used the knowledge I learnt from them in other situations
- N/A

Question 19: Have you experienced video modelling as a support?

- Yes
- No

Question 20: What is your experience with video modelling?

- Not helpful
- A bit helpful
- Helpful sometimes but not other times
- All the video models were helpful
- Video models were very helpful and I used the knowledge I learnt from them in other situations
- N/A

Question 21: Have you used technology to communicate?

- Yes
- No

Question 22: What is your experience with technology to communicate?

- Not helpful
- A bit helpful
- Helpful sometimes but not other times
- Technology is helpful
- Technology is very helpful and I can use it in a range of situations
- N/A

Question 23: Have you used technology to support your access to learning or study or the wider community?

- Yes
- No

Question 24: What is your experience with technology to support your access to learning or study or the wider community?

- Not helpful
- A bit helpful
- Helpful sometimes but not other times
- Technology was helpful
- Technology is very helpful and I can use it in a range of situations
- N/A

Question 25: Have you used robots to support your access to learning or study or the wider community?

- Yes
- No

Question 26: What is your experience with robots to support your access to learning or study or the wider community?

- Not helpful
- A bit helpful
- Helpful sometimes but not other times
- The robot is always helpful
- The robot is very helpful and I can use it to help in a range of situations
- N/A

Question 27: Have you used coloured overlays or irlen lenses?

- Yes
- No

Question 28: What is your experience with coloured overlays or irlen lenses?

- Uncomfortable and/or useless
- Not helpful
- A bit helpful
- Helpful sometimes but not other times
- Helpful all the time
- N/A

Question 29: Have you personally had/used an assistance or therapy dog?

- Yes, my own therapy dog
- Yes, my own assistance dog
- Yes, a therapy dog that came to my school/work or a group that I attend
- No

Question 30: How was your experience of a therapy or assistance dog?

- Did not enjoy or find useful
- Enjoyed but did not find useful
- Did not enjoy but found useful
- Enjoyed and found useful
- Enjoyed, found useful, and was able to be more confident or confident even without the dog
- N/A

Question 31: Have you personally experienced equine therapy (horse riding as a therapy for autism)?

- Yes, more than ten times
- Yes, between two and ten times
- Yes, once
- No

Question 32: How was your experience of an equine therapy (horse riding as a therapy for autism)?

- Did not enjoy or find useful
- Enjoyed but did not find useful
- Did not enjoy but found useful
- Enjoyed and found useful
- Enjoyed, found useful and was able to be more confident, or felt confident after riding
- N/A

Question 33: Have you personally experienced dolphin-assisted therapy (swimming with dolphins as a therapy for autism)?

- Yes, more than ten times
- Yes, between two and ten times
- Yes, once
- No

Question 34: How was your experience of a dolphin assisted therapy (swimming with dolphins as a therapy for autism)?

- Did not enjoy or find useful
- Enjoyed but did not find useful
- Did not enjoy but found useful
- Enjoyed and found useful
- Enjoyed, found useful, and was able to be more confident
- N/A

Question 35: Have you personally experienced any other animal therapy (interacting with an animal of any type as a therapy for autism)?

- Yes, a variety of animals
- Yes, one animal
- Yes, once
- No

Question 36: How was your experience of an animal assisted therapy (from q35) as a therapy for autism?

- Did not enjoy or find useful
- Enjoyed but did not find useful
- Did not enjoy but found useful
- Enjoyed and found useful
- Enjoyed, found useful, and was able to be more confident
- N/A

Question 37: Have you personally used weighted blankets and/or weighted vests?

- Yes, both
- Yes, weighted blankets only
- Yes, weighted vest only
- No

Question 38: How was your experience of using weighted blankets?

- Did not enjoy or find useful
- Enjoyed but did not find useful
- Did not enjoy but found useful
- Enjoyed and found useful
- Enjoyed, found useful, and was able to be more confident or confident after using
- N/A

Question 39: How was your experience using weighted vests?

- Did not enjoy or find useful
- Enjoyed but did not find useful
- Did not enjoy but found useful
- Enjoyed and found useful
- Enjoyed, found useful, and was able to be more confident or confident after using
- N/A

Question 40: Have you personally used aromatherapy and/or aromatherapy massage to manage anything related to your autism?

- Yes, both
- Yes, aromatherapy only
- Yes, aromatherapy massage only
- No

Question 41: How was your experience of aromatherapy as an autism therapy?

- Did not enjoy or find useful
- Enjoyed but did not find useful
- Did not enjoy but found useful
- Enjoyed and found useful
- Enjoyed, found useful, and was able to be more confident or confident after using
- N/A

Question 42: How was your experience of aromatherapy massage as an autism therapy?

- Did not enjoy or find useful
- Enjoyed but did not find useful
- Did not enjoy but found useful
- Enjoyed and found useful
- Enjoyed, found useful, and was able to be more confident or confident after having
- N/A

Question 43: Have you personally used acupuncture to manage anything related to your autism?

- Yes
- I have used acupuncture but not for anything related to my autism
- No

Question 44: How was your experience of acupuncture as an autism therapy?

- Did not enjoy or find useful
- Enjoyed but did not find useful
- Did not enjoy but found useful
- Enjoyed and found useful
- Enjoyed, found useful, and was able to be more confident or confident after having
- N/A

Question 45: Have you personally experienced holding therapy?

- Yes
- No

Question 46: How was your experience of holding therapy?

- Did not enjoy or find useful
- Enjoyed but did not find useful
- Did not enjoy but found useful
- Enjoyed and found useful
- Enjoyed, found useful, and was able to be more confident or confident after having
- N/A

Question 47: Have you personally used Sensory Integration therapy (SIT) and/or Auditory Integration therapy (AIT) to manage anything related to your autism?

- Yes, both
- Yes, sensory integration therapy only
- Yes, auditory integration therapy only
- No

Question 48: How was your experience of Sensory Integration therapy as an autism therapy?

- Did not enjoy or find useful
- Enjoyed but did not find useful
- Did not enjoy but found useful
- Enjoyed and found useful
- Enjoyed, found useful, and was able to be more confident or confident after participating
- N/A

Question 49: How was your experience of Auditory Integration therapy as an autism therapy?

- Did not enjoy or find useful
- Enjoyed but did not find useful
- Did not enjoy but found useful
- Enjoyed and found useful
- Enjoyed, found useful, and was able to be more confident or confident after participating
- N/A

Question 50: Have you personally taken part in music therapy as an autism therapy?

- Yes
- Yes, I have taken part but it was not an autism therapy
- No

Question 51: How was your experience of music therapy?

- Did not enjoy or find useful
- Enjoyed but did not find useful
- Did not enjoy but found useful
- Enjoyed and found useful
- Enjoyed, found useful, and was able to be more confident or confident after participating
- N/A

Question 52: Have you personally taken part in art/drawing therapy as an autism therapy?

- Yes
- Yes, I have taken part but it was not an autism therapy
- No

Question 53: How was your experience of art/drawing therapy?

- Did not enjoy or find useful
- Enjoyed but did not find useful
- Did not enjoy but found useful
- Enjoyed and found useful
- Enjoyed, found useful, and was able to be more confident or confident after participating
- N/A

Question 54: Have you ever used a specific type of diet to manage any symptoms related to your autism?

- Ketogenic (keto) diet
- Gluten free (GF) diet
- Casein free (CS) diet
- No, but I have a restricted diet of preferred foods
- No, I eat pretty much whatever I want
- Vegan/vegetarian
- FODMAP
- Other (please specify)

Question 55: How did you find using a particular diet to help you manage symptoms related to your autism?

- Did not enjoy or find useful
- Enjoyed but did not find useful
- Did not enjoy but found useful
- Enjoyed and found useful
- Enjoyed, found useful, and found that my wellbeing and mood were improved
- N/A

Question 56: Have you ever used any type of physical therapy or activity to manage any aspect of your autism?

- Sport therapy or team sports
- Physical therapy or physical exercise program
- Dance or movement therapy
- Yoga and/or pilates
- Walking and/or running
- No
- Other (please specify)

Question 57: How did you find using a particular physical activity or therapy to manage symptoms related to your autism?

- Did not enjoy or find useful
- Enjoyed but did not find useful
- Did not enjoy but found useful
- Enjoyed and found useful
- Enjoyed, found useful, and found that my wellbeing and mood were improved
- N/A

Question 58: Have you ever used any type of prescribed medication to manage any aspect of your autism under the direction of a health profession?

- Psychotropic (mental health medication)
- Other prescribed medication
- No

Question 59: Have you ever used any type of non-prescribed or recreational drugs or alcohol to self-medicate or self-manage any aspect of your autism?

- Psychotropic (mental health medication)
- Other medication that can be prescribed
- Recreational drugs
- Alcohol
- No

Question 60: Have you personally used trans-cranial magnetic stimulation to manage anything related to your autism?

- Yes
- I have used it but not in relation to my autism
- No

Question 61: How was your experience of Trans-Cranial Magnetic stimulation as an autism therapy?

- Did not enjoy or find useful
- Enjoyed but did not find useful
- Did not enjoy but found useful
- Enjoyed and found useful
- Enjoyed, found useful, and was able to be more confident or confident after participating
- N/A

Question 62: Have you personally used hyperbaric oxygen therapy to manage anything related to your autism?

- Yes
- I have used it but not in relation to my autism
- No

Question 63: How was your experience of hyperbaric oxygen therapy as an autism therapy?

- Did not enjoy or find useful
- Enjoyed but did not find useful
- Did not enjoy but found useful
- Enjoyed and found useful
- Enjoyed, found useful and was able to be more confident or confident after participating
- N/A

Question 64: Have you personally experienced medical interventions or supports to manage anything related to your autism?

- Yes
- No

Question 65: How did you find using a particular medical intervention or support (from Q64) to manage symptoms related to your autism?

- Did not enjoy or find useful
- Enjoyed but did not find useful
- Did not enjoy but found useful
- Enjoyed and found useful
- Enjoyed, found useful, and found that my well-being and mood were improved
- N/A

Question 66: Have you ever used meditation and/or mindfulness and/or interoception to manage any aspect of your autism?

- Meditation
- Mindfulness
- Interoception
- No

Question 67: How did you find using meditation to manage any aspects of your autism?

- Did not enjoy or find useful
- Enjoyed but did not find useful
- Did not enjoy but found useful
- Enjoyed and found useful
- Enjoyed, found useful, and found that my well-being and mood were improved
- N/A

Question 68: How did you find using mindfulness to manage any aspects of your autism?

- Did not enjoy or find useful
- Enjoyed but did not find useful
- Did not enjoy but found useful
- Enjoyed and found useful
- Enjoyed, found useful, and found that my well-being and mood were improved
- N/A

Question 69: How did you find using interoception to manage any aspects of your autism?

- Did not enjoy or find useful
- Enjoyed but did not find useful
- Did not enjoy but found useful
- Enjoyed and found useful
- Enjoyed, found useful, and found that my well-being and mood were improved
- N/A

Question 70: Have you personally used cognitive behaviour therapy (CBT) to manage anything related to your autism?

- Yes
- No

Question 71: How did you find using cognitive behaviour therapy (CBT) to manage anything related to your autism?

- Did not enjoy or find useful
- Enjoyed but did not find useful
- Did not enjoy but found useful
- Enjoyed and found useful
- Enjoyed, found useful, and found that my well-being and mood were improved
- N/A

Question 72: Have you personally used any other psychological supports or strategies to manage anything related to your autism?

- Yes
- No

Question 73: How did you find using a particular psychological support or strategy (from Q72) to manage symptoms related to your autism?

- Did not enjoy or find useful
- Enjoyed but did not find useful
- Did not enjoy but found useful
- Enjoyed and found useful
- Enjoyed, found useful, and found that my well-being and mood were improved
- N/A

Question 74: Have you personally used any other supports or strategies to manage anything related to your autism?

- Yes
- No

Index

Locators in **bold** refer to tables.

For Product Safety Concerns and Information please contact our EU representative GPSR@taylorandfrancis.com
Taylor & Francis Verlag GmbH, Kaufingerstraße 24, 80331 München, Germany

www.ingramcontent.com/pod-product-compliance
Ingram Content Group UK Ltd.
Pitfield, Milton Keynes, MK11 3LW, UK
UKHW052225190926
475702UK00007B/1203
* 9 7 8 0 3 6 7 4 2 1 2 6 7 *